Management of Menopause

Ruchika Garg
Editor

Management of Menopause

A Guide for Practitioners

Springer

Editor
Ruchika Garg
Department of Obstetrics and Gynecology
Sarojini Naidu Medical College
Agra, Uttar Pradesh, India

ISBN 978-981-96-0238-4 ISBN 978-981-96-0239-1 (eBook)
https://doi.org/10.1007/978-981-96-0239-1

This Springer imprint is published by the registered company Springer Nature Singapore Pte Ltd.
The registered company address is: 152 Beach Road, #21-01/04 Gateway East, Singapore 189721, Singapore

Foreword

Menopause is a natural and inevitable stage in every woman's life, yet it remains a topic that is often shrouded in mystery and misinformation. As healthcare practitioners, it is our duty to provide our patients with accurate information, effective treatment options, and compassionate care during this important phase of their lives.

Ruchika Garg's book, *Management of Menopause*, is a comprehensive guide for healthcare practitioners who want to deepen their knowledge and understanding of menopause. Drawing from the latest research, clinical experience, and patient stories, Garg provides a clear and concise overview of the physiology of menopause, common symptoms, and evidence-based treatment options.

What sets this book apart is its practical and patient-centered approach. Garg emphasizes the importance of personalized care, informed consent, and shared decision-making. She also addresses the unique challenges that menopause presents for women from diverse backgrounds and cultures, highlighting the need for cultural humility and sensitivity in clinical practice.

As a healthcare practitioner myself, I highly recommend this book to anyone who wants to provide high-quality care for women during menopause. Whether you are a primary care physician, gynecologist, nurse practitioner, or any other healthcare professional who works with women, "Management of Menopause" will provide you with the knowledge, skills, and confidence to support your patients through this important life transition.

Trustee FIGO Asia Oceania Region
D Y Patil University, Navi Mumbai, India

Prof Hrishikesh Pai

Preface

Management of Menopause by Prof Ruchika Garg with Springer Nature Singapore Publishers is a valuable addition to the field of menopause healthcare. This book is an essential resource for healthcare practitioners who are looking to expand their knowledge of menopause and provide better care for their patients.

What makes this book particularly noteworthy is its comprehensive and evidence-based approach. We have compiled a wealth of information on the physiology of menopause, common symptoms, and available treatment options. The book also explores the impact of menopause on a woman's overall health and wellbeing, including the risk of cardiovascular disease, osteoporosis, and depression. Starting from physiology to psychological problems at menopause, and the place of complementary and cognitive behavioral therapy, all have been described in detail. The book covers extensive chapters on the effect of menopause on memory, cardiovascular system, skin, and eye. Contraception, premature ovarian failure, and postmenopausal bleeding have been well described. All the authors have vast clinical experience and are academicians.

Another strength of this book is its practical guidance for healthcare practitioners. The book provides clear and concise recommendations for the management of menopausal symptoms, including hormonal and non-hormonal treatment options. The book also covers the importance of lifestyle modifications, such as exercise and a healthy diet, in managing menopause symptoms.

Overall, *Management of Menopause* is a must-read for anyone involved in menopause healthcare. It provides a thorough and up-to-date understanding of menopause and its management, and will undoubtedly be a valuable resource for healthcare practitioners looking to provide the best possible care for their patients. I highly recommend this book to anyone interested in women's health or menopause care. This book will be a useful guide for postgraduate students pursuing specialization in gynecology.

I would like to thank my husband Professor Prabhat Agrawal and my kids Pratham and Palakshi for their love and support throughout the journey. I would also thank Jagjeet Kaur Saini, Kumar Athiappan, Dhanushya Vijayakandeepan, and the entire team of Springer for this herculean task.

Happy Reading

Agra, Uttar Pradesh, India Prof Ruchika Garg

Contents

About the Editor

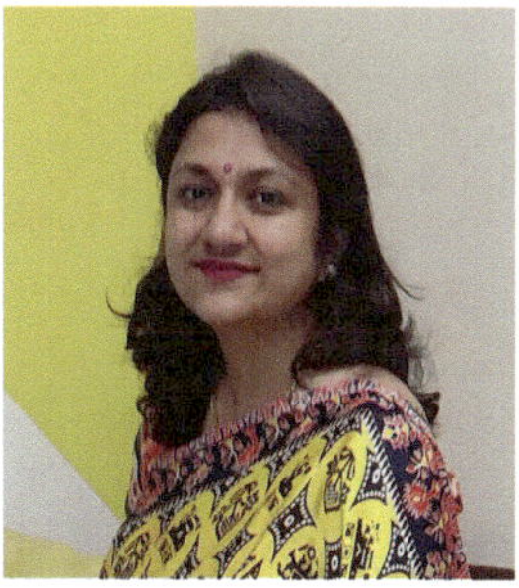

Ruchika Garg, MD (Obs Gyne) she has more than 200 scientific publications in national and international journals and has H index of 11 and has many citations to her credit. She has edited many books including, *Labour and Delivery: Updated Guide, Medical Disorders in Pregnancy, Multiple Choice Questions in Obstetrics and Gynaecology*, and *Clinical Focus on PCOS*. She has authored and coauthored around 100 book chapters. She is a peer reviewer of many international journals. Dr Garg, the editor-in-chief of *Journal of Midlife Health* (2023–2025), has been an associate editor of *Journal of SAFOG* (South Asian Federation of Obstetrics and Gynecology) and editorial board member of Pan Asian Journal Obstetrics and Gynecology.

Dr. Garg is currently national chairperson of rural committee, ISOPARB, and founder secretary Agra chapter, ISOPARB. She has received several prestigious awards to her credit. She is committed to social cause of raising awareness about cervical cancer and conducts camps for anemia prevention in India.

Department of Obstetrics and Gynecology, SN Medical College, Agra, Uttar Pradesh, India.

Physiology of Menopause

1

Pavika Lal, Divya Dwivedi, and Ruchika Garg

1.1 Background

Menopause is a phenomenon that occurs universally and with increased life expectancy many females in most parts of the world tend to spend almost one-third of their lifetime beyond 50 years of age. The world's elderly population will be more than double from 1998 to 2025, rising from 264 million in 2009 to 416 million in 2050 [1]. In 1990, it was estimated that there were almost 500 million women aged 50 years or over worldwide, and this number is expected to increase to 1.2 billion by 2030. By that time, 76% will be living in developing countries. About 50 million women worldwide reach menopause each year [2]. The term menopause relates to permanent cessation of menses that marks the end of a woman's reproductive years due to loss of ovarian follicular activity and is a retrospective diagnosis. The event is said to have occurred after 12 consecutive months of amenorrhea for which no physiological or pathological cause have been ascertained. The term climacteric or perimenopausal phase has been replaced by menopausal transition and begins 4–7 years preceding menopause during which the endocrinological, biological, and clinical features of declining ovarian activity appear.

The average or median age of menopause globally is between 50 and 52 years [3], and in India it is approximately 47 years of age [4]. Various demographic (race, ethnicity, education, employment), menstrual and reproductive history (parity and OCP use), and familial and genetic lifestyle (e.g., smoking, weight, physical activity, and diet) are important determinants of the age at which menopause is attained [4]. Age at natural menopause may be a surrogate marker of overall health and general well-being as late age of menopause (52 and beyond) has been associated with the following:

P. Lal (✉) · D. Dwivedi
Department of Obstetrics and Gynaecology, GSVM Medical College, Kanpur, India

R. Garg
Department Obstetrics and Gynaecology SN Medical College, Agra, India

R. Garg (ed.), *Management of Menopause*,
https://doi.org/10.1007/978-981-96-0239-1_1

- Improved overall survival and life expectancy along with decrease in overall mortality [5, 6]
- Decreased risk of cardiovascular diseases (ischemic heart diseases), stroke, and atherosclerosis [7–11]
- Decreased risk of osteoporosis and fractures [12, 13]
- Slight increased risk of endometrial, breast, and ovarian cancers [14, 15]

Although menopause is a ubiquitous event occurring in all women, the timing of onset and duration of menopausal transition and the attainment of final menstrual period is unique to every female.

Premature menopause also known as premature ovarian insufficiency (POI) refers to cessation of menses before 40 years of age, and it has been observed that the incidence of POI, i.e., 1% has been on a rising trend [4]. Surgical menopause is the term which is used in females when they have undergone hysterectomy with or without bilateral oophorectomy before the attainment of natural menopause. Females who have undergone hysterectomy before the age of 45 years for benign and malignant conditions are at increased risk of mortality especially from ischemic heart disease if not treated with HRT [16].

1.2 Classification and Staging of Menopausal Transition and Menopause

There were many classification systems but the most accepted is the Stages of Reproductive Aging Workshop (STRAW) classification which was proposed in 2001 after extensive and thorough research. STRAW describes the various stages of reproductive life in females as well as it brings uniformity in nomenclature and the characteristic transformation at every stage across the studies conducted [17]. It was revised in 2010 and was renamed as Re STRAW +10 which was upgraded to incorporate the biochemical or hormonal changes along with ultrasound findings throughout the reproductive aging.

The Stages of Reproductive Aging Workshop (STRAW) proposed a system that divides female reproductive aging into five stages before the final menstrual period, and two afterward. Each of these stages is divided into substages on the basis of menstrual cycle pattern and investigations (serum levels of follicle-stimulating hormone [FSH], anti-Mullerian hormone [AMHI], and ultrasound-based ovarian antral follicle count [AFC] (Fig. 1.1).

1.3 Hormonal and Menstrual Changes Across the Menopausal Transition

(a) **Ovarian Changes**: The size of ovary in postmenopausal females 10 cm^3 compared to 20 cm^3 in reproductive age females. The functional unit of ovary is the ovarian follicle and approximately 30 follicles are recruited in each menstrual

REPRODUCTIVE PERIOD			MENOPAUSAL TRANSITION		FINAL MENSTRUAL PERIOD	POST MENOPAUSAL	
EARLY	PEAK	LATE	EARLY	LATE	FMP	EARLY	LATE
-5	-4	-3a, b	-2	-1	0	+1a,b,c	+2

Fig. 1.1 Phases of female reproductive life span. Three stages (early (−5), peak (−4), and late (−3) reproductive) describe the years before the perimenopause. Stage −3 is characterized by regular cycles but elevated levels of follicle-stimulating hormone (FSH) in the follicular phase. Stage −3 has been subdivided into substages −3b and −3a. In substage −3b, the menstrual cycle remains unchanged along with normal serum levels of FSH in early follicular phases but AFC and AMH tend to become low. The only difference between substages −3b and −3a is that in −3a early follicular phase, FSH level increases leading to shorter menstrual cycles. Stage −2 (early menopause transition) is characterized by variable cycle length. Stage −1 (late menopause transition) is characterized by two or more stopped cycles and 60 or more days of amenorrhea. Stage +1 is the first 5 years after the final menstrual period. Stage +2 is the late postmenopause

cycle out of which 1 becomes a dominant follicle surrounded by granulosa cells along with theca cells. All the follicles develop from the population of primordial follicles which are maximum during the intra-uterine life (six million), one to two million at birth and 500,000 at puberty. There is substantial acceleration/exponential loss of follicles when the female reaches beyond 40 years of age. By the time menopause is attained, only 1000 follicles remain which are atretic and of substandard quality, and also they become less responsive to gonadotrophins as compared to the reproductive age period.

(b) **Hormonal Changes**: The endocrinology of menopause can be summarized as a sequence of events that results in replacement of the cyclical secretory pattern of gonadotropins (FSH, LH) and gonadal steroids (estrogen, progesterone) and peptides (inhibin) by a monophasic pattern of increased levels of gonadotropins along with decreased levels of estrogen, progesterone, and inhibins. Secretion of androgens particularly testosterone is not affected by the event of menopause.

1. Follicle-Stimulating Hormone (FSH) [7]

   As the ovarian function declines, the pituitary gland increases FSH release in an attempt to stimulate the ovaries to produce more estrogen. Monotropic rise in FSH (>40 IU/L) is the hallmark of MT and is often used as a diagnostic marker for menopause. It is more indicative of egg quantity rather than quality especially during the early transition. Significant changes in central neural processes that produce LH surge in mid-reproductive life also become dysfunctional leading to irregular cycle (skipping of menstrual cycles or intermenstrual interval >7 days) during early transition. FSH rises are more sustained over time during the late menopausal transition when there is amenorrhea for more than 3 months, and the rise is most remarkable in the years preceding FMP.
2. Gonadal Steroids [8–10]

The two gonadal steroids involved in physiology of menopause are estrogen and progesterone out of which estrogen levels fluctuate and more closely resemble the various stages of menopausal transition as well as postmenopause. The four major naturally occurring estrogens are esterone (E1), estradiol (E2), estriol (E3), and estetrol (E4). Estradiol is the predominant estrogen during reproductive years both in terms of absolute serum levels and in terms of estrogenic activity. During menopause, esterone is the predominant circulating estrogen and has the weakest estrogenic activity. In early menopausal transition, estradiol levels are initially elevated in early follicular phase as a result of accelerated folliculogenesis and shortening of the follicular phase. There occurs a rapid decline beginning 2 years before the FMP followed by reaching a plateau level 2 years thereafter; therefore, it is the last biomarker from MT to FMP. Progesterone levels do not show marked fluctuations during menopausal transition but eventually become undetectable during menopause; therefore, progesterone cannot be used as a marker. The hormonal changes during menopause can lead to various physical and emotional symptoms.

3. Inhibin [18]

   Inhibin B is the product of granulosa cells of the cohort of follicles, and in a normal ovarian cycle, its level is highest in early follicular phase followed by peak in mid-cycle and declines thereafter. It represents the overall quality of the follicle along with its numbers. Inhibin-B becomes undetectable in the preceding 4–5 years before complete cessation which is consistent with a decrease in both the size of primordial follicle pool and the cohort of follicles recruited from that pool in each menstrual cycle. The fall in Inhibin-B parallels the rise in FSH which supports the evidence that inhibin-B plays an important role in negative feedback regulation of FSH secretion.

   Inhibin A is the product of the dominant follicle as well as also produced by corpus luteum; therefore its levels are highest during mid-cycle and also detected during luteal phase. The inhibin levels eventually vanish after the attainment of menopause. The measurement of inhibin B is more important than inhibin-A as it is one of the earliest harbingers of menopausal transition.

4. Anti-Mullerian Hormone (AMH)/MIS

   AMH is produced by primary, secondary, and early antral follicles and more closely correlate with the follicle cohort, and therefore its concentration declines throughout the reproductive life with minimal inter-cycle variations and constitute the earliest and the most efficient way to predict the women's progress toward menopause. It can be hoped in near future that AMH becomes a menopause test with the development of a comprehensive sensitive assay.

5. Testosterone and DHEA-S [19]

   Both testosterone and dehydroepiandrosterone (DHEA) metabolites show age-related decline as ovarian androgen production decreases, but there has been an increase in adrenal-derived androgens during the MT in majority of females. Due to falling estrogen levels, there is decline in SHBG leading to rise in free testosterone besides being contributed by adrenals in postmenopausal females. The complimentary contributions of DHEA metabolites to total androgenicity should not be ignored, but DHEA-S levels across the MT are still under research, and no conclusions can be made.

1.4 Menstrual Changes [20]

During the menopausal transition, the pattern of menstrual bleeding changes with respect to regularity, timing, as well as nature, i.e., cycles may become irregular in length and flow along with periods of heavier or lighter bleeding and missed periods. Eventually, menstruation stops completely, and menopause is confirmed when a woman has not had a menstrual period for 12 consecutive months. The nature and timing of bleeding vary within an individual and also among different women:

- During the STRAW stage −2, i.e., early menopausal transition, there is increase in irregularity of the cycles which is defined as recurrence of 7-day difference in cycle length over a period of 10 consecutive cycles. The duration of the follicular phase is the major determinant of cycle length.
- Menstrual cycles become increasingly irregular due to (short/inadequate luteal phase or anovulation). Insufficient FSH responsiveness results in decreased luteal phase estrogen and progesterone secretion leading to lack of corpus luteum which results in only estrogen secretion (hyper-estrogenic states) without progesterone secretion eventually resulting in profuse bleeding.
- During late menopausal transition, STRAW stage −1 is characterized by amenorrhea lasting for 3 months due to increased chances of anovulation during this period.
- Early postmenopause STRAW stage +1a, b, and c includes post-1 year beyond FMP, and early postmenopause which spans a total of 5–8 years.

1.5 Symptoms [21]

The SWAN ((Study of Women's Health Across the Nation) multicentric, multiethnic longitudinal study across 7 clinical sites with 3302 females enrolled between 42 and 52 years of age were followed with the effects of menopause on their health and various risk factors for age-related disease) is the most comprehensive characterization till date about the various physiological and psychological changes during the menopausal transition along with postmenopause [22, 23]. The most consistent observation of SWAN was that most of the symptomatology along with detectable physiological changes coincides with late perimenopause (3 months of amenorrhea).

Clinical consequences of profound hormonal deprivation of estrogen leads to various symptoms affecting almost every organ of the body which maybe bothersome and troublesome and may even require expert advice from the physicians and pharmacological interventions along with life behavioral modifications.

- **Vasomotor Symptoms (VMS)**: Approximately 75% of the females experience VMS (hot flashes, night sweats) which is most marked during early postmenopausal period, which usually lasts up to 5 years and very rarely 15 years. The exact pathophysiology is unclear, but it has been speculated that the central thermoregulatory zone narrows down toward menopausal transition so that vasodilatation and sweating are triggered at a lower temperature. Transition of late perimenopause was the strongest predictor of VMS.
- **Genitourinary Syndrome of Menopause (GSM)**: is most concerning issue after VMS but occurs more commonly during the late menopause as compared to early menopause and gradually worsens over a period of time. The term vulvovaginal atrophy (VVA) has been replaced by GSM which is a constellation of symptoms complex involving atrophy of the vulva, vagina, urogenital atrophy, and sexual dissatisfaction due to loss of estrogen and progesterone receptors which lines the lower genital tract along with the bladder and urethra:
  - Osteoporosis
  - Metabolic syndrome
  - Ischemic heart diseases
  - Dementia/stroke
  - Cancers
  - Aging of skin
  - Loss of libido
  - Centripetal fat distribution due to increased androgen estrogen ratio and insulin resistance
  - Psychological symptoms (anxiety, depression, cognitive decline, impaired concentration)

1.6 Conclusion [24]

The following points should be considered during management of perimenopausal and postmenopausal females:

- Provide reassurance that reproductive aging is a natural phenomenon and menopause is not a disorder.
- Provide guidance and education to facilitate a patient's decision-making regarding MHT if the symptoms are bothersome.
- Be involved in community with the help of awareness camps for bone, mental, and cardiovascular health.

Regardless of chronological age, women should undergo annual medical evaluations that should include a thorough medical history as well as physical examination.

Annual visits should include assessment of vitals (blood pressure and pulse), body weight, and body mass index (BMI), breast and pelvic examinations, and screening for sexually transmitted infections when appropriate. Thyroid function

(TSH) should be assessed in the 40's and annually beginning at age 60 increases with aging and is more common in women).

- Annual screening mammography should begin at age 40.
- At each visit, appropriate testing is scheduled for specific chronic conditions (including abnormal lipids), indicated immunizations are provided, and counselling covers changing nutritional needs; physical activities; injury prevention; occupational, sexual, marital, and parental problems; urinary function; and use of tobacco, alcohol, and drugs. Stool hemoccult testing should be performed annually after age 50.
- For low-risk individuals without a family history of colon cancer, screening colonoscopy is recommended starting at age 50, and then every 10 years through age 75.

Menopause is a naturally occurring transition in a women's life with significant bodily changes as well as change in attitude and behavior toward the perception of life. Therefore, it becomes important to consult a healthcare provider for personalized counselling, advice, and support for a smooth and comfortable adaptation during this period to lead a healthy life.

References

1. Fritz MA, Speroff L. Chapter 17. Clinical gynecologic endocrinology and infertility, 9th ed. p. 693.
2. Burger HG. Physiology and endocrinology of the menopause. Medicine. 2006;34(1):27–30. issn:1357-3039. https://doi.org/10.1383/medc.2006.34.1.27.
3. Fritz MA, Speroff L. Chapter 17. Clinical gynecologic endocrinology and infertility, 9th ed. p. 692.
4. Ahuja M. Age of menopause and determinants of menopause age: a PAN India survey by IMS. J Midlife Health. 2016;7(3):126–31. https://doi.org/10.4103/0976-7800.191012. PMID: 27721640; PMCID: PMC5051232.
5. Ossewaarde ME, Bots ML, Verbeek ALM, et al. Age at menopause, cause-specific mortality and total life expectancy. Epidemiology. 2005;16:556–62.
6. Jacobsen BK, Heuch I, Kvale G. Age at natural menopause and all-cause mortality: a 37-year follow-up of 19,731 Norwegian women. Am J Epidemiol. 2003;157:923–9.
7. Jansen SC, Temme EH, Schouten EG. Lifetime estrogen exposure versus age at menopause as mortality predictor. Maturitas. 2002;43:105–12.
8. Jacobsen BK, Knutson SF, Fraser GE. Age at natural menopause and total mortality and mortality from ischemic heart disease: the Adventist Health Study. J Clin Epidemiol. 1999;52:303–7.
9. Lisabeth LD, Beiser AS, Brown DL, et al. Age at natural menopause and risk of ischemic stroke: the Framingham Heart Study. Stroke. 2009;40:1044–9.
10. Parashar S, Reid KJ, Spertus JA, et al. Early menopause predicts angina after myocardial infarction. Menopause. 2010;17(5):938–45.
11. Joakimsen O, Bonaa KR Stensland-Bugge E, et al. Population-based study of age myocardial infarction.
12. Parazzini F, Bidoli E, Franceschi S, et al. Menopause, menstrual and reproductive his and bone density in northern Italy. J Clin Epidemiol. 2000;53:525–30.
13. Kritz-Silverstein D, Barrett-Connor E. Early menopause, number of reproductive years, and bone mineral density in postmenopausal women. Am J Public Health. 1993;83(7):983–8.

14. Monninkhof EM, van der Schouw YT, Peeters PH. Early age at menopause and breast cancer: are leaner women more protected? A prospective analysis of the Dutch DOM cohort. Breast Cancer Res Treat. 1999;55:285–91.
15. De Graaff J, Stolte LA. Age at menarche and menopause of uterine cancer patients. Eur J Obstet Gynecol Reprod Biol. 1978;8:187–93.
16. Xu WH, Xiang YB, Ruan ZX, et al. Menstrual and reproductive factors and endometrial cancer risk: results from a population-based case-control study in urban Shanghai. Int J Cancer. 2004;108(4):613–9.
17. Harlow SD, Gass M, Hall JE, Lobo R, Maki P, Rebar RW, Sherman S, Sluss PM, de Villiers TJ, STRAW +10 Collaborative Group. Executive summary of the stages of reproductive aging workshop + 10: addressing the unfinished agenda of staging reproductive aging. J Clin Endocrinol Metab. 2012;97(4):1159–68.
18. Overlie I, Mørkrid L, Andersson A-M, Skakkebaek NE, Moen MH, Holte A. Inhibin A and B as markers of menopause: a five-year prospective longitudinal study of hormonal changes during the menopausal transition. Acta Obstet Gynecol Scand. 2005;84:281–5.
19. McConnell DS, Stanczyk FZ, Sowers MR, Randolph JF Jr, Lasley BL. Menopausal transition stage-specific changes in circulating adrenal androgens. Menopause. 2012;19(6):658–63. https://doi.org/10.1097/gme.0b013e31823fe274. PMID: 22415570; PMCID: PMC3366025.
20. Peacock K, Ketvertis KM. Menopause [Updated 2022 Aug 11]. In: StatPearls [Internet]. Treasure Island: StatPearls Publishing; 2023. https://www.ncbi.nlm.nih.gov/books/NBK507826/.
21. Dennerstein L. Well-being, symptoms and the menopausal transition. Maturitas. 1996;23(2):147–57.
22. Avis NE, Colvin A, Bromberger JT, et al. Change in health-related quality of life over the menopausal transition in a multiethnic cohort of middle-aged women: Study of Women's Health Across the Nation (SWAN). Menopause. 2009;16:860–9.
23. Avis NE, Ory M, Matthews KA, et al. Health-related quality of life in a multiethnic sample of middle- aged women: Study of Women's Health Across the Nation (SWAN). Med Care. 2003;41:1262–76.
24. Fritz MA, Speroff L. Chapter 17. Clinical gynecologic endocrinology and infertility, 9th ed. pp. 701–702.

Diagnosis of Menopause

2

Shehla Jamal and Natasha Singh

India being the world's most populous country has witnessed a dramatic demographic transition in past 50 years owing to tripling in size in the geriatric population (over 60 years). In India, where there are 1.2 billion people, 96 million of them are women, and by 2026, that number is expected to rise to 401 million. Women in India currently have an average life expectancy of 70.3 years, and by 2050, that figure is predicted to rise to 77 years (World Health Organization, 2018) [1]. Future issues posed by this group will be significant for both public and private healthcare providers. Such large population that will be in menopausal group raises an alarm to have a precise knowledge about the diagnosis of menopause so that early interventions can be done to improve the quality of life index and prevent osteoporosis and vasomotor and genitourinary symptoms.

As women get closer to reproductive senescence, there are physiologic changes throughout the menopausal transition. Evidence backs up the clinical significance of the transition for many women as a time of temporal changes in health and quality of life (such as vasomotor symptoms, sleep problems, and depression) and longer-term changes in several health outcomes (such as urogenital symptoms, bone, and lipids), which may affect women's quality of life and likelihood of healthy aging.

There are various stages and definitions associated to menopause, that include the following (Fig. 2.1):

Premenopause: Reproductive period prior to menopause.

Perimenopause: 3–5 years before and 1 year after menopause.

Menopause transition: Disturbed menstrual cycle, endocrine changes.

Postmenopause: It is the span of time dating from the final menstrual period, regardless of whether menopause was spontaneous or iatrogenic.

Senescence: It is the period after the age of 60 years.

S. Jamal (✉) · N. Singh
Department of Obstetrics and Gynecology, RMRI, Bareilly, India

R. Garg (ed.), *Management of Menopause*,
https://doi.org/10.1007/978-981-96-0239-1_2

	Menarche ↓					Final Menstrual Period(0) ↓				
STAGE	-5	-4	-3b	-3a	-2	-1	+1a	+1b	+1c	+2
Terminology	REPRODUCTIVE				MENOPAUSAL TRANSITIONS		POSTMENOPAUSE			
	EARLY	PEAK	LATE		EARLY	LATE	EARLY		LATE	
				PERIMENOPAUSE						
DURATION	Variable				Variable	1-3 years	2 years (1+1)		3-6 years	Remaining life span
PRINCIPAL CRITERIA										
Menstrual cycle	Variable to regular	Regular	Regular	Subtle changes in Flow/ length	Variable length persistant ≥ - day difference in length of consecutive cycles	Interval of amenorrhea of ≥ 60 days				
SUPPORTIVE CRITERIA										
Endocrine FSH AMH Inhibin B			Normal Low Low	Variable Low Low	Variable Low low	>25 IU/L Low Low	Variable Low low		Stabilizes Very low Very low	
Antral Follicle count 2-10 mm			Low	Low	Low	Low	Very low		Very low	
Symptoms						Vaso –motor symptom likely	Vaso –motor symptom most Likely			Increasing symptoms of urogenital atrophy

Fig. 2.1 The STRAW +10 staging system for reproductive aging in women

Premature menopause: Spontaneous menopause occurring two standard deviations below the mean estimated age for the reference population. It is traditionally considered to be below the age of 40 years.

Early menopause: It is the time span between the spontaneous or iatrogenic menopause occurring between the age of 40 years and the accepted typical age of menopause for a given population.

Delayed menopause: It is not defined but may be important in terms of the increased problems associated with the hyperestrogenism. It is two standard deviations above from the natural average age of menopause in a given population (beyond 54 years).

Induced menopause: Cessation of menstruation that follows bilateral oophorectomy or iatrogenic ablation of ovarian function.

Temporary menopause: It is a term preferably not to be used, since definition of menopause is complete cessation of menstruation. Rarely, ovarian function is interrupted for a period of time and later resumes.

Diagnosis of menopause is mainly clinical and post facto. In 2001 the Stages of Reproductive Aging Workshop (STRAW) criteria was given, but in 2011 STRAW+10 workshop [2] reviewed advances in understanding of the critical changes in hypothalamic-pituitary-ovarian function that occur before and after the final menstrual period (FMP).

Also Anklesaria's staging is used for the staging of menopause and may be utilized for clinical purposes and treatment of menopause (Fig. 2.2).

Genitourinary syndrome of menopause (GSM) is defined as a collection of symptoms and signs caused by hypoestrogenic changes to the labia majora/minora, clitoris, vestibule/introitus, vagina, urethra, and bladder that occur in menopausal patients. The syndrome may include, but is not limited to, genital symptoms of dryness, burning, and irritation; sexual symptoms of lack of lubrication, discomfort or pain, and impaired function; and urinary symptoms of urgency, dysuria, and recurrent urinary tract infections.

Diagnosis of menopause is made by history, examination followed by laboratory parameters.

History includes irregularity in menstruation (amenorrhea, scanty menses, prolonged menses, intermenstrual bleeding), mood disturbances, sleep disturbances, vasomotor symptoms (hot flashes), genitourinary symptoms.

All menopausal symptoms were more common and more severe in postmenopausal women. The most common menopausal symptoms in premenopausal women are mental tiredness (49.5%), joint and muscle pain (48.5%), and irritation (41.3%). The most common menopausal symptoms in postmenopausal women are reported as hot flushes (42.2%), irritability (48.2%), physical and mental weariness (53%), and irritation.

Menopause			
Stage I	Stage II A	Stage II B	Stage III
Roughly 2 years before menopause Early (Premenopausal symptoms): IA Vasomotor instability IB Early psychosomatic symptoms Menstrual problems	1 year after last period Atrophic changes Genitourinary Vasomotor Weight gain Osteopenia	Up to 5 years after menopause Intermediate (postmenopausal symptoms): Late psychosomatic and genital symptoms Sexual disorders Residual changes from stage II A osteopenia or osteoporosis	From 5 years postmenopausal till Late (postmenopausal) complications: Residual changes from stage II Ischemic heart changes Other late complications, e.g. Alzheimer's disease, Osteoporosis
PREVENT	TREAT	TREAT	PALLIATE
	Window of Opportunity		

Fig. 2.2 Modified Anklesaria's IMS consensus group staging [3]

2.1 Vasomotor Symptoms

Vasomotor symptoms are experienced by about 75% of women. Hot flashes, nocturnal sweats, palpitations, and migraines are a few of these signs. Hot flashes frequently occur at random intervals and last 3–4 min. Alcohol, food, mental stress, and physical exercise can all make them worse. The degree and intensity of migraines might fluctuate. Migraines without aura are more frequent than aura-filled migraines. Stroke risk is higher in migraines with aura, particularly in women who smoke or use oral contraceptives. Changes in hormone levels may also result in a rise in headaches of other sorts, such as cluster and tension headaches.

2.2 Genitourinary Symptoms

Sixty percent of women report having urogenital symptoms. These signs include urethral atrophy, sexual dysfunction (such as a drop in desire), and vaginal atrophy. Dryness, pruritus, and dyspareunia (painful intercourse) are the outcomes of vaginal atrophy. Stress incontinence, frequency, urgency, and dysuria are the outcomes of urethral atrophy.

2.3 Psychological Symptoms

Psychogenic symptoms are experienced by about 45% of women. These signs and symptoms include rage/irritability, tension/anxiety, sadness, disturbed sleep, loss of focus, and low self-esteem/confidence.

Along with that other history like medical history and risk factors for breast cancer, cardiovascular disease, thromboembolic disease, and osteoporosis has to be taken. Also absolute or relative contraindications to menopausal hormonal therapy (MHT) (uncontrolled hypertension, undiagnosed abnormal bleeding, previous breast or endometrial cancer, and personal history or high inherited risk of thromboembolic disease) have to be asked.

For symptom score, the Australian Menopause Society has given a score, *The Modified Greene Scale* [4], that includes following symptoms like hot flushes, light-headed feelings, headaches, irritability, depression, unloved feelings, anxiety, mood changes, sleeplessness, unusual tiredness, backache, joint pains, muscle pains, new facial hair, dry skin, crawling feelings under the skin, less sexual feelings, dry vagina, uncomfortable intercourse, and urinary frequency. Each symptom has given score before MHT, 3 months after starting MHT and 6 months after MHT.

Severity of problem is scored as follows score: None = 0; Mild = 1; Moderate = 2; Severe = 3.

The symptoms are grouped into four categories: vasomotor, psychological, locomotor, and urogenital. If one group does not respond to MHT, look for other causes and specific treatments for that group.

Other scales used for diagnosis of menopause by symptoms include *Modified Kupperman Index*

Raw score, severity score of each symptom; weighted score, raw score × weighting factor; total score, sum of the weighted score. Classification of the modified Kupperman index is "no complaint" (total score 0–6), "mild" (total score 7–15), "moderate" (total score 16–30), or "severe" (total score > 30) (Fig. 2.3).

Other score is menopause rating scale.

Physical examination: after making diagnosis of menopause clinically, physical examination should be performed for associated comorbidities, if present. It should include measurement of blood pressure, weight and height, breast palpation, vaginal examination, and Pap smear.

Blood pressure: Elevated blood pressure may be noted due to arterial vasoconstriction.

Weight and height: Weight gain may be noted, as many women report some degree of weight gain during menopause. Additionally, a decrease in height may be noted, associated with osteoporosis and spine fractures.

Breast and vagina: Breast palpation usually notes decreased breast size. The vaginal examination notes dryness and urogenital atrophy. Abnormal uterine bleeding is an indication to perform a Papanicolaou (Pap) smear.

Laboratory parameters: usually testing is not required for making the diagnosis of menopause, but for premature menopause, testing is necessary for diagnosis, and they include serum day 3 follicle-stimulating hormone (FSH) levels, estradiol levels, anti mullerian hormone (AMH), inhibin B, antral follicle count, ovarian volume, ovarian blood flow, ovarian biopsy, clomiphene citrate challenge test,

Symptoms	Weighting Factor	Severity scale				Score	
		0	1	2	3	Raw score	Weighted score
Sweating/ hot flashes	x4	None	<3 times a day	3-9 times a day	≥ 10 times/day		
Parasthesia	x2	None	Relationship with climate	Feel tingling, pricking, Or numbness frequently	Lose sense of warm and pain		
Insomnia	x2	None	Once in a while	Frequent need sleeping pill	Affects life and work		
Nervousness	x2	None	Once in a while	Frequent	Frequent, cannot control		

Fig. 2.3 Modified Kupperman index [5]

exogenous follicle-stimulating hormone ovarian reserve test, gonadotrophin-releasing hormone agonist stimulation test.

Other ancillary tests include DEXA scan, Frax score, S.TSH, mammography, Pap smear, lipid profile, echocardiography, complete blood picture, urine test routine, fasting blood glucose level, serum thyroid-stimulating hormone, Papanicolaou (Pap) smear, transvaginal ultrasound, and mammogram.

For the purpose of ease and handy learning, *Shehla's Rule of 4* can be used for making the diagnosis of menopause that includes the following:

1. >40 years of age
2. >40 m IU/mL FSH
3. <4 antral follicle count
4. <40/2–20 pg/mL estradiol levels

2.4 Differential Diagnosis of Menopause

The most frequent ailments that can co-occur are thyroid problems, anemia, and depression. Hot flushes can be brought on by hyperthyroidism and intractable diabetes. Hot flushes can also be brought on by medication, including antidepressants from the selective serotonin reuptake inhibitor (SSRI) family.

The diagnosis is typically made by performing a blood count, ferritin test, and/or TSH level. However, if a woman exhibits signs of poor mood or worry, it is important to determine if this is a natural anxiety or depression or one that has been made worse by estrogen deficiency. Making the distinction between the two may be aided by a prior history of depression or an increased FSH. In contrast to menopause, iron deficiency or hypothyroidism may be the cause of hair loss.

Key Points

- Menopause is defined as the final/last menstrual period.
- Menopause is a retrospective clinical diagnosis as the final menstrual period can only be defined if followed by 12 months of amenorrhea.
- Menopause is a natural and inevitable event that happens on average at age 51 in white Caucasians, with ethnic and regional variations.
- Menopause before age 40 is considered to be premature.
- Accurate staging of reproductive aging is important from a clinical and research perspectives.
- Large population that will be in menopausal group by 2030 raises an alarm to have a precise knowledge about the diagnosis of menopause so that early interventions can be done to improve the quality of life index, prevent osteoporosis and vasomotor and genitourinary symptoms.
- Diagnosis of menopause is mainly clinical and post facto.
- Various staging systems are used for staging menopause; they include STRAW +10 and Modified Anklesaria's IMS Consensus Group Staging.

- For diagnosing menopause, various classification systems on the basis of symptoms are used like Modified Greene Scale, Modified Kupperman Index, and Menopause Rating Scale.
- For the purpose of ease and handy learning, *Shehla's Rule of 4* can be used for making the diagnosis of menopause.

References

1. World Health Organization. Regional framework on healthy ageing (2018–2022).
2. Harlow SD, Gass M, Hall JE, Lobo R, Maki P, Rebar RW, Sherman S, Sluss PM, De Villiers TJ, STRAW +10 Collaborative Group. Executive summary of the Stages of Reproductive Aging Workshop + 10: addressing the unfinished agenda of staging reproductive aging. Climacteric. 2012;15(2):105–14.
3. Meeta M, Digumarti L, Agarwal N, Vaze N, Shah R, Malik S. Clinical practice guidelines on menopause: *an executive summary and recommendations: Indian menopause society 2019–2020. J Midlife Health. 2020;11(2):55.
4. Greene JG. Constructing a standard climacteric scale. Maturitas. 2008;61(1–2):78–84.
5. Alder E. The Blatt-Kupperman menopausal index: a critique. Maturitas. 1998;29(1):19–24.

Hot Flushes

3

Vibha Rani Pipal, Shikha Seth, and Prabhat Agrawal

3.1 Introduction

Hot flashes, often spelled as hot flushes, as it is like irrational feelings of sudden onset, transient episodes of heat and sweating, typically accompanied by feelings of palpitations and anxiety. These are collectively described as vasomotor symptoms (VMS) [1].

Hot flashes vary among individuals in terms of frequency, duration, and severity. It shows an increasing trend, starting from the transition phase to menopause and lasting for 6 months to several years. The duration of its persistence typically falls below 5 min on average, but its frequency might range from ten occurrences per day to multiple instances per week. The average duration subsequent to menopause is 4 years [2]. A significant proportion of women, approximately one-third, continue to have hot flashes even after a decade has passed since the onset of menopause [3].

It was discovered that 88% of women going through a natural menopause and 92% of those going through a surgical menopause experienced hot flashes [4]. Based on a recent cross-sectional study, it has been shown that women within the age range of 40–60 years have hot flashes and sweating at a rate of 43.05% [5].

An Indian data showed that 87.7% of women reported having menopausal symptoms, of which anxiety (80%) was most common, followed by general weakness (71.5%), sleep disturbance (61.2%), irritability (60.7%), musculoskeletal symptoms (56%), and cardiovascular symptoms (54%). The foremost symptom, hot flushes, was reported in 36.7% of cases [6].

V. R. Pipal (✉) · S. Seth
Department of Obstetrics and Gynaecology, All India Institute of Medical Sciences, Gorakhpur, Uttar Pradesh, India

P. Agrawal
PG Department of Medicine, SN Medical College, Agra, India

R. Garg (ed.), *Management of Menopause*,
https://doi.org/10.1007/978-981-96-0239-1_3

3.2 Predisposing Factors

Hot flashes are found more often in women who attained menarche at ≤11 years and were overweight or obese than in normal-weight women and menarche age of ≥14 years [7].

Its occurrence is associated with increased body mass index (BMI), lower socioeconomic position, sedentary lifestyle, smoking, and African American origin [8].

The utilization of single-nucleotide polymorphisms (SNPs) within the tachykinin receptor 3 gene, responsible for encoding neurokinin B (NKB), has been employed to demonstrate a genetic association. It was shown that NKB gene expression and neurons expressing NKB increase in postmenopausal women. Further evidence to support the efficacy of drugs serving as neurokinin 3 receptor antagonists in the management of vasomotor symptoms comes from randomized controlled trials [9–11].

3.3 Etiopathogenesis

The most typical symptom encountered throughout the perimenopausal and menopausal transition is hot flashes. Although multiple processes have been described, the precise etiopathogenesis remains unclear. The characteristic features of this phenomenon include perspiration, vasodilatation in the skin, and an increased heart rate [12].

Hot flashes are believed to be caused by high plasma levels of 3-methoxy-4-hydroxy-phenylglycol (MHPG), the primary metabolic agent of brain norepinephrine. This results in an increase in core body temperature (Tc), basal metabolic rate, and skin temperature [13, 14].

An essential function of estrogen is to modulate the brain's adrenergic receptor. Though the precise mechanism is not known, it is hypothesized that its withdrawal along with an increased level of norepinephrine leads to the occurrence of vasomotor symptoms during menopause [15].

- **Conditions other than menopause producing hot flushes** [16]:
  - Hyperthyroidism
  - Carcinoid tumors
  - Pheochromocytoma
  - Acromegaly
  - Medullary carcinoma of the thyroid
  - Idiopathic anaphylaxis
- **A few drugs may potentially be the cause of hot flushes** [16]:
  - Clomiphene
  - Tamoxifen
  - Raloxifene
  - Tricyclic antidepressants
  - Calcium channel blocker
  - Monoamine oxidase inhibitor
  - Chemotherapy

3.4 Treatment (Table 3.1)

Among the multiple treatment options, only a few are FDA-approved. Systemic estrogen therapy is widely recognized as the most effective therapeutic option as it yields a substantial 75% decrease in the occurrence of vasomotor symptoms. The US Food and

Table 3.1 Hormonal and nonhormonal pharmacologic measures for vasomotor symptoms [22–24]

Hormone preparations		
1. Estrogens		
Formulation	**Route of administration**	**Dosing**
17β-estradiol Conjugated equine estrogen	Oral Transdermal Topical Vaginal cream Intravaginal ring Oral Vaginal cream	1–2 mg/day 0.05 mg–0.1 mg; one patch/3–7 days 1.74 gm/day 500 mg–1000 mg every day × 14 days, 1–3 × weekly 0.05 mg/day for 3 months 0.3 mg–1.25 mg/day 0.5 g daily × 2 weeks then twice a week
Esterone	Injectable	0.10–0.50 mg 2–3 times a week
Esterified estrogen	Oral	0.30–1.25 mg once a day
Ethinylestradiol	Oral	20–50 mcg 1–3 times a day
2. Progestogens		
Medroxyprogesterone (MPA)	Oral	5–10 mg daily for 10–14 days or 2.5–5 mg once a day in a 30 day cycle
Micronized progesterone	Oral	200 mg daily for 12 days 100 mg/day in 28-day cycle
Norethindrone acetate	Oral Transdermal	5 mg/day 0.0.14 mg 2× weekly
Dydrogesterone	Oral	10 mg/day in 28-day cycle
3. Synthetic steroid		
Tibolone	Oral	2.5 mg/day
4. Nonhormonal pharmacologic treatments for vasomotor symptoms		
Pharmacologic drug	**Category**	**Suggested dosing**
Paroxetine	Selective serotonin reuptake inhibitor (SSRI)	Paroxetine mesylate 7.5 mg once a day Paroxetine hydrochloride 10–20 mg once a day
Venlafaxine	Serotonin-norepinephrine reuptake inhibitors (SNRI)	37.5–150 mg/day
Gabapentin	Analogue of gamma-aminobutyric acid	100–300 mg thrice a day
Oxybutynin	Anticholinergic, antimuscarinic	2.5–5 mg bd/day max dose—15 mg

Drug Administration (FDA) has granted approval for the utilization of low-dose paroxetine as a nonhormonal medication in a daily dosage of 7.5 mg over a 4-week period; it has been seen that there is a 33% decrease in vasomotor symptoms (VMS) without any accompanying adverse effects such as gain in weight or diminished libido [17, 18]. According to the position statement of the North American Menopause Society 2023, for vasomotor symptoms hormone therapy (HT) is the most effective treatment within a decade of the final menstrual periods. Hormone treatment is contraindicated in certain situations such as in the case of women with malignancies that are estrogen-dependent or cardiovascular disease or who are not willing to take it, different nonhormonal treatment options can be prescribed. Some of the options recommended based on evidence searches in different literature are selective serotonin reuptake inhibitors (SSRI), serotonin-norepinephrine reuptake inhibitors (SNRI), gabapentin, fezolinetant, oxybutynin, stellate ganglion block, loss of weight, cognitive-behavioral therapy, and clinical hypnosis [19]. Postmenopausal women with a uterus can be prescribed estrogen in different formulations depending upon the route of administration such as, oral, transdermal preparations alone, or combined with progestogens and vaginal rings. Progestogen can be administered by several routes, including oral, injectable, intrauterine device, and vaginal [20]. Bijuva 1mg/100mg, a single oral capsule in a soft-gel form containing combined 17β-estradiol and progesterone, is now available to treat moderate to severe postmenopausal vasomotor symptomatology [21].

3.5 Replacement of HT

SSRIs and SNRIs can be considered as replacement therapy for menopausal hot flashes where HT is contraindicated or compliance is poor due to the side effects [25].

3.6 Hot Flashes in Individuals with Prostate and Breast Malignancy

Patients diagnosed with prostate and breast cancer commonly encounter distressing episodes of hot flashes as a result of targeted therapy that reduces the production of testosterone and estrogen. Hot flashes can differ greatly in frequency, intensity, and length across patients; nonetheless, it is reported by over 65% of breast cancer survivors using tamoxifen and 80% of men undergoing androgen deprivation therapy (ADT) for prostate cancer. Comparing venlafaxine, paroxetine, clonidine, and electroacupuncture versus a placebo dramatically decreased the hot flash in these patients [26–28].

Another study has claimed that women experiencing hot flashes brought on by tamoxifen should not use paroxetine or other SSRIs as they interfere with drug metabolism by inhibiting the enzyme CYP2D6. SNRIs (venlafaxine), gabapentin, and clonidine can be other options for these women [29].

3.7 Other Nonhormonal Treatment Options: Block of Stellate Ganglions

For VMS, this is a nonhormonal therapy alternative. A collection of sympathetic nerves from the upper thoracic and lower cervical regions, which are located in the C6 area of the anterior cervical spine, make up the stellate ganglion.

Administration of local anesthetics such as lidocaine or bupivacaine under ultrasonographic or fluoroscopic view has been used for treating pain, migraine, and upper extremity pain. Different randomized controlled trials exhibited a decrease in the occurrence of moderate to severe vasomotor symptoms (VMS) by a maximum of 52%, and its efficacy was shown to be comparable to that of Paroxetine [30, 31].

3.8 Contraindications for Hormone Therapy [32]

- Prior history of ischemic heart disease, cerebrovascular accident, myocardial infarction, and venous thromboembolic episodes
- Unexplained vaginal bleeding
- Malignancies responsive to estrogen such as breast cancer

A multicenter, double-blind, placebo-controlled study involving women aged 50–79 revealed a higher risk of venous thrombosis, coronary heart disease, stroke, and gallstones with hormone therapy. Therefore, the lowest dose of HT should be provided or an alternate non-hormonal therapy can be given [33].

- **Mind-Body Techniques**
  - **Lifestyle modification**
  - A Cochrane analysis of the research revealed insufficient support for the benefit of exercise or physical activity in lowering the severity of VMS [34].
  - **Cognitive-behavioral therapy**
  - Research findings have indicated that the use of cognitive-behavioral therapy (CBT) has resulted in a notable reduction in occurrences of hot flashes and night sweats, as well as an improvement in sexual activity among those who have undergone breast cancer treatment [35].
  - **Clinical hypnosis**
  - A randomized controlled trial has provided evidence supporting the efficacy of clinical hypnosis in dramatically reducing the frequency of hot flashes by up to 56.86% [36].

3.9 New Research/New Therapy

- **Phytoestrogens**
- Genistein, daidzein, and S-equol are phytoestrogens that belong to the class of selective estrogen receptor beta (ERβ) modulators known as phyto-SERM. They

have been demonstrated to increase brain estrogenic activity but to have no or minimal effect on reproductive tissue. For women going through menopause-related hot flashes and cognitive decline, this group may be a safe and useful alternative to hormone therapy. More investigation and advancement are required [37].

- Different randomized controlled trials have evaluated the therapeutic role of newer agents such as estetrol (E4) and neurokinin 3 receptor antagonists (NK3R antagonists) [38, 39].
- **Antagonist of the neurokinin 3/NK3 receptor**
- It has been discovered that fezolinetant, the first neurokinin/NK3 receptor antagonist, works well to treat menopausal vasomotor symptoms (VMS) ranging from moderate to severe at doses of 30 and 45 mg [40]. The US Food and Drug Administration has authorized the brand name "Veozah" (fezolinetant) for the management of moderate to severe hot flashes associated with menopause. It works by attaching to and inhibiting the brain's NK3 receptors, which are thermoregulators (FDA news release on May 12, 2023) [41].

3.10 Drug Update: Fezolinetant—Newer Nonhormonal Treatment of Vasomotor Symptoms

It is the first nonhormonal drug.

3.10.1 Mechanism of Action

Fezolinetant blocks neurokinin B (NKB) binding on the kisspeptin/neurokinin B/dynorphin (KNDy) neuron to modulate neuronal activity in the thermoregulatory center. The thermoregulatory center (median preoptic nucleus) in the hypothalamus has nerve supply from KNDy neurons. These are inhibited by estrogen through the nuclear estrogen receptor (ERα) and stimulated by neurokinin B via the NK3 receptor. So, normal cooling will happen in the periphery as there is a balance. This occurs before menopause. At menopause, low estrogen results in the unopposed activity of neurokinin B and hypertrophy of KNDy neurons. signals to the thermoregulatory.

The recommended dose is a single 45-mg tablet orally once daily and can be given irrespective of food. A missed dose should be taken as soon as possible, up to 12 h before the next dose. Follow the usual schedule the next day. Baseline liver function tests should be done and to be followed up at 3, 6, and 9 months after treatment and when symptoms of liver injury are suspected.

The following adverse drug reactions were reported when the drug effect was studied for 52 weeks:

- Abdominal pain
- Diarrhea
- Insomnia

- Back pain
- Hot flush
- Hepatic transaminase elevation

3.10.2 Contraindications

- Known cirrhosis
- Severe renal impairment or end-stage renal disease
- Concomitant use with CYP1A2 inhibitors (e.g., ciprofloxacin, fluvoxamine, etc.)

3.10.3 Drug Interactions

Fezolinetant is a substrate of CYP1A2. The use of fezolinetant with drugs that are weak, moderate, or strong CYP1A2 inhibitors can increase the plasma Cmax (maximum concentration) and AUC (area under the curve) of fezolinetant. Hence, its use is contraindicated in persons taking CYP1A2 inhibitors.

Cautious use is recommended in renal impairment.

Contraindicated in patients with severe renal impairment (eGFR 15 to less than 30 mL/min/1.73 m^2) or end-stage renal disease (eGFR less than 15 mL/min/1.73 m^2). No dose adjustment is required for individuals with mild or moderate renal impairment.

- Hepatic transaminase. Alanine aminotransferase and/or aspartate transaminase levels were elevated and greater than three times the upper limit of normal. Women with raised hepatic transaminases were generally asymptomatic. These high levels came back to pretreatment levels without any sequelae despite continuation of dose or dose interruption or discontinuation. No elevations in serum total bilirubin were found.

3.11 Conclusion

Hot flashes or flushes are very common in women undergoing menopause and in patients of breast malignancy receiving tamoxifen therapy. If VMS is not treated, it degrades quality of life. It can last for several months to 4 years, or within a third of postmenopausal women, it can last for 10 years. When there are no contraindications, hormone therapy is the best option, but it should be used cautiously on older women.

References

1. Mohyi D, et al. Differential diagnosis of hot flashes. Maturitas. 1997;27:203–14.
2. Politi MC, Schleinitz MD, Col NF. Revisiting the duration of vasomotor symptoms of menopause: a meta-analysis. J Gen Intern Med. 2008;23(9):1507–13. https://doi.org/10.1007/s11606-008-0655-4. Epub 2008 Jun 3. PMID: 18521690; PMCID: PMC2518020.

3. Freeman EW, Sammel MD, Sanders RJ. Risk of long-term hot flashes after natural menopause: evidence from the Penn Ovarian Aging Study cohort. Menopause. 2014;21(9):924–32. https://doi.org/10.1097/GME.0000000000000196. PMID: 24473530; PMCID: PMC4574289.
4. Feldman BM, Voda A, Gronseth E. The prevalence of hot flash and associated variables among perimenopausal women. Res Nurs Health. 1985;8(3):261–8. https://doi.org/10.1002/nur.4770080308. PMID: 3852361.
5. Lu J, Li K, Zheng X, et al. Prevalence of menopausal symptoms and attitudes towards menopausal hormone therapy in women aged 40–60 years: a cross-sectional study. BMC Womens Health. 2023;23:472. https://doi.org/10.1186/s12905-023-02621-8.
6. Kalhan M, Singhania K, Choudhary P, Verma S, Kaushal P, Singh T. Prevalence of menopausal symptoms and its effect on quality of life among rural middle aged women (40–60 years) of Haryana, India. Int J Appl Basic Med Res. 2020;10(3):183–8. https://doi.org/10.4103/ijabmr.IJABMR_428_19. Epub 2020 Jul 11. PMID: 33088741; PMCID: PMC7534715.
7. Chung H-F, Zhu D, Dobson AJ, Kuh D, Gold EB, Crawford SL, Avis NE, Mitchell ES, Woods NF, Anderson DJ, Mishra GD. Age at menarche and risk of vasomotor menopausal symptoms: a pooled analysis of six studies. BJOG. 2021;128:603. https://doi.org/10.1111/1471-0528.16393.
8. Gold EB, Sternfeld B, Kelsey JL, Brown C, Mouton C, Reame N, Salamone L, Stellato R. Relation of demographic and lifestyle factors to symptoms in a multi-racial/ethnic population of women 40-55 years of age. Am J Epidemiol. 2000;152(5):463–73. https://doi.org/10.1093/aje/152.5.463. PMID: 10981461.
9. Crandall CJ, Diamant AL, Maglione M, Thurston RC, Sinsheimer J. Genetic variation and hot flashes: a systematic review. J Clin Endocrinol Metab. 2020;105(12):e4907–57. https://doi.org/10.1210/clinem/dgaa536. PMID: 32797194; PMCID: PMC7538102.
10. Rance NE, Krajewski SJ, Smith MA, Cholanian M, Dacks PA. Neurokinin B and the hypothalamic regulation of reproduction. Brain Res. 2010;1364:116–28. https://doi.org/10.1016/j.brainres.2010.08.059. Epub 2010 Aug 25. PMID: 20800582; PMCID: PMC2992576.
11. Depypere H, Timmerman D, Donders G, Sieprath P, Ramael S, Combalbert J, Hoveyda HR, Fraser GL. Treatment of menopausal vasomotor symptoms with Fezolinetant, a neurokinin 3 receptor antagonist: a phase 2a trial. J Clin Endocrinol Metab. 2019;104(12):5893–905. https://doi.org/10.1210/jc.2019-00677. PMID: 31415087.
12. Freedman RR. Laboratory and ambulatory monitoring of menopausal hot flashes. Psychophysiology. 1989;26(5):573–9. https://doi.org/10.1111/j.1469-8986.1989.tb00712.x. PMID: 2616704.
13. Freedman RR, Woodward SU. Elevated α2-adrenergic responsiveness in menopausal hot flushes: pharmacologic and biochemical studies. Thermoregulation: the pathophysiological basis of clinical disorders. Basel: Karger; 1992. p. 6–9.
14. Freedman RR. Biochemical, metabolic, and vascular mechanisms in menopausal hot flashes. Fertil Steril. 1998;70(2):332–7. https://doi.org/10.1016/s0015-0282(98)00137-x. PMID: 9696230.
15. Etgen AM, Ansonoff MA, Quesada A. Mechanisms of ovarian steroid regulation of norepinephrine receptor-mediated signal transduction in the hypothalamus: implications for female reproductive physiology. Horm Behav. 2001;40(2):169–77. https://doi.org/10.1006/hbeh.2001.1676. PMID: 11534978.
16. Izikson L, English JC 3rd, Zirwas MJ. The flushing patient: differential diagnosis, workup, and treatment. J Am Acad Dermatol. 2006;55(2):193–208. https://doi.org/10.1016/j.jaad.2005.07.057. PMID: 16844500.
17. Maclennan AH, Broadbent JL, Lester S, Moore V. Oral oestrogen and combined oestrogen/progestogen therapy versus placebo for hot flushes. Cochrane Database Syst Rev. 2004;2004(4):CD002978. https://doi.org/10.1002/14651858.CD002978.pub2. PMID: 15495039; PMCID: PMC7004247.
18. Simon JA, Portman DJ, Kaunitz AM, Mekonnen H, Kazempour K, Bhaskar S, Lippman J. Low-dose paroxetine 7.5 mg for menopausal vasomotor symptoms: two randomized controlled trials. Menopause. 2013;20(10):1027–35. https://doi.org/10.1097/GME.0b013e3182a66aa7.

19. "The 2023 Nonhormone Therapy Position Statement of The North American Menopause Society" Advisory Panel. The 2023 nonhormone therapy position statement of The North American Menopause Society. Menopause. 2023;30(6):573–590. https://doi.org/10.1097/GME.0000000000002200. PMID: 37252752.
20. The NAMS 2017 Hormone Therapy Position Statement Advisory Panel. The 2017 hormone therapy position statement of The North American Menopause Society. Menopause. 2017;24(7):728–53. https://doi.org/10.1097/GME.0000000000000921. PMID: 28650869.
21. Kaunitz AM, Bitner D, Constantine GD, Bernick B, Graham S, Mirkin S. 17β-estradiol/progesterone in a single, oral, softgel capsule (TX-001HR) significantly increased the number of vasomotor symptom-free days in the REPLENISH trial. Menopause. 2020;27(12):1382–7. https://doi.org/10.1097/GME.0000000000001615. PMID: 32740481; PMCID: PMC7709918.
22. Santoro N, Roeca C, Peters BA, Neal-Perry G. The menopause transition: signs, symptoms, and management options. J Clin Endocrinol Metabol. 2021;106(1):1–15. https://doi.org/10.1210/clinem/dgaa764.
23. Mehta J, Kling JM, Manson JE. Risks, benefits, and treatment modalities of menopausal hormone therapy: current concepts. Front Endocrinol (Lausanne). 2021;12:564781. https://doi.org/10.3389/fendo.2021.564781. PMID: 33841322; PMCID: PMC8034540.
24. David PS, Smith TL, Nordhues HC, Kling JM. A clinical review on paroxetine and emerging therapies for the treatment of vasomotor symptoms. Int J Womens Health. 2022;14:353–61. https://doi.org/10.2147/IJWH.S282396. PMID: 35300283; PMCID: PMC8921794.
25. Azizi M, Khani S, Kamali M, Elyasi F. The efficacy and safety of selective serotonin reuptake inhibitors and serotonin-norepinephrine reuptake inhibitors in the treatment of menopausal hot flashes: a systematic review of clinical trials. Iran J Med Sci. 2022;47(3):173–93. https://doi.org/10.30476/ijms.2020.87687.1817. PMID: 35634530; PMCID: PMC9126898.
26. Chang HY, Jotwani AC, Lai YH, Jensen MP, Syrjala KL, Fann JR, Gralow J. Hot flashes in breast cancer survivors: frequency, severity and impact. Breast. 2016;27:116–21. https://doi.org/10.1016/j.breast.2016.02.013. Epub 2016 Apr 8. PMID: 27065357; PMCID: PMC5893329.
27. Frisk J. Managing hot flushes in men after prostate cancer—a systematic review. Maturitas. 2010;65(1):15–22. https://doi.org/10.1016/j.maturitas.2009.10.017. Epub 2009 Dec 4. PMID: 19962840.
28. Hutton B, Hersi M, Cheng W, Pratt M, Barbeau P, Mazzarello S, Ahmadzai N, Skidmore B, Morgan SC, Bordeleau L, Ginex PK, Sadeghirad B, Morgan RL, Cole KM, Clemons M. Comparing interventions for management of hot flashes in patients with breast and prostate cancer: a systematic review with meta-analyses. Oncol Nurs Forum. 2020;47(4):E86–E106. https://doi.org/10.1188/20.ONF.E86-E106. PMID: 32555553; PMCID: PMC7891229.
29. Desmarais JE, Looper KJ. Managing menopausal symptoms and depression in tamoxifen users: implications of drug and medicinal interactions. Maturitas. 2010;67(4):296–308. https://doi.org/10.1016/j.maturitas.2010.08.005. Epub 2010 Sep 28. PMID: 20880642.
30. Walega DR, Rubin LH, Banuvar S, Shulman LP, Maki PM. Effects of stellate ganglion block on vasomotor symptoms: findings from a randomized controlled clinical trial in postmenopausal women. Menopause. 2014;21(8):807–14. https://doi.org/10.1097/GME.0000000000000194. PMID: 24496086; PMCID: PMC4110158.
31. Rahimzadeh P, Imani F, Nafissi N, Ebrahimi B, Faiz SHR. Comparison of the effects of stellate ganglion block and paroxetine on hot flashes and sleep disturbance in breast cancer survivors. Cancer Manag Res. 2018;10:4831–7. https://doi.org/10.2147/CMAR.S173511. PMID: 30464591; PMCID: PMC6208490.
32. "The 2022 Hormone Therapy Position Statement of The North American Menopause Society" Advisory Panel. The 2022 hormone therapy position statement of The North American Menopause Society. Menopause. 2022;29(7):767–794. https://doi.org/10.1097/GME.0000000000002028. PMID: 35797481.
33. Manson JE, Chlebowski RT, Stefanick ML, et al. Menopausal hormone therapy and health outcomes during the intervention and extended poststopping phases of the Women's Health

Initiative randomized trials. JAMA. 2013;310(13):1353–68. https://doi.org/10.1001/jama.2013.278040.
34. Daley A, Stokes-Lampard H, Thomas A, MacArthur C. Exercise for vasomotor menopausal symptoms. Cochrane Database Syst Rev. 2014;2014(11):CD006108. https://doi.org/10.1002/14651858.CD006108.pub4. PMID: 25431132; PMCID: PMC10116337.
35. Duijts SF, van Beurden M, Oldenburg HS, Hunter MS, Kieffer JM, Stuiver MM, Gerritsma MA, Menke-Pluymers MB, Plaisier PW, Rijna H, Lopes Cardozo AM, Timmers G, van der Meij S, van der Veen H, Bijker N, de Widt-Levert LM, Geenen MM, Heuff G, van Dulken EJ, Boven E, Aaronson NK. Efficacy of cognitive behavioral therapy and physical exercise in alleviating treatment-induced menopausal symptoms in patients with breast cancer: results of a randomized, controlled, multicenter trial. J Clin Oncol. 2012;30(33):4124–33. https://doi.org/10.1200/JCO.2012.41.8525. Epub 2012 Oct 8. PMID: 23045575.
36. Elkins GR, Fisher WI, Johnson AK, Carpenter JS, Keith TZ. Clinical hypnosis in the treatment of postmenopausal hot flashes: a randomized controlled trial. Menopause. 2013;20(3):291–8. https://doi.org/10.1097/gme.0b013e31826ce3ed. PMID: 23435026; PMCID: PMC3556367.
37. Wang Y, Hernandez G, Mack WJ, Schneider LS, Yin F, Brinton RD. Retrospective analysis of phytoSERM for management of menopause-associated vasomotor symptoms and cognitive decline: a pilot study on pharmacogenomic effects of mitochondrial haplogroup and APOE genotype on therapeutic efficacy. Menopause. 2020;27(1):57–65. https://doi.org/10.1097/GME.0000000000001418. PMID: 31567873; PMCID: PMC7100617.
38. Gaspard U, Taziaux M, Mawet M, Jost M, Gordenne V, Coelingh Bennink HJT, Lobo RA, Utian WH, Foidart JM. A multicenter, randomized study to select the minimum effective dose of estetrol (E4) in postmenopausal women (E4Relief): part 1. Vasomotor symptoms and overall safety. Menopause. 2020;27(8):848–57. https://doi.org/10.1097/GME.0000000000001561. PMID: 32379217; PMCID: PMC7386865.
39. Trower M, Anderson RA, Ballantyne E, Joffe H, Kerr M, Pawsey S. Effects of NT-814, a dual neurokinin 1 and 3 receptor antagonist, on vasomotor symptoms in postmenopausal women: a placebo-controlled, randomized trial. Menopause. 2020;27(5):498–505. https://doi.org/10.1097/GME.0000000000001500. PMID: 32068688; PMCID: PMC7188053.
40. Johnson KA, Martin N, Nappi RE, Neal-Perry G, Shapiro M, Stute P, Thurston RC, Wolfman W, English M, Franklin C, Lee M, Santoro N. Efficacy and safety of fezolinetant in moderate to severe vasomotor symptoms associated with menopause: a phase 3 RCT. J Clin Endocrinol Metab. 2023;108(8):1981–97. https://doi.org/10.1210/clinem/dgad058. PMID: 36734148; PMCID: PMC10348473.
41. https://www.fda.gov/news-events/press-announcements/fda-approves-novel-drug-treat-moderate-severe-hot-flashes-caused-menopause#:~:text=Veozah%20is%20the%20first%20neurokinin,brain%27s%20regulation%20of%20body%20temperature. Accessed 14 Oct 2023.

Sleep and Menopause

4

Gehanath Baral and Reetu Sharma

4.1 Menopause

Menopause itself is not the issue of menstruation but a vulnerable stage in the life cycle of every woman. This stage of the life cycle needs utmost care because of multisystem dysfunction requiring preventive and promotive intervention since its transition—called a climacteric period. Different degrees of vasomotor, physical, urogenital, or psychosexual manifestations occur that may require multiple interventions; and a woman will be labeled as a sick person if this condition is not understood appropriately [1]. The literal meaning of menopause is a cessation of menstruation. Amenorrhoea could be temporary or reversible like in hypothalamic-pituitary-ovarian suppression from hormonal intake, pregnancy, lactation, drug-induced, and anxiety-depression-like disorder. It may also be a permanent event due to ovarian destruction or excision. Permanent cessation of menstruation due to ovarian failure is considered natural menopause, and it is operationalized by the cutoff of 1 year from the last natural cycle. However, surgical menopause doesn't require this cutoff as this is an abrupt event. Chemotherapeutic and radiotherapeutic destruction of the ovary also lead to the gradual onset of amenorrhoea.

4.2 Menopausal Physiology

The hypothalamus controls the circadian rhythm and internal homeostasis of several neurotransmitters that influence the sleep pattern and mental status. The role of progesterone is to produce non-rapid eye movement (NREM) sleep by stimulating

G. Baral (✉) · R. Sharma
Kathmandu University, Nobel Medical College, Biratnagar, Nepal
e-mail: gehanath.baral@nmcth.edu.np

R. Garg (ed.), *Management of Menopause*,
https://doi.org/10.1007/978-981-96-0239-1_4

benzodiazepine receptors associated with GABA receptors. It also stimulates the respiratory centre and helps to mitigate mild forms of obstructive sleep apnoea.

There are different ways to influence sleep structure by oestrogen. It promotes the metabolism of norepinephrine, serotonin, and acetylcholine neurotransmitters that affect sleep patterns, decreases sleep latency and frequency of awakening or arousals, and increases total sleep time.

It acts as a thermostat to decrease night sweats stabilizes the mood by increasing norepinephrine and serotonin uptake and acts as an antidepressant agent. Vasomotor symptoms and insomnia occur either due to sex hormone deficiency or their rapidly changing level in the body.

Thus, hormone replacement therapy in peri-or post-menopause helps a woman in her sleep quality, vasomotor flush, mood, and bone health. Both hot flashes and insomnia cause depression and oestrogen therapy can ameliorate most of these symptoms [2, 3].

4.3 Sleep

Around one-third of our life is spent asleep which is an internally regulated universal biological function of life. It is required for survival, energy conservation, neural development, learning, memory, and vital functions [4].

Sleep is considered healthy for an adult if it is adequate, timely, regular, and without disturbances. There is a risk of adverse health outcomes if the duration of sleep is less than 7 h such as weight gain and obesity, diabetes, hypertension, heart disease, stroke, depression, impaired performance, and increased errors [5].

There are four stages of a sleep cycle composed of NREM, REM, and wake stages; and the typical sleep cycles are illustrated with varied stages in each cycle. In insomnia, the probability of moving from NREM 2 to NREM 1 appears to be higher leading to more frequent awakenings and lighter total sleep. NREM stage 3 is the most important physiologic need that needs to be compensated for good health [6].

The relative time spent in each stage of sleep is N1 (stage 1, NREM, light sleep), 5%; N2 (stage 2, NREM, deeper sleep), 45%; N3 (stage 3, NREM, deepest sleep), 25%; and REM (stage 4, dream), 25%. There are four to five sleep cycles in a typical night's sleep and the sleep progresses in the order of N1 → N2 → N3 → N2 → REM. There is a progressive reduction in N3 (slow wave sleep or deepest sleep) as age advances. Adults in contrast to children spend less time in REM sleep; alcohol intake also decreases REM stage, but as its effect wears off, there is rebound prolongation of REM sleep (Fig. 4.1). The sleep-wake cycle is controlled by different brain structures like the *hypothalamus*, which controls the onset of sleep; the *hippocampus*, a memory region active during dreaming; the *amygdala*, an emotion centre active during dreaming; the *thalamus*, which prevents sensory signals from reaching the cortex; *reticular formation*, regulates the transition between sleep and wakefulness; and *pons*, helps initiate REM sleep. The extraocular movements during REM are due to the activity of paramedian pontine reticular formation/conjugate gaze center [7].

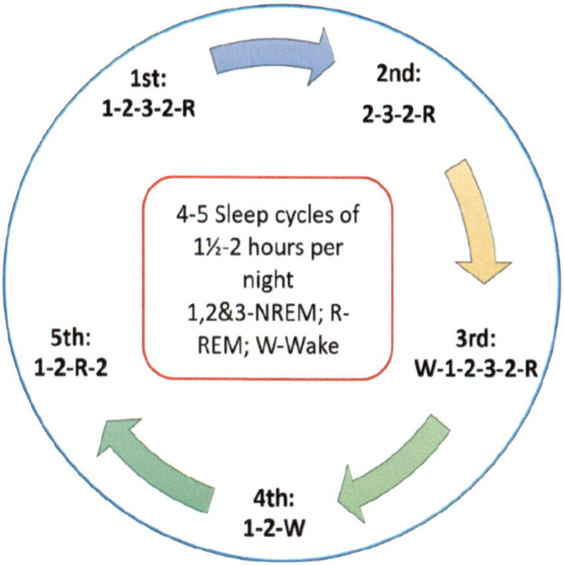

Fig. 4.1 Typical night sleep cycles (Created by author)

4.4 Sleep Dysfunction

Sleep disorders are hormone-specific concerning the phases of reproductive life like the luteal phase of menstruation, pregnancy, and menopause. Increasing nocturnal awakenings or wake-after-sleep onset (WASO) is common. There is an increased risk for insomnia in the luteal phase; an increased risk of restless legs syndrome (RLS) and sleep apnoea in the third trimester of pregnancy; and a high prevalence of insomnia and sleep-disordered breathing (SDB) in menopause [8].

The most common sleep disorder is insomnia which presents in 10–30% of the adult population, and one of the common predisposing non-modifiable factors for this and its persistence is female sex, especially at menopause. Insomnia is the difficulty in initiating or maintaining sleep with impaired daytime functioning.

Insomnia of menopause is the chronic insomnia disorder characterized by chronic sleep-onset or sleep maintenance complaints with an associated daytime impairment that occurs at least three times a week persisting for at least 3 months and is not due to other morbid conditions [9].

Insomnia of menopause may fall into the psychophysiological type of primary insomnia. Psychophysiological insomnia is characterized primarily by heightened arousal and learned sleep-preventing associations that result in a complaint of insomnia. Patients who presumed to have this type of insomnia often have sleep difficulty when trying to sleep in their usual sleep setting at home but may fall asleep easily in a novel sleep setting or when not trying to sleep. They also demonstrate excessive focus on and worry about sleep and suffer from elevated levels of cognitive and somatic arousal, particularly at bedtime.

Sleep can be evaluated by multiple sleep latency tests and sleep logs. "The sleep latency usually is in the range of 10–15 min. Sleep logs typically show a long sleep latency, reduced TST (Total Sleep Time), increased WASO, and frequent nocturnal awakenings. Poor sleep quality is often reported. Typically, there is considerable night-to-night variability in sleep quality. There may also be evidence of poor sleep hygiene with prolonged time in bed, napping, and variability in wake times." There is a reduction in an inhibitory neurotransmitter like gamma-aminobutyric acid (GABA) in non-medicated patients with primary insomnia leading to impaired sleep. Thus, the pharmacotherapy will be decided accordingly [10].

The prevalence of insomnia is 6–10% and higher in women, older age, and lonely people. At least 6–7 h of sleep is considered a normal sleep duration, and the odds of associated diabetes and hypertension are 3 and 5, respectively, for the short sleep duration. Chronic insomnia of three nights a week for 3 months or more may result in reduced work efficiency, attention, and stability.

Variations in sleep stages occur in other conditions like narcolepsy (REM sleep is reached much more quickly than usual), sleep apnoea (pauses in breathing during sleep especially interrupt REM sleep) [11], depression (less time appears to be spent in NREM 3, and REM sleep may be reached earlier than is typical) [12], and schizophrenia (less time appears to be spent in NREM phases, especially NREM 3. REM sleep may be reached earlier than is typical, but this could be due to the high rates of depression in people with schizophrenia [13].

4.5 Management of Insomnia

The American Academy of Sleep Medicine (AASM) considers stimulus control therapy, relaxation training, and cognitive behavioural therapy (CBT-I) as the standard treatments for insomnia. CBT for insomnia and pharmacotherapy are treatment options. *Cognitive behavioural therapy for insomnia* (standard): cognitive behavioural therapy (CBT) for insomnia is also sometimes termed *CBTI.* This technique combines cognitive therapy with behavioural techniques. The behavioural component may include stimulus control therapy and/or sleep restriction therapy with or without the use of relaxation therapy. Sleep hygiene education is often included.

$GABA_A$ receptor modulators bind to the GABA-benzodiazepine-chloride ionophore complex (GBC) and act as the GABA-BZ receptor agonist (BZRAs) action to promote sleep. Benzodiazepines like triazolam (0.125–0.25 mg HS), estazolam (1–2 mg HS), temazepam (15–30 mg HS), flurazepam (15–30 mg HS), clonazepam (0.25–0.5 mg HS), and lorazepam (0.5–1 mg HS); nonbenzodiazepines like zaleplon (5–10 mg HS), zolpidem (5–10 mg HS), and eszopiclone (1–3 mg HS); or melatonin (MT) receptor agonist like ramelteon (8 mg HS) can be used as the pharmacotherapeutic agents as the hypnotic medication.

Short-acting medications work for sleep-onset insomnia but may not help with sleep-maintenance insomnia. Triazolam has a short duration of action but is associated with significant rebound insomnia and is no longer considered a first-line agent for insomnia. Zaleplon has a very short duration of action and may be useful as a "rescue medication" for middle-of-the-night dosing (as long as 4–6 h of potential sleep remains) [14, 15].

4.6 Clinical Evaluation

The hypnotic treatment algorithm is to be followed for the clinical management of insomnia requiring hypnotic agents (Fig. 4.2).

4.7 Menopausal Insomnia

Three out of five menopausal women experience insomnia. Hot flush is the prominent menopausal symptom, and at night it produces night sweats that may also contribute to insomnia. Chronic insomnia brings sleep deprivation-related symptoms and mental disturbances as well (Fig. 4.3).

Preventive measures to deal with menopausal insomnia are optimizing weight; following a sleep schedule; minimizing hot flashes by avoiding large evening meals

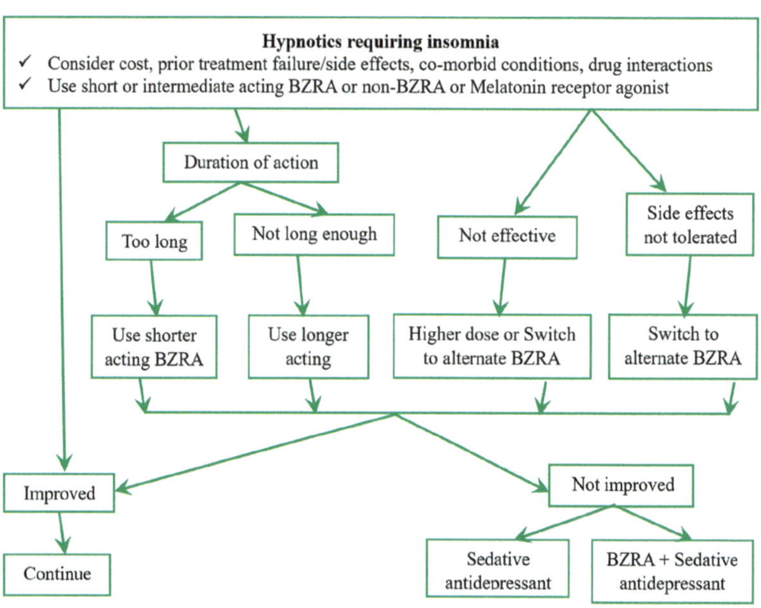

[BZRA = benzodiazepine receptor agonist; SMI = sleep-maintenance insomnia; SOI = sleep onset insomnia]

Fig. 4.2 Clinical pathway for hypnotic treatment of insomnia. (Created by the author based on Schutte-Rodin, 2008 [16]). *BZRA* benzodiazepine receptor agonist, *SMI* sleep-maintenance insomnia, *SOI* sleep onset insomnia

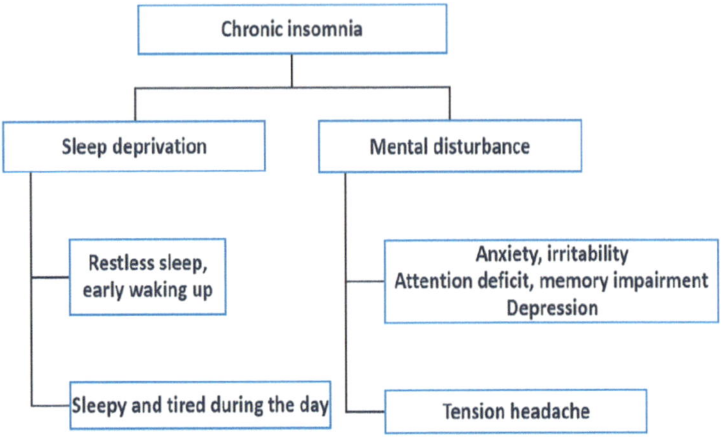

Fig. 4.3 Presentation of chronic insomnia (Created by author)

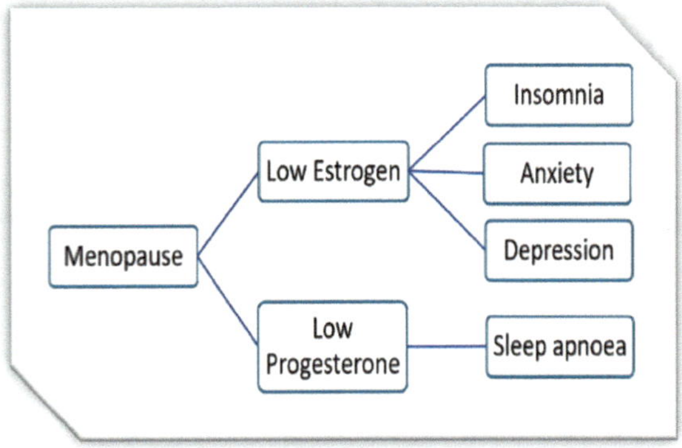

Fig. 4.4 Hormone deficiency in menopause (Created by author)

and spicy or acidic foods; stopping drinking before bedtime; preserving sleep quality by avoiding nicotine, caffeine, and alcohol in the late afternoon and early evening; using the restroom before going to bed; lowering stress by massage, exercise, yoga, and evening bath; meditation or deep breathing; minimizing daytime nap and bedtime and maximizing sleep time; and keeping room temperature at reasonably cool and wear light night dress [17, 18].

There is significant sleep electrical activity in the brain of women on HRT with increased frequency of REM sleep and reduced awake time. Combining both oestrogen and progesterone yields improved sleep quality and cognitive function, lesser sleep latency and wake-up frequency, and increased REM sleep. Obstructive sleep apnoea (OSA) occurs in 2% of women, and its annual increased risk is 4% per annum from perimenopausal age (Fig. 4.4). However, it will be less if hormone replacement therapy is begun earlier. This is because progesterone acts as a respiratory stimulant to prevent both central and obstructive sleep apnoea by preventing the relaxation of the upper airways [19].

4.8 Management Principle

International sleep guidelines from the World Sleep Society are the endorsement of insomnia treatment from European guidelines as the primary intervention of Cognitive-Behavioural Therapy (CBT-I) and second-line pharmacological therapy. CBT-I includes sleep hygiene education, behavioural sleep scheduling interventions such as sleep restriction and stimulus control procedures, cognitive restructuring therapy, and relaxation-based interventions. Pharmacological therapy as a second-line intervention includes benzodiazepines and other GABA-A receptor agonists (zolpidem, eszopiclone, zopiclone), sedating antidepressants, orexin antagonists, antihistamines, antipsychotics, melatonin (MT) receptor agonists, and phyto-therapeutic substances (valerian, medicinal cannabis). For adults with primary insomnia treated for any duration or secondary insomnia in which underlying comorbidities are managed, the antipsychotics should be stopped without tapering [20].

European guidelines detail the diagnostic procedure for insomnia, and its comorbidities, such as a clinical sleep history, questionnaires, and diaries, psychosomatic history, physical examination, and diagnostic tests like blood tests, ECG, and EEG. If there is clinically significant nocturnal and diurnal sleep impairment with maintained synchrony but having sleep affecting substance intake, then, a change of medication is advised. If it is associated with comorbid somatic or mental disorders, then, the respective treatment is advised; but in its absence, the first-line treatment option is CBT-I or short-term medications like BZ, BZRA, or sedating antidepressants. If there is no clinically significant sleep impairment and sleep synchrony is maintained, then psychoeducation would be sufficient [21, 22].

Insomnia of menopause is managed by hormone replacement therapy especially oestrogen which helps treat anxiety, depression, insomnia, mood swings, and hot flashes. It has beneficial effects on skin and bone health as well as lipid metabolism. Progesterone can help to minimize sleep apnoea as well. Hormone replacement therapy can usually be continued for 7–10 years to minimize vasomotor symptoms and osteoporosis; at the same time, it helps to minimize menopause-related insomnia, but other conditions leading to insomnia should be dealt with simultaneously.

Thus, insomnia at menopause is the disequilibrium in post-reproductive life due to the inadequacy of sex hormones. It has a cause-effect relationship. This hormonal imbalance produces multiorgan symptoms and may result in multiple symptomatic medical interventions. Therefore, treating the cause is the first line of intervention, and the remaining symptoms are to be managed accordingly. Causal intervention would be either hormone replacement therapy or hormone modulator-rich foodstuff. Promotive lifestyle modification interventions will be supportive of the quality of life.

References

1. Baral G. Menopause rating scale: validation and applicability in Nepalese women. J Nepal Health Res Counc. 2019;17(42):9–14. https://doi.org/10.33314/jnhrc.v17i01.1770.
2. Lee J, Han Y, Cho HH, Kim MR. Sleep disorders and menopause. J Menopausal Med. 2019;25(2):83–7. https://doi.org/10.6118/jmm.19192.
3. Joffe H, Petrillo LF, Koukopoulos A, Viguera AC, Hirschberg A, Nonacs R, et al. Increased estradiol and improved sleep, but not hot flashes, predict enhanced mood during the menopausal transition. J Clin Endocrinol Metab. 2011;96(7):E1044–54. https://doi.org/10.1210/jc.2010-2503.
4. Mukherjee S, Patel SR, Kales SN, Ayas NT, Strohl KP, Gozal D, et al. An official American Thoracic Society statement: the importance of healthy sleep. Recommendations and future priorities. Am J Respir Crit Care Med. 2015;191(12):1450–8. https://doi.org/10.1164/rccm.201504-0767ST.
5. Watson NF, Badr MS, Belenky G, Bliwise DL, Buxton OM, Buysse D, et al. The recommended amount of sleep for a healthy adult: a joint consensus statement of the American Academy of Sleep Medicine and Sleep Research Society. J Clin Sleep Med. 2015;11(6):591–2.
6. Wei Y, Colombo MA, Ramautar JR, Blanken TF, Werf YD, Spiegelhalder K, et al. Sleep stage transition dynamics reveal specific stage 2 vulnerability in insomnia. Sleep. 2017;40(9). https://doi.org/10.1093/sleep/zsx117.
7. Patel AK, Reddy V, Shumway KR, Araujo JF. Physiology, sleep stages. [Updated 2022 Sep 7]. In: StatPearls [Internet]. Treasure Island: StatPearls Publishing; 2023. https://www.ncbi.nlm.nih.gov/books/NBK526132/.
8. Dorsey A, de Lecea L, Jennings KJ. Neurobiological and hormonal mechanisms regulating women's sleep. Front Neurosci. 2020;14:625397. https://doi.org/10.3389/fnins.2020.625397.
9. ICSD-3-TR. International classification of sleep disorders, 3rd ed., text revision. American Academy of Sleep Medicine; 2023.
10. Darien IL. International classification of sleep disorders, 3rd ed. American Academy of Sleep Medicine; 2014.
11. Fraigne JJ, Grace KP, Horner RL, Peever J. Mechanisms of REM sleep in health and disease. Curr Opin Pulm Med. 2014;20(6):527–32. https://doi.org/10.1097/MCP.0000000000000103.
12. Wang YQ, Li R, Zhang MQ, Zhang Z, Qu WM, Huang ZL. The neurobiological mechanisms and treatments of REM sleep disturbances in depression. Curr Neuropharmacol. 2015;13(4):543–53. https://doi.org/10.2174/1570159x13666150310002540.
13. Baglioni C, Nanovska S, Regen W, Spiegelhalder K, Feige B, Nissen C, et al. Sleep and mental disorders: a meta-analysis of polysomnographic research. Psychol Bull. 2016;142(9):969–90. https://doi.org/10.1037/bul0000053.
14. Berry RB. Fundamental of sleep medicine. Elsevier; 2012.
15. Leschziner G. Oxford handbook of sleep medicine, 1st ed.; 2022. isbn:978-0-19-284825-3. https://doi.org/10.1093/med/9780192848253.001.0001.
16. Schutte-Rodin S, Broch L, Buysee D, Dorsey C, Sateia M. Clinical guideline for the evaluation and management of chronic insomnia in adults. J Clin Sleep Med. 2008;4:487–504.
17. Pacheco D, Callender E. Menopause and sleep (internet journal). 2022. https://www.sleepfoundation.org/women-sleep/menopause-and-sleep.
18. U.S. Department of Health & Human Services (HHS), National Institutes of Health (NIH), National Institute of Aging 2021. https://www.nia.nih.gov/health/sleep-problems-and-menopause-what-can-i-do.
19. Belcher NL. Winona (internet journal). Correlation between estrogen and sleep disturbances 2023. https://bywinona.com/journal/estrogen-and-sleep-disturbances.
20. Bjerre LM, Farrell B, Hogel M, Graham L, Lemay G, McCarthy L. Deprescribing antipsychotics for behavioural and psychological symptoms of dementia and insomnia. Evidence-based clinical practice guideline. Can Fam Physician. 2018;64:17–27.

21. Riemann D, Baglioni C, Bassett C, Bjorvatn B, Groselj LD, Ellis JG, et al. European guidelines for the diagnosis and treatment of insomnia. J Sleep Res. 2017;26:675–700. https://doi.org/10.1111/jsr.12594.
22. Morin CM, Inoue Y, Kushida C, Poyares D, Winkelman J, Guidelines Committee Members; Governing Council of the World Sleep Society. Endorsement of European guidelines for the diagnosis and treatment of insomnia by the World Sleep Society. Sleep Med. 2021;81:124–6. https://doi.org/10.1016/j.sleep.2021.01.023. Epub 2021 Jan 21. PMID: 33667998.

Psychological Problems and Menopause

5

Radhika Chetan, Jyothi G. Seshadri, and Prabhat Agrawal

5.1 Introduction [1]

- Menopausal transition, though a normal physiological phase in women, is considered as a critical milestone, with changes in physical status, hormonal fluctuations, menstrual pattern, mood, and emotions, having significant effect on quality of life. Majority of women undergo smooth transition through pre-menopause to menopause, but some women face the "window of vulnerability" when they develop increased mood changes, irritability, anxiety issues, and depressive episodes (DE), and few may even develop major depressive disorders (MDDs) which require therapy [1, 2]. Data is evolving in favour of perimenopausal hormonal changes and its influence on mood disorders.
- About 20% of women in menopausal transition experience depression [3]. About one in four women seek care for menopausal mood changes in the United States. This can be due to aggravation of previous psychological condition or a new-onset mood disorder. Perimenopause (period before attaining menopause and just after last menses) has more psychological effects than postmenopause phase [4]. Suicide rates are known to be highest among women in their midlife as per data from the United States and Australia [5, 6]. It is important to screen women for suicidal tendencies whenever they present with DE or MDD in midlife.

R. Chetan (✉)
Department of Obstetrics and Gynaecology, Bangalore Medical College and Research Institute, Bengaluru, India

J. G. Seshadri
Department of Obstetrics and Gynaecology, Ramaiah Medical College and Hospitals, Bengaluru, India

P. Agrawal
PG Department of Medicine, SN Medical College, Agra, India

R. Garg (ed.), *Management of Menopause*,
https://doi.org/10.1007/978-981-96-0239-1_5

- Menopausal vasomotor symptoms (VMS) like hot flushes, sleep disturbance, and irritability may overlap with mood changes, making diagnosis difficult or may aggravate psychological effects of menopause. Differentiating severe menopausal vasomotor symptoms from DE may be challenging. Other features of menopause such as genitourinary syndrome of menopause (GSM) may affect sexuality and predispose to depression. Midlife stressors like professional career stages, family issues, taking care of elderly parents, and empty nest syndrome (children leaving home) may precipitate pre-existing depression or have effect on new-onset depression [2]. VMS, GSM, weight gain, physical fatigue, and change in sexual practice associated with menopause may further accentuate mood disorders in women. Guidelines on clinical presentation, recognition, and management of depression around menopause transition are lacking [2, 3].
- It is vital to know the psychological changes during and after menopausal transition for managing these cases and also to refer to psychiatrist/counsellors by primary care physicians.

5.2 Epidemiology [1, 2, 5–20]

- Compared to men, women are 1.7 times more prone to develop MDD during lifetime [7, 8]. About 50% of women aged 18–65 years had mood disorder at some point in life, as per national survey 2017 [8]. Women in midlife are two to four times more likely to experience DE and MDD compared to younger women [2, 9, 10].
- Around 20% perimenopausal women present with mood disorders to healthcare providers. Risk of depression is higher after surgical menopause, about 20% higher, after only hysterectomy and 44% higher risk after hysterectomy with ovary removal. Early menopause due to premature ovarian insufficiency also carries 20% higher risk of MDD [11, 12].
- Premenstrual phase, postpartum, and perimenopause are windows of vulnerability for mood disorders and may be related to phases of reproductive hormonal fluctuations. Menopausal transition in particular may be a more significant phase as it is affected by multiple factors other than hormonal changes, including changes in physical appearance, VMS, and GSM with changes in sexuality, family, and career pressures.
- There is evolving evidence that menopause is an independent risk factor for depressive disorders. Overlapping of VMS, sleep disturbances, self-reported symptoms, and nonavailability of standardised questionnaires for menopausal depression made evidence generation difficult. Earlier data suggested women with pre-existing mood disorder are more likely to develop psychological disorders during menopause; however, new longitudinal population based data suggest that pre-menopause and menopausal transition have a significant effect on mood disorders than menopause per se [13–15]. *Psychological effects are seen more in menopausal transition phase, more than post-menopausal women* [4].
- The Structured Clinical Interview for Depression (SWAN) study concluded that there is two to four times increased risk of women experiencing MDD during

menopausal transition and early postmenopause, but the Primary Care Evaluation of Mental Disorders (POAS) study reported no such increased risk during these periods [16, 17]. SWAN study also reflected on ethnic variations in VMS and mood disorders. VMS and mood changes were more common in African-American and Hispanic population compared to Japanese and Chinese women [18].
- Study on Norway population using Hospital Anxiety and Depression Scale (HADS) revealed a higher depressive score among perimenopausal women than in pre-menopausal and post-menopausal women [9].
- Swedish study concluded that psychological effects were strongly related to social status, attitude towards menopause, and lifestyle. Menopause is not an independent risk factor for mood changes [19]. Psychological effects are also affected by partner views on menopause. Spouses support during menopause may have positive impact on quality of life [20].

5.3 Aetiology [2, 3, 10, 21–25]

Hormonal changes around menopause transition, life stressors, lifestyle, and psychosocial factors play a major role in mood disorders, both new-onset and precipitating existing disorders [21]:

- *Hormonal causes*: Women have more mood disorders compared to men, and windows of vulnerability (premenstrual, puerperal, and perimenopausal) point towards hormonal aetiology. Mental illnesses are usually seen between menarche and menopause suggesting reproductive hormone aetiology.
- There are no abnormal values for hormone levels associated with depression. Fluctuating hormone levels and sensitivity to these levels seem to be the underlying cause in certain women [22, 23]. Perimenopausal phase has higher risk of menopausal mood disorders than post-menopausal women. Also, women with hypogonadism (Turner's syndrome -XO) with constant low estrogenic levels do not have a significant risk of depression. History of premenstrual symptoms (PMS) and postpartum depression appears to be strongly associated with MDD during menopausal transition.
- *Stressors*: Lifestyle, family responsibilities, career, and social roles contribute to psychological effects around menopausal transition [24, 25]. These life stressors are enumerated in Table 5.1. Nonsmoker, high income, and educational status are associated with positive menopause attitudes and less mood disorders.
- *Psychological conditions*: Pre-existing psychological disorders may get precipitated during menopausal transition. Women with bipolar disorders are known to have more DE during menopausal transition. Empty nest syndrome, when children leave home, may predispose women to DE; however, this is not seen in recent population-based longitudinal studies. Women assume new social responsibilities and take this as opportunity to indulge in social responsibilities.
- *Others*: Weight gain (androgenic obesity) during menopausal transition, VMS, and GSM contribute to aggravation of mood disorders. Mood changes may hap-

Table 5.1 Factors contributing for menopausal mood disorders

Factors affecting mood disorders	
Unemployment, low socio-economic status, financial difficulties	Increased body weight/weight gain
Lack of social support	Negative attitude towards menopause
Poor general health—metabolic or systemic disease	Pre-existing PMS, puerperal depression or previous psychological disorders
Smoking, alcohol, illicit drug use	Co-existing menopausal symptoms like VMS, GSM
Sedentary life style	Loss of fertility
Major social event like loss of partner	Society attitude towards young vs menopausal women
Family—care demanding parents, empty nest syndrome	Negative feelings by partner towards menopause
History of DE while taking hormonal contraceptives	

pen independently of VMS, though VMS is known to precipitate MDD. Society and partner attitude towards menopause also affect mood disorders during menopausal transition. Family history of MDD is also a risk factor. History of DE while taking hormonal contraception is shown to be a risk factor.

- However, perimenopausal depression can happen without any previous history suggestive of psychological disorders.
- Social role, employment, active life style, exercises, improvement of general health, and positive attitude towards menopause are known to improve psychological effects during menopausal transition.

5.4 Pathophysiology

- Neurobiology of menopausal mental illnesses is poorly understood. There are no specific biomarkers indicating menopausal mood disorders. Neurotransmitters involved in depressive disorders—dopamine, serotonin, and norepinephrine and their effects—are shown in Fig. 5.1.
- *Oestrogen and neuronal function*: Oestrogen has positive effect on neuronal cells in the brain, independent of age. Oestrogen is known to affect neurosignalling of dopamine-serotonergic pathway. It reduces monoamine oxidase (MAO) which facilitates breakdown of dopamine and serotonin [26]. Synthesis of serotonin and upregulation of 5-hydroxy-tryptamine receptors are mediated by oestrogen. Oestrogen also increases norepinephrine levels by reducing degradation through inhibition of MAO and catechol-o-methyl transferase [27]
- Oestrogen maintains neuronal growth factors, neuropeptides like dehydroepiandrosterone (DHEA) and gamma-aminobutyric acid (GABA). MDD models have shown a decline in serotonin and dopamine and lower levels of DHEA and GABA [28, 29].
- Oestrogen facilitates glucose uptake by augmenting receptors and improves glucose utilisation by the brain [30]. It improves blood supply to brain and prevents

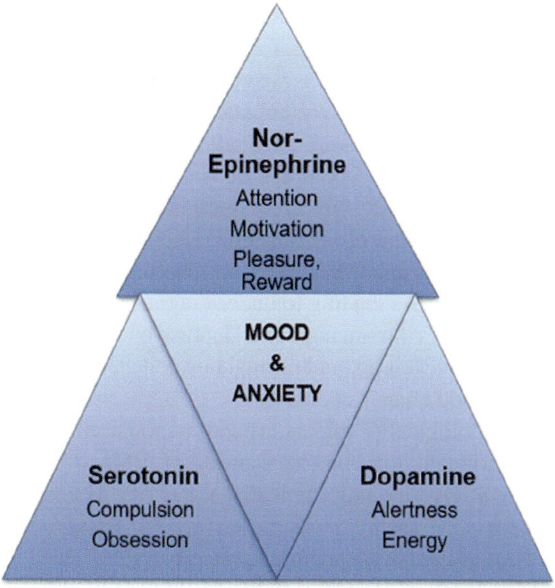

Fig. 5.1 Neurotransmitters involved in depressive disorders

hippocampal atrophy and loss of grey matter [31]. Depletion of oestrogen in the postmenopause phase is associated with increased amyloid deposition, loss of hippocampal volume, and decreased glucose utilisation [32].

- Reduced brain-derived neurotrophic factor (BDNF) is associated with depression and bipolar disorder. Expression of BDNF gene is regulated by oestrogen.
- Progesterone is known for sleep-inducing activity and with mood changes.
- Though both hormones decrease in post-menopausal phase, mood disorders return to general population levels during late menopause. *Fluctuations in the reproductive hormones (oestrogen and progesterone) and sensitivity of cortical centres to these fluctuations in subset of women is known to be associated with mood disorders.* Low levels after menopausal phase have less psychological effects on mental illness [1–4].
- Other factors implicated in perimenopausal mood disorders are diet (increased saturated fatty acid intake, reduced polyunsaturated fat intake), gut dysbiosis, inflammation, high cortisol levels, and low testosterone levels [33].

5.5 Clinical Presentation and Diagnosis [2, 10, 21]

- Menopausal mood disorders may present for the first time in a woman's life or as relapse of pre-existing psychological disorders. Perimenopausal psychological effects include altered sleep, irritability, anxiety, DE, MDD, obsessive-compulsive disorder, bipolar disorder, and rarely frank psychosis (schizophrenia). This spectrum may represent pre-existing tendency of women for mood disorders or a new developing disorder.

- Cognitive disorders associated with menopause include reduced attention span, reduction in processing, forgetfulness, and effect on verbal fluency (difficulty in finding words).
- It is essential to take complete history of psychological events including PMS, postpartum depression, DE after hormonal contraceptive intake, or any other mood changes to be noted down. History of smoking, alcohol, drugs, physical activity, and lifestyle are essential. History of endocrine dysfunction (thyroid disorders, hyperprolactinaemia) also to be elicited.
- Mood disorders may present well before stoppage of menses and typical features of menopause leading to under-diagnosis. There are no specific investigations or biomarkers for menopausal depression. Generally fluctuating hormonal levels are not picked up, and normal hormone levels are seen before menopause, when the mood changes peak.
- Psychological problems around menopausal transition may often be missed or contributed for clinical features of VMS, GSM, and disturbed sleep due to VMS. Overlapping clinical features of DE and perimenopause include weight gain, sleep disturbances, lack of energy, impaired attention, and altered libido.
- Features of MDD are enumerated in Table 5.2.
- Examination of mental status reveal the following:
  - Slow thought process
  - Late response time for questions
  - Motor retardation
  - Reduced speech
  - Not maintaining eye contact
  - Poor hygiene/grooming (due to loss of interest in daily activities. Indicates advanced stages of depression)
- Patient health questionnaire-9 (PHQ-9) and menopause-related quality of life questionnaire are available for screening and assessment of mood disorders in these groups of women. A validated questionnaire "Meno-D" has been developed for clinical practice, which is useful to screen for specific symptoms of menopause. It includes detailed questionnaire regarding 12 items graded 0–4;

Table 5.2 Features of perimenopausal mood disorders

Essential features	Additional features
1. Depressed mood Sadness/empty mood	Suicidal/homicidal ideation/plans
2. Loss of interest in activities/ social isolation	Reduced or excessive sleep
	Reduced concentration, Impaired memory, verbal memory loss
	Reduced self-esteem, feeling of guilt/grief/ worthlessness/feeling hopeless
	Weight changes, increased or decreased appetite, reduced libido
	Anxiety, irritability/easily angered

low energy, paranoid thinking, irritability, self-esteem, isolation, anxiety, somatic symptoms, sleep disturbances, weight, sexual interest, memory, and concentration [34].
- Blood tests include screening for anaemia (haemoglobin and haematocrit) and thyroid disorders (serum TSH). Screening for diabetes, breast malignancies, and cervical cancer screening and screening for bone mineral density testing are done as per local guidelines or as opportunistic screening.

5.6 Management

- Screening midlife women for mood disorders is essential for primary care physicians or gynaecologists. Simple questionnaires like PHQ-9 can be used to assess mood disorders. Women should be referred for psychiatrist and counsellor management whenever required.
- Individual tailored approach is recommended for managing menopausal mood disorders. Standard guidelines are available for guiding therapy [2, 35–37]:
  - Lifestyle changes
  - Psychological therapy-cognitive behavioural therapy
  - Anti-depressant medications
  - Menopausal hormone therapy
- *Lifestyle changes*: Adoption of healthy lifestyle brings positive outlook and reduction in mood disorders. Improving nutrition (increase polyunsaturated fat intake); reducing intake of alcohol, caffeine, and smoking; and low to moderate intensity exercises are known to reduce DE and help MDD in midlife [38]. Weight reduction and management of associated symptoms like VMS and GSM improve depressed mood.
- *Psychological therapy*
- Cognitive behavioural therapy (CBT) is efficacious in DE and MDD [2, 35–37]. It is a structured psychotherapy with timed sessions addressing the thought patterns and emotions. Patients and therapists work together to identify and modify thought process leading to cognitive distortion. Strategies like goal-setting, breathing techniques, and mindful behaviour to reduce emotional distress are included. CBT can be done in person or online based on patient comfort and understanding. Both individual and group counselling are done as preferred by patient. CBT may be used alone or in conjunction with medications to improve outcome. This can be used at all stages of MDD management, either as first-line or second-line. CBT also helps in reducing relapses in MDD.
- *Anti-depressants* [2, 35–37]
- Management with antipsychotics remains the first line of care. Pharmacotherapy may be indicated during MDD. Selective serotonin reuptake inhibitors (SSRI) and serotonin-noradrenaline reuptake inhibitors (SNRI) are used commonly as first-line agents. Tricyclic anti-depressants are also used during DE or MDD as second-line agents. Response to anti-depressants is not altered by menopausal status.

- Desvenlafaxine, a SNRI is a commonly used and recommended agent in midlife women. Desvenlafaxine is well studied and supported by randomised controlled trials in peri- and post-menopausal depression.
- Anti-depressant benefits are seen within 4–5 weeks of therapy, and relapses are reduced when continued for at least 6–12 months. Duration of therapy is not supported by evidence. Side effects like sweating, weight gain, and sexual dysfunction associated with these agents may preclude long-term use.
- For women with history of previous MDD presenting with recurrence, therapy is guided by the previous successful drugs in the management.
- Many of SSRI and SNRI have additional advantage of improving VMS and pain symptoms associated with menopause.
- *Menopausal hormone herapy (MHT)* [2, 35–37]
- Oestrogen therapy improves mood and sleep quality for perimenopausal women. Women with mild depression associated with VMS or GSM are benefitted by MHT. It is not recommended as first-line therapy for MDD. However; associated VMS, GSM, or side effects for SSRI/SNRI indicate MHT use. Evidence shows benefits of oestrogen in perimenopausal than in post-menopausal women, suggesting window of opportunity for starting MHT.
- Oestrogen therapy is not FDA-approved for management of mood disorders. There is insufficient data for using MHT for prevention of depression in midlife women.
- Progesterone therapy needs to be added along with oestrogen in women with intact uterus, whenever MHT is considered.
- Table 5.3 shows treatment options for menopausal mood disorders.

Table 5.3 Management of menopausal depressive episodes and major depressive disorders

	Treatment	Group	Recommendation	Effects
1.	Cognitive behavioural therapy	Psychotherapy	First line and adjunct to pharmacotherapy	Improved cognitive thinking for positive attitude
2.	Desvenlafaxine	SNRI	First line	Effective as monotherapy
3.	Escitalopram, citalopram	SSRI	Second line	Effective as monotherapy
4.	Duloxetine	SNRI	Second line	
5.	Mirtazapine, nortriptyline	TCA	Second line	
6.	Oestrogen Oral/transdermal (with or without progestin)	MHT	Second line	Effective as mono or adjunctive treatment
7.	Tibolone	STEAR (selective tissue estrogenic activity regulator)	–	Effective as adjunctive therapy
8.	Vortioxetine	Serotonin modulator	Second line	Effective as monotherapy

- There is no sufficient evidence to support herbal or botanical preparations and alternative medications in the management of mood disorders in midlife. Phyto-oestrogens, black cohosh, ginseng, and St. John's wort are not shown to be beneficial.

5.7 Summary

- Mood disorders are common in perimenopausal women than in post-menopausal women, which serves as opportunity for primary care physicians to screen midlife women.
- Fluctuating hormone levels contribute to mood changes rather than deficiency state of reproductive hormones. VMS, GSM, and multiple stressors increase depressive scores in DE and MDD.
- Lifestyle modification, CBT, and pharmacotherapy are used in management. MHT is shown to be effective in mood elevation and used as a second-line agent. MHT is preferred in women with mild depression associated with VMS and GSM.

Key Points

- Women experience more mood disorders compared to men. Menopausal transition is considered as a window of vulnerability for development of mood disorders similar to premenstrual and postpartum phase. One in four women seek supportive treatment for mood disorders during midlife.
- Mood disorders are common in pre-menopause than in post-menopausal women.
- Features of menopause like VMS leading to irritability and disturbed sleep may overlap with mood disorders making diagnosis difficult. Many stressors including lifestyle, general health, social support, income, smoking, and attitude towards menopause contribute to menopausal mood disorders.
- Screening for mood disorders is done using PHQ-9 or Meno-D tools. Women are managed in consultation with psychiatrists and counsellors by individualised approach.
- Cognitive behavioural therapy and anti-depressant medications are used as first-line agents. MHT is preferred in perimenopausal women with associated VMS and GSM symptoms. Weight gain and sexual dysfunction preclude the use of anti-depressants for long term.

References

1. Minuzzi L, Frey BN, Soares CN. Depression during the menopausal transition: an update on epidemiology and biological treatments. FOCUS. 2012;10:22–7. https://doi.org/10.1176/appi.focus.10.1.22.

2. Maki PM, Kornstein SG, Joffe H, Bromberger JT, Freeman EW, Athappilly G, Bobo WV, Rubin LH, Koleva HK, Cohen LS, Soares CN. Guidelines for the evaluation and treatment of perimenopausal depression: summary and recommendations. J Womens Health (Larchmt). 2019;28(2):117–34. https://doi.org/10.1089/jwh.2018.27099.mensocrec. Epub 2018 Sep 5. PMID: 30182804.
3. Soares CN. Perimenopause-related mood disturbance: an update on risk factors and novel treatment strategies available. Meeting program and abstracts. Psychopharmacology and reproductive transitions symposium. American Psychiatric Association 157th annual meeting; May 1–6, 2004; New York, NY. Arlington: American Psychiatric Publishing; 2004. p. 51–61.
4. Harlow BL, Wise LA, Otto MW, Soares CN, Cohen LS. Depression and its influence on reproductive endocrine and menstrual cycle markers associated with perimenopause: the Harvard Study of Moods and Cycles. Arch Gen Psychiatry. 2003;60(1):29–36. https://doi.org/10.1001/archpsyc.60.1.29. PMID: 12511170.
5. Curtin SC, Warner M, Hedegaard H. Increase in suicide in the United States, 1999-2014. NCHS Data Brief. 2016;241:1–8.
6. Australian Bureau of Statistics (ABS). Causes of death, Australia 2020. Canberra, ABS; 2021. https://www.abs.gov.au/statistics/health/causes-death/causes-death-australia/2020. Accessed September 2022.
7. Bebbington P, Dunn G, Jenkins R, Lewis G, Brugha T, Farrell M, Meltzer H. The influence of age and sex on the prevalence of depressive conditions: report from the National Survey of Psychiatric Morbidity. Int Rev Psychiatry. 2003;15:74–83.
8. Australian Bureau of Statistics. National Survey of Mental Health and Well-Being: summary of results, 2007. Canberra: ABS; 2009.
9. Tangen T, Mykletun A. Depression and anxiety through the climacteric period: an epidemiologic study (HUNT-II). J Psychosom Obstet Gynecol. 2008;29:125–231.
10. Kulkarni J. Depression: a major challenge of the menopause transition. Med Today. 2022;23(10):16–22.
11. Wilson L, Pandeya N, Byles J, Mishra G. Hysterectomy and incidence of depressive symptoms in midlife women: the Australian Longitudinal Study on Women's Health. Epidemiol Psychiatr Sci. 2018;27(4):381–92. https://doi.org/10.1017/S2045796016001220. Epub 2017 Feb 13. PMID: 28190411; PMCID: PMC6998864.
12. Schmidt PJ, Luff JA, Haq NA, Vanderhoof VH, Koziol DE, Calis KA, Rubinow DR, Nelson LM. Depression in women with spontaneous 46, XX primary ovarian insufficiency. J Clin Endocrinol Metab. 2011;96(2):E278–87. https://doi.org/10.1210/jc.2010-0613. Epub 2010 Nov 3. PMID: 21047929; PMCID: PMC3048327.
13. National Institutes of Health National Institutes of Health State-of-the-Science. Conference statement: management of menopausal-related symptoms. Ann Intern Med. 2005;142: 1003–1013.
14. Vesco KK, Haney EM, Humphrey L, Fu R, Nelson HD. Influence of menopause on mood: a systematic review of cohort studies. Climacteric. 2007;10(6):448–65.
15. Freeman EW. Associations of depression with the transition to menopause. Menopause. 2010;17(4):823–7.
16. Bromberger JT, Kravitz HM, Chang YF, Cyranowski JM, Brown C, Matthews KA. Major depression during and after the menopausal transition: study of Women's Health Across the Nation (SWAN). Psychol Med. 2011;41:1879–88.
17. Freeman EW, Sammel MD, Liu L, Gracia CR, Nelson DB, Hollander L. Hormones and menopausal status as predictors of depression in women in transition to menopause. Arch Gen Psychiatry. 2004;61:62–70.
18. Bromberger JT, Kravitz HM, Wei HL, Brown C, Youk AO, Cordal A, Powell LH, Matthews KA. History of depression and women's current health and functioning during midlife. Gen Hosp Psychiatry. 2005;27(3):200–8. https://doi.org/10.1016/j.genhosppsych.2005.01.007. PMID: 15882767.
19. Olofsson AS, Collins A. Psychosocial factors, attitude to menopause and symptoms in Swedish perimenopausal women. Climacteric. 2000;3(1):33–42. https://doi.org/10.3109/13697130009167597. PMID: 11910608.

20. Zhang X, Wang G, Wang H, Wang X, Ji T, Hou D, Wu J, Sun J, Zhu B. Spouses' perceptions of and attitudes toward female menopause: a mixed-methods systematic review. Climacteric. 2020;23(2):148–57. https://doi.org/10.1080/13697137.2019.1703937. Epub 2020 Jan 14. PMID: 31933386.
21. Emedicine Medscape. Bhatt NV, editor. Menopause and mood disorders. Hategan A, Chief Editor. https://emedicine.medscape.com/article/295382-overview#showall?&icd=login_success_email_match_fpf.
22. Charney DA, Stewart DE. Psychiatric aspects. In: Steward DE, Robinson GE, editors. A clinician's guide to menopause. Washington: Health Press International; 1997. p. 129–44.
23. Payne JL. The role of estrogen in mood disorders in women. Int Rev Psychiatry. 2003;15(3):280–90.
24. Bromberger JT, Assmann SF, Avis NE, Schocken M, Kravitz HM, Cordal A. Persistent mood symptoms in a multiethnic community cohort of pre- and perimenopausal women. Am J Epidemiol. 2003;158(4):347–56.
25. Dennerstein L, Lehert P, Burger H, Dudley E. Mood and the menopausal transition. J Nerv Ment Dis. 1999;187(11):685–91.
26. Spinelli MG. Depression and hormone therapy. Clin Obstet Gynecol. 2004;47(2):428–36.
27. Halbreich U. Role of estrogen in postmenopausal depression. Neurology. 1997;48(5 Suppl 7):S16–9.
28. Morrison MF, Ten Have T, Freeman EW, Sammel MD, Grisso JA. DHEA-S levels and depressive symptoms in a cohort of African American and Caucasian women in the late reproductive years. Biol Psychiatry. 2001;50:705–11.
29. Wang Z, Zhang A, Zhao B, et al. GABA+ levels in postmenopausal women with mild-to-moderate depression. A preliminary study. Medicine (Baltimore). 2016;95:e4918.
30. Cheng CM, Cohen M, Wang J, Bondy CA. Estrogen augments glucose transporter and IGF1 expression in primate cerebral cortex. FASEB J. 2001;15:907–15.
31. Eberling JL, Wu C, Haan MN, Mungas D, Buonocore M, Jagust WJ. Preliminary evidence that estrogen protects against age-related hippocampal atrophy. Neurobiol Aging. 2003;24:725–32.
32. Mosconi L, Rahman A, Diaz I, et al. Increased Alzheimer's risk during the menopause transition: a 3-year longitudinal brain imaging study. PLoS One. 2018;13:e0207885.
33. Musial N, Ali Z, Grbevski J, Veerakumar A, Sharma P. Perimenopause and first-onset mood disorders: a closer look. Focus (Am Psychiatr Publ). 2021;19(3):330–7. https://doi.org/10.1176/appi.focus.20200041. Epub 2021 Jul 9. PMID: 34690602; PMCID: PMC8475932.
34. Kulkarni J, Gavrilidis E, Hudaib AR, Bleeker C, Worsley R, Gurvich C. Development and validation of a new rating scale for perimenopausal depression-the Meno-D. Transl Psychiatry. 2018;8(1):123. https://doi.org/10.1038/s41398-018-0172-0. PMID: 29955034; PMCID: PMC6023883.
35. MacQueen GM, Frey BN, Ismail Z, Jaworska N, Steiner M, Lieshout RJ, Kennedy SH, Lam RW, Milev RV, Parikh SV, Ravindran AV, CANMAT Depression Work Group. Canadian Network for Mood and Anxiety Treatments (CANMAT) 2016 clinical guidelines for the management of adults with major depressive disorder: section 6. Special populations: youth, women, and the elderly. Can J Psychiatry. 2016;61(9):588–603. https://doi.org/10.1177/0706743716659276. Epub 2016 Aug 2. Erratum in: Can J Psychiatry. 2017 May;62(5):356. PMID: 27486149; PMCID: PMC4994788.
36. NICE guideline menopause: diagnosis and management (NG23), 2015. https://www.nice.org.uk/guidance/ng23/resources/menopause-diagnosis-and-management-pdf-1837330217413.
37. Australian Menopause Society guidelines on mood and menopause. https://www.menopause.org.au/images/stories/infosheets/docs/AMS_Mood_and_the_menopause_2023.pdf.
38. Pérez-López FR, Martínez-Domínguez SJ, Lajusticia H, Chedraui P, Health Outcomes Systematic Analyses Project. Effects of programmed exercise on depressive symptoms in midlife and older women: a meta-analysis of randomized controlled trials. Maturitas. 2017;106:38–47. https://doi.org/10.1016/j.maturitas.2017.09.001. Epub 2017 Sep 4. PMID: 29150165.

Menopause and Bone Health

6

Jyothi G. Seshadri and Radhika Chetan

6.1 Introduction/Background of Osteoporosis [1–10]

- Osteoporosis is progressive, multifactorial systemic skeletal disease characterised by loss of bone strength, due to reduced bone mineral density (BMD) and microarchitectural deterioration [1, 2]. This results in increase in fragility fractures and other types of fractures of bones more commonly in the hip, vertebra (spine), and wrist [2]. Menopause is associated with accelerated bone loss resulting in osteoporosis. Figure 6.1 shows comparison between normal bone architecture and osteoporotic bone.
- Osteomalacia refers to impaired bone mineralisation. In osteoporosis the ratio of mineral content to matrix content is maintained, and in osteomalacia, the ratio is altered. Osteomalacia is due to vitamin D deficiency, either reduced intake or altered absorption.
- Osteoporosis occurs three times more in females than males. This is attributable to low peak bone mass (PBM) in women compared to men and accelerated bone loss after menopause. Life expectancy and longevity of women also make them susceptible for bone loss and an increased number of osteoporotic fractures are seen in them [1–6]. Among osteoporotic fractures, about 80% of fore arm, 70% of hip, and 58% of spine fractures occur in women. *One in three women are affected by osteoporotic fracture after the age of 50 years* [7]. Most of them remain undiagnosed and untreated.

J. G. Seshadri (✉)
Department of Obstetrics and Gynaecology, Ramaiah Medical College and Hospitals, Bengaluru, India

R. Chetan
Department of Obstetrics and Gynaecology, Bangalore Medical College and Research Institute, Bengaluru, India

R. Garg (ed.), *Management of Menopause*,
https://doi.org/10.1007/978-981-96-0239-1_6

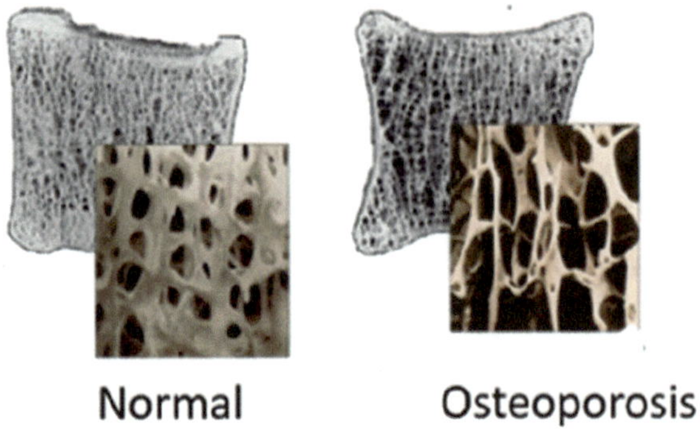

Fig. 6.1 Normal vs osteoporotic bone

- More than ten million Americans are affected by osteoporosis and two million suffer fractures. Seventy percent of them occur in females. The cost of managing fractures is a huge burden for country's healthcare, same as that of coronary artery disease and stroke in this age group [3, 4].
- About 61 million suffer from osteoporosis in India, 80% of them are women. More than 30% of postmenopausal women suffer from osteoporosis in India [5, 6]. Risk of osteoporosis is similar to other conditions like coronary artery disease and stroke. However, osteoporosis is often not evaluated unless women present with acute incident like fracture.
- Mortality may occur in 20% women within 1 year of hip fracture, and many do not regain functional capacity of ambulation [8]. They are also more prone for repeat fracture incidents in the following years.
- Osteoporosis is recognised as a public health problem by the World Health Organisation (WHO) and many international organisations, as often it is under-looked and under-treated owing to its asymptomatic nature [1, 9–11]. National osteoporosis foundation has stated that only 23% of hip fractures in the elderly are treated for osteoporosis.
- Fragility fracture due to osteoporosis is preventable and, when treated early, restores functional ability of bones. Fragility fracture is defined as fracture due to trivial trauma like fall from standing from height or less, which in routine circumstances does not cause injury to normal bone [1, 9, 10].
- Sarcopenia which is reduced muscle mass and strength is usually co-existent with osteoporosis in elderly, when it is termed osteo-sarcopenia [12]. Sarcopenia may increase the risk of fall and fractures.

6.2 Bone Remodelling: Physiology of Bone Formation and Role of Oestrogen [1, 2, 8, 12–16]

- The human bone consists of mainly calcium hydroxyapatite (65%) and collagen matrix (35%).
- Adults have both cortical and trabecular (cancellous) bone. The composition of these components vary based on various parts of the body. Lumbar vertebrae

have 70% of trabecular bone vs 50% in femur neck and only 5% in radius diaphysis.

- Bones are live dynamic structure, which undergo constant change throughout the life time. Old or damaged bone is replaced by formation of new bone tissue. About 25% of trabecular bone and 3% of cortical bone is remodelled every year. Around 10% of bone is getting remodelled at any one point of time. New remodelled bone is at risk of fracture, as mineralisation is not dense and complete.
- Different types of cells in bone remodelling are the following:
- *Osteocytes*: Derived from osteoblasts, which interconnects solid matrix of bone by canalicular network. They recognise micro trauma and regulate both location and rate of bone turn-over or remodelling. Osteocytes are regulated by hormones: parathyroid hormone (PTH) and oestrogen and mechanical load (bones bearing load undergo remodelling at a faster rate).
- *Osteoclasts*: Derived from haematopoietic stem cells. They cause resorption of bone. This usually takes weeks.
- *Osteoblasts*: Derived from mesenchymal cells. They help in rebuilding the bone site after action of osteoclasts. This process happens over months.
- All these cells are interdependent on each other for remodelling procedure.
- Hormones and cytokines act on the precursor cell of osteoclast, with cell surface molecule called as RANK ligand (RANKL), receptor activator of nuclear factor kappa-β ligand) and surface receptor, osteoprotegerin (OPG). RANKL initiates bone remodelling by activating osteoclasts, and OPG turns off remodelling by inhibiting osteoclast cells.
- *Oestrogen on bone physiology* [1, 15, 16]: All three types of bone cells possess oestrogen receptors. Oestrogen stimulates bone formation by suppression of osteoclast cells. Also, oestrogen affects bone quality through influence on cytokines and local bone growth factors. Oestrogen inhibits interleukin 6 (IL 6) which activates osteoclast recruitment. Oestrogen reduces bone resorption and decreases remodelling rate. Bone mineral density (BMD) is higher when serum oestradiol levels exceed 15 pg/mL, and when level drops to ˂5 pg/mL, fracture risk is higher [17].
- *Peak Bone Mass (PBM)*: Refers to the amount of bone tissue present at the end of skeletal maturation. For the spine and hip, PBM is reached in mid-20s; for other bones (like—radius) PBM is reached by 40s [18, 19]. At skeletal maturity PBM in women is lesser compared to men. Asian women have lesser PBM compared to Caucasians [19]. Low calcium intake and nutritional factors during childhood and adolescence contribute to low PBM in women, particularly in India. PBM is affected by factors such as genetic potential, racial, hormonal, nutritional, and lifestyle. During perimenopause and menopausal years, there is accelerated bone loss, starting 1–3 years before menopause till 4–8 years after menopause. Bone loss happens at the rate of 2.5%/year following menopause, compared to 0.13%/year before menopause. Loss in BMD during menopause transition phase is around 10%, which may be more in Asian population. If PBM acquired during skeletal maturation is less, then these women develop osteoporosis rapidly during menopause and develop fragility fractures, in their 50s.

Table 6.1 Risk factors for osteoporosis

Primary risk factors (Used in FRAX—fracture risk assessment tool)	Others
Age: 40 years onwards. Main risk factor	Peak bone mass
Race/ethnicity: Asians and Caucasian are high-risk group Country of origin	Nutrition: calcium, protein intake
Sex: females are prone	Sunlight exposure: vitamin D
BMI: ˂20, thin tall people at risk	Physical activity: sedentary lifestyle increases osteoporosis
Family history: parent history of osteoporosis	Pregnancy, lactation
Systemic steroids (glucocorticoids)use	Previous history of fracture
Rheumatoid arthritis	Risk of falling/loss of balance: vision, ear abnormalities
Smoking	Early menopause (less than 45 years)
Alcohol	Delayed puberty
Secondary osteoporosis (Table 6.3)	

- There is reduction in total body calcium during menopause about 200 mg/day in the initial 3–4 years followed by 45 mg/day in the next 5–10 years after menopause [17, 18]. Though oestrogen deficiency causes more bone turnover, other factors such as reduced calcium absorption from gut due to ageing and due to decreased formation of 1,25 dihydroxy vitamin D by kidneys in elderly are contributory factors [18].
- Osteoporosis is affected by many factors. Age is the significant risk factor. Peak bone mass, hormone status, and activity are the other non-modifiable factors affecting remodelling and osteoporosis.
- Risk factors for osteoporosis are given in Table 6.1 [1, 9–11].

6.3 Aetiology of Osteoporosis: [1, 9–11, 20, 21]

- Osteoporosis can be generalised or localised.
- Generalised: Most of the skeletal structure has reduced BMD, for example, age-related and hormonal-related.
- Localised: One part of the bone may be affected due to malignancy, infection/inflammation.
- Osteoporosis is *classified* as *primary or secondary.*
- Causes of primary osteoporosis are summarised in Table 6.2 [21].
- Secondary osteoporosis caused by specific conditions, tabulated in Table 6.3 [21].

Table 6.2 Primary osteoporosis causes and presentation

Causes	Features
Juvenile osteoporosis	• In children/young adolescents (8–14 years) • Normal gonadal function • Abrupt bone pain or fracture following trivial trauma
Type 1 osteoporosis	• Women with oestrogen deficiency • Accelerated bone loss during menopause transition • Fractures in vertebra and wrist are common type
Type 2 osteoporosis	• Age-related osteoporosis in both sexes, generally after 65 years • Fragility fractures both in cortical and trabecular bone • Fractures in hip, vertebra, and wrist are common

Table 6.3 Secondary osteoporosis—causes

Causes	Conditions
Congenital/ metabolic or genetic causes	Renal hypercalciuria—most common secondary cause managed using thiazide diuretics Hypogonadal states—ovarian insufficiency, osteogenesis imperfecta, cystic fibrosis, Marfan's syndrome, idiopathic hypercalciuria, Ehlers-Danlos syndrome, homocystinuria, Riley-Day syndrome, Gaucher's disease
Hypogonadal causes	Congenital: Turners, Klinefelter syndrome, androgen insensitivity, pan hypopituitarism Acquired: anorexia nervosa, female athlete triad, hyper-prolactinaemia, radiation, chemotherapy
Endocrine diseases	Hyperparathyroidism, hyperthyroidism, Cushing's syndrome, diabetes, acromegaly, porphyria, adrenal/oestrogen insufficiency
Nutritional/ malabsorption	Alcohol Malnutrition: calcium, vitamin D, magnesium, protein deficiency Obesity surgeries Chronic liver, renal diseases Gastrectomy, parenteral nutrition
Inflammatory causes	Bowel diseases; Crohn's disease, Rheumatoid arthritis, ankylosing spondylitis, systemic lupus erythematosus
Haematologic causes and malignancies	Leukaemia, multiple myeloma, lymphoma haemophilia, thalassemia, sickle cell anaemia Hemochromatosis Metastatic disease
Drugs/medications	Systemic glucocorticoids (more than 3 months of use) Furosemide Chemotherapy drugs Anti-convulsant, anti-psychotics (lithium, selective serotonin reuptake inhibitors) Anti-retroviral drugs Aromatase inhibitors Long-term heparin use Hormones—GnRh agonists, depot medroxyprogesterone Proton pump inhibitors Thiazolidinediones
Miscellaneous	Immobility, loss of weight Amyloidosis, sarcoidosis, multiple sclerosis, COPD, HIV Organ transplantation

6.4 Screening and Diagnosis of Osteoporosis [1, 9–11]

- Detection of BMD is the cornerstone for screening and diagnosis. It is also essential to take clinical details to know the additional risk factors and conditions causing loss of balance (reduced vision), gait disorders (decreased body balance), and conditions leading to secondary osteoporosis. This will help in individualising the prevention and management approach.
- Osteoporosis is often asymptomatic unless present with fractures. However, fractures being painful condition lead to prolonged hospital stay and functional disability and may cause death. Vertebral fractures are relatively painless and can be suspected in women with loss of height, kyphosis, or when they present with backache. Type 1 osteoporosis is common in hip and fore arm (radius, wrist) bones. Vertebra and other bones are involved after 65 years.
- Secondary osteoporosis (Table 6.3) conditions are ruled out by age of onset, medication history, and other associated clinical features.
- Comprehensive history taken regarding age of menopause, recent fall, loss of balance, parental history (maternal) of fragility fractures, nutrition (protein, calcium intake), sunlight exposure (vitamin D), physical activity, smoking, and alcohol intake, which are essential to guide nutrition therapy.
- Physical examination to include:
  - Annual measurement of height and weight. Height loss by >1.5 inches or 4 cm indicates vertebral fracture. Weight less than 57.8 kg is a risk factor for osteoporosis.
  - Kyphosis: unable to touch occiput to wall in standing position
  - Gait, speed of walking, and balance while walking
  - Getting up from chair without use of arms
  - Hand grip test
  - Gait, balance while walking, speed of walking, and hand grip strength point towards osteo-sarcopenia.
- Assessment of fracture risk can be done using standardised charts available online.

FRAX (Fracture Risk Assessment Tool), OSTA (Osteoporosis Self-Assessment Tool for Asians), and SCORE (Simple Calculated Risk Estimation) systems:

- FRAX—is commonly used tool. It is devised by the WHO (World health Organisation). Clinical risk factors used in FRAX assessment tool are mentioned in Table 6.1. BMD obtained by double-energy X-ray absorptiometry (DXA) is added in the score if available [9, 10]. FRAX scoring is available for Indian ethnicity group also, through online link. FRAX is interpreted as percentage of risk or probability of fracture for different sites over 10 years. Cut-offs are taken based on country-specific thresholds.

Generally major osteoporotic fracture probability *risk more than 20% and hip fracture risk more than 3% over 10 years* are taken as threshold for treatment.

FRAX score under estimates Type 2 diabetes, multiple fractures related to osteoporosis, recent fractures, and those with secondary osteoporosis [10]. It also does not include falls. Garvan fracture risk method may be used for calculating fracture risk in women with history of falls [10]. An example of FRAX risk assessment using bone mineral density report is shown in Fig. 6.2.

- OSTA (Osteoporosis Self-Assessment Tool for Asians): Developed by the WHO. It is calculated using the *formula: 0.2 (weight in kg—age in year).* Low risk is more than 1, moderate risk is −1 to −4, and high risk ˂−4. It has good sensitivity as a screening test [1, 22, 23].

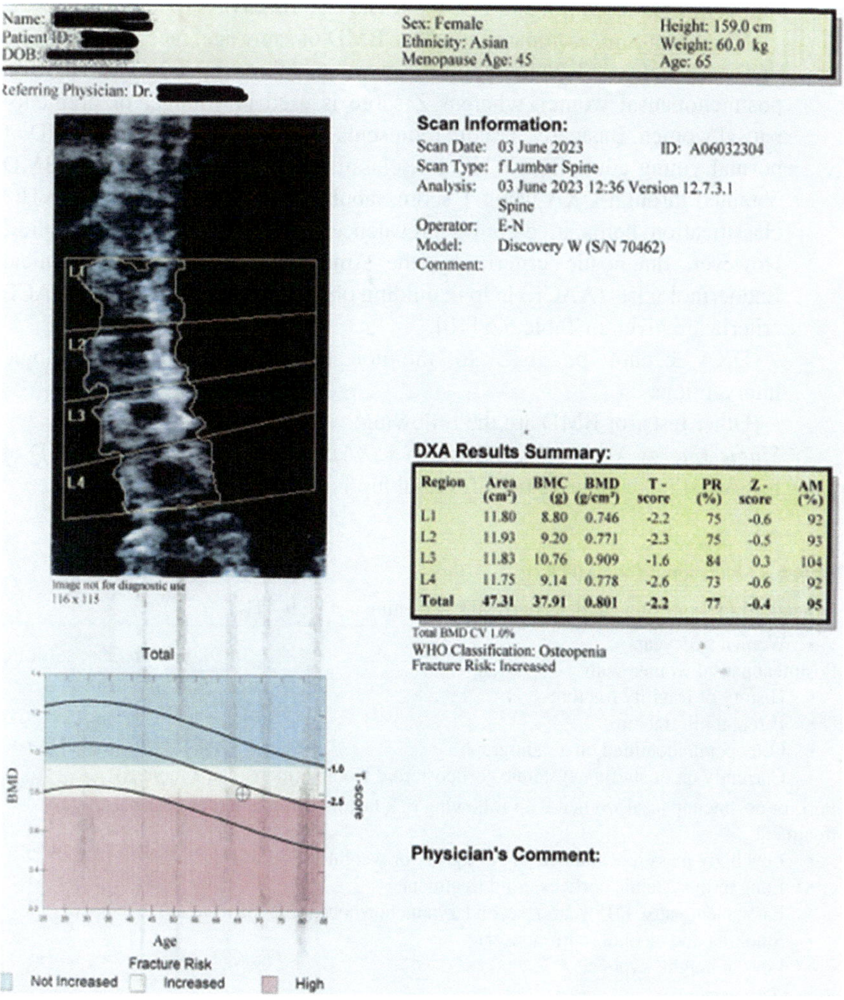
Name: [redacted]
Patient ID: [redacted]
DOB: [redacted]
Sex: Female
Ethnicity: Asian
Menopause Age: 45
Height: 159.0 cm
Weight: 60.0 kg
Age: 65

Referring Physician: Dr. [redacted]

Scan Information:
Scan Date: 03 June 2023 ID: A06032304
Scan Type: f Lumbar Spine
Analysis: 03 June 2023 12:36 Version 12.7.3.1
Spine
Operator: E-N
Model: Discovery W (S/N 70462)
Comment:

Image not for diagnostic use
116 x 115

DXA Results Summary:

Region	Area (cm^2)	BMC (g)	BMD (g/cm^2)	T-score	PR (%)	Z-score	AM (%)
L1	11.80	8.80	0.746	-2.2	75	-0.6	92
L2	11.93	9.20	0.771	-2.3	75	-0.5	93
L3	11.83	10.76	0.909	-1.6	84	0.3	104
L4	11.75	9.14	0.778	-2.6	73	-0.6	92
Total	**47.31**	**37.91**	**0.801**	**-2.2**	**77**	**-0.4**	**95**

Total BMD CV 1.0%
WHO Classification: Osteopenia
Fracture Risk: Increased

Physician's Comment:

Fig. 6.2 DXA report

- SCORE (Simple Calculated Risk Estimation): Calculated using six risk factors: age, race, weight, oestrogen use, rheumatoid arthritis, and past history of fractures [23].
- *Assessment of Bone Mineral Density*: Evaluation of BMD periodically can detect osteopenia. Indications for testing BMD are described in Table 6.4 [9, 10]. BMD evaluation is done by various diagnostic tests, as mentioned below [1, 21].
  1. *Double Energy X-ray Absorptiometry (DXA)*: *Considered as* "gold-standard" test for BMD assessment. Bone mineral content per surface area is calculated in Single-energy X-ray absorptiometry (SXA) and DXA which gives BMD. Commonly used sites are total hip, femur neck, lumbar spine, and distal 1/3 radius. Images of commonly used sites are shown in Fig. 6.3 *(hip)*, Fig. 6.4 *(lumbar spine)*, and Fig. 6.5 *(distal 1/3 radius)*.

     BMD scores are compared to either BMD of same age, race, and ethnicity (Z score) *or* normal young adult mean values (T score). T score is used in postmenopausal women whereas Z score is used in younger or premenopausal women. Basically, T score represents standard deviation from BMD of normal young adult. The WHO has classified osteoporosis based on BMD obtained through DXA using T score, tabulated in Table 6.5 [1]. The WHO classification helps in defining prevalence, guiding public health policy. However, diagnostic criteria by the American Association of Clinical Endocrinologists (AACE) help in guiding pharmacologic therapy. The AACE criteria are given in Table 6.6 [10].

     DXA cannot be used to monitor the effects of pharmacologic interventions.

     Other tests for BMD are the following:
  2. *Single-Energy X-ray Absorptiometry (SXA)*: is useful in assessing BMD at heel/wrist but cannot be used for total hip/femur or spine.

Table 6.4 Indications for BMD test

Indications for bone mineral density (BMD) screening test [1, 9–11]
• Women ≥65 years Postmenopausal women with • History of fragility fracture • Parental hip fracture • Osteopenia identified on a radiograph • Currently on or starting systemic corticosteroid therapy (more than 3 months)
Peri- or postmenopausal women with following risk factors and willing for pharmacologic treatment • Low body mass index (BMI) of <19 kg/m^2, or weight <57.8 kg) [1] • Long term systemic corticosteroid treatment • Early menopause (<45 years), secondary amenorrhoea more than 1 year • Smoking and alcohol (current user) • Loss of height, kyphosis
Secondary osteoporosis
Assess response to pharmacologic therapy

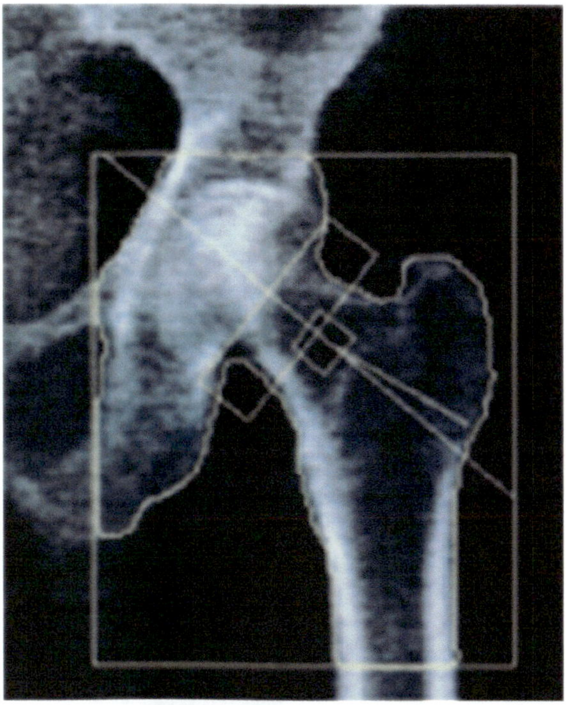

Fig. 6.3 DXA of hip showing osteoporosis

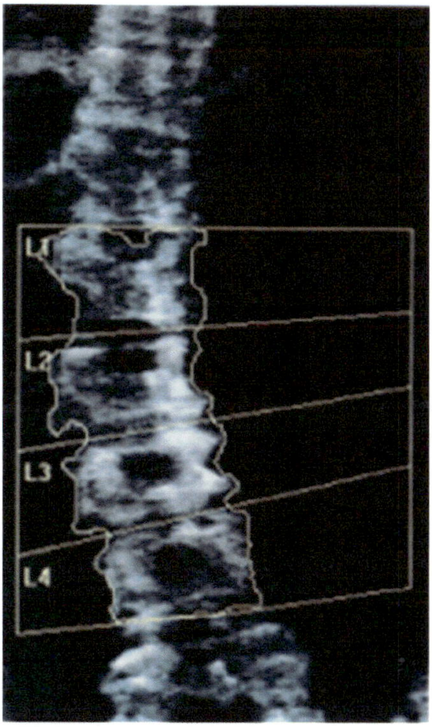

Fig. 6.4 DXA of lumbar spine showing osteoporosis

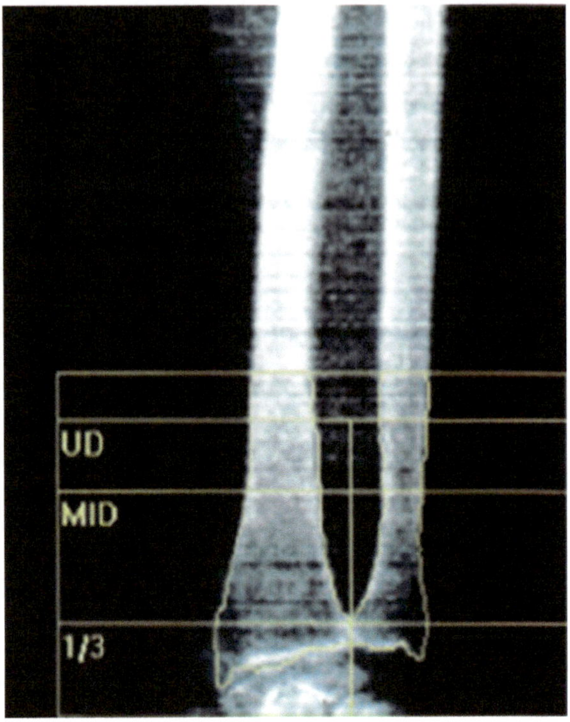

Fig. 6.5 DXA of distal 1/3 radius showing osteoporosis

Table 6.5 Osteoporosis definition by the WHO [1] based on DXA—T score

T score	Classification
−1 or above	Normal BMD
−1 to −2.5	Osteopenia or low BMD
≤−2.5	Osteoporosis
≤−2.5 with fragility fracture	Severe osteoporosis/established osteoporosis

Table 6.6 Osteoporosis diagnosis of the American Association of Clnical Endocrinologists (AACE) [10]

Criteria by the AACE—diagnosis of postmenopausal osteoporosis
1. T score ≤−2.5 in lumbar vertebra, femur neck, proximal femur or 1/3 of radius
2. Fragility/low trauma fracture (regardless of BMD)
3. T score −1 to −2.5 and fragility fracture of proximal humerus, pelvis, or distal forearm
4. T score −1 to −2.5 with high FRAX fracture probability

3. *Quantitative Ultrasound (QUS)*: is a low-cost tool, without the risk of radiation, but accuracy is low for detecting osteoporosis. Preferred site for BMD testing is calcaneus. T score based on WHO classification cannot be applied to QUS.
4. *Quantitative computed tomography (QCT)*: most sensitive method in detecting osteoporosis in spine as it measures trabecular content in vertebrae. QCT requires higher radiation dose than DXA.
5. *Magnetic Resonance Imaging (MRI)*: useful in identifying acute vs chronic vertebral fractures, also in assessment of occult fractures of femur. But test is not widely available.
6. *Plain radiograph*: Though simple assessment BMD may be done by radiographs, they are not sensitive indicator. BMD may be assessed using morphometric measurements—cortical thickness of meta carpal bones. They are useful in diagnosing established fractures with osteoporosis.

   However, these tests are not standardised for evaluation of BMD. DXA is the preferred test and evaluated for efficacy in studies [1, 24, 25].

- Other investigations as required are done based on clinical picture, to rule out secondary causes of osteoporosis as described in Table 6.7 [9, 10].
- *Bone Turnover Markers (BTM)*: Two markers, serum C-terminal telopeptide Type 1 collagen (CTX) and serum-carboxy terminal propeptide (PINP), indicate higher bone turnover and suggest osteoporosis. CTX, a resorption marker, and

Table 6.7 Laboratory tests for evaluation of osteoporosis [9]

Tests	Remark
Complete blood count (CBC)	In all cases
Serum calcium	Hyperparathyroidism Vitamin D deficiency, malabsorption, hypoparathyroidism
Serum phosphate	Renal failure patients will have high levels Hyperparathyroidism, renal wasting will demonstrate lower levels
Serum creatinine	Renal failure, osteodystrophy. Bisphosphonates are contraindicated
Serum alkaline phosphatase	Vitamin D deficiency, malabsorption, liver disease, Paget's disease will have elevated levels Hypophosphataemia will have decreased
Serum vitamin 25-hydroxy D3	Lower levels may be due to deficiency or malabsorption
Serum PTH (parathyroid hormone)	Hyperparathyroidism will have increased levels
24-h urinary calcium	Vitamin deficiency, malabsorption Renal, multiple myeloma, hyperthyroidism, hyperparathyroidism
24-h urinary cortisol	Cushing's syndrome
Serum TSH (Thyroid-stimulating hormone (TSH)	Hyperthyroidism
Serum transglutaminase	Celiac disease
Bone marrow biopsy	Haematological, bone malignancies

PINP, a bone formation marker, are useful markers for skeletal assessment but cannot be used for diagnosis of osteoporosis. Clinical trials for pharmacotherapy use BTMs as a marker for drug compliance, absorption, and efficacy of the drug. Practically BTMs are useful to provide feedback to patients on pharmacotherapy regarding efficacy. However, they are not indicated in all cases requiring pharmacotherapy [9, 10]. They are costly, lack availability, and are influenced by renal insufficiency which restrict their applicability.

6.5 Management of Osteoporosis: [1, 9–11, 26]

Includes the following:

- Non-pharmacological interventions for both prevention and treatment of osteoporosis.
- Pharmacological interventions for prevention for osteoporosis.
- Pharmacological intervention for management of osteoporosis.
- Surgery—usually indicated for management of fractures. Kyphoplasty and vertebroplasty—for collapse of vertebrae (bone cement is injected). Rarely done.

Fracture risks are stratified based on risk assessment tool and BMD measurement, as described by the International Menopause Society to guide management [26]. Risk stratification of osteoporotic women into low risk, high risk, and very high risk for fracture and their recommended management is described in Table 6.8.

- **Non-pharmacological Interventions for Prevention and Treatment of Osteoporosis** [1, 9–11, 26–29]
  - Lifestyle modifications involving diet and exercise regimes are cornerstone for management of chronic noncommunicable diseases like osteoporosis.
  - Calcium and vitamin D intake: adequate intake of these to meet daily allowance is necessary for skeletal growth. Recommended daily intake of calcium is 1200 mg/day in postmenopausal women. Vitamin D intake recommended is about 600 IU/day in women between 51 and 70 years and 800 IU after 70 years [27].
  - Calcium and vitamin D together reduce fall episodes and prevent both hip, non-vertebral fractures [28, 29].
  - Dietary calcium is the best way to meet daily demands. Emphasise on nutrition rich in protein and calcium and sun exposure for 20–30 min between 10 a.m. and 3 p.m.
  - Supplements should be prescribed only in cases of deficiency. Supra-physiological doses of vitamin D (weekly doses) are less effective than daily doses.
  - Cholecalciferol preparation (D3) is preferred over ergocalciferol (D2) as it is shown to correct deficiencies adequately.

Table 6.8 Fracture risk stratification and plan of management by the IMS (International Menopause Society)

Risk of fracture	Criteria	Treatment plan
Low risk (all must be present)	• No fragility fracture • T score <-1 to >-2.5 on DXA • 10 year probability on FRAX Major osteoporotic fracture risk $<20\%$ Hip fracture risk $<3\%$	• **MHT**—if woman has menopausal symptoms • Adequate protein, calcium, and vitamin D3 and exercises for bone health like walking, resistance training, and yoga and avoiding falls
High risk (any one)	• Fragility fracture is present • T score ≤-2.5 • 10 year probability on FRAX Major osteoporotic fracture risk $>20\%$ Hip fracture risk $>3\%$	• ***Anti-resorptive*** therapy along with adequate protein, calcium, and vitamin D3 and exercises for bone health like walking, resistance training, and yoga and avoiding falls
Very high risk (any one)	• Recent fracture • Fracture on corticosteroid therapy or other drugs • T score <-3. • 10 year probability on FRAX Major osteoporotic fracture risk $>30\%$ Hip fracture risk $>4.5\%$ Women who have high risk of fall	• ***Anabolic therapy***—for 1–1.5 years followed by anti-resorptive therapy and adequate protein, calcium, and vitamin D3 and exercises for bone health like walking, resistance training, and yoga and avoiding falls

– Calcium carbonate has high absorption (40%) compared to calcium citrate (21%). However, calcium citrate does not need gastric acid for absorption and is associated with less gastrointestinal side effects like constipation and flatulence. 24-h urinary calcium is a good method to assess calcium intake and absorption.
– Protein: Higher protein intake is associated with improved skeletal growth and reduced fall frequency. Intake of 1 g per kg per day is recommended for adults.
– Cessation of smoking and alcohol intake.
– Other trace elements required for bone growth include magnesium, zinc, and copper. Routine supplementation of these is not recommended in osteoporosis.

- Physical activity and exercises: Younger children and adults less than 45 years will have improved peak bone density with high-impact load exercises which reduces risk of osteoporosis. Exercises also improve muscle strength and balance and reduce the risk of falls. All types of physical activity (weight bearing, resistance exercises—dance, aerobics, Tai-chi, swimming) improve skeletal health. Exercises reduce bone loss, improve balance, and prevent falls.
- However, elderly with osteopenia and osteoporosis should avoid lifting activities, spine flexion—rotation movements and slouching movements. They can follow simple weight bearing or muscle-strengthening exercises with support, initially using trained physiotherapist. Balance and posture exercises should be done every day. Weight bearing and strengthening exercises are done at least 3–4 days/week for 30 min. Physiotherapist help is essential in elderly with severe osteoporosis and tendency for loss of balance.
- Fall prevention: is highly recommended to prevent fragility fractures.
- Improving vision (eye check-ups, adequate light in the walking areas), avoiding slippery floors, well-lit corridor/walkways, non-slippery shoes, keeping the medications (benzodiazepines, anti-depressants, neuroleptics) to the minimum effective dose, and control of neuromuscular diseases (Parkinsonism, myositis) are essential in preventing fragility fractures.

- **Pharmacotherapy for Prevention of Postmenopausal Osteoporosis** [1, 9–11, 26, 28]
- Prevention of osteoporosis is often underlooked and not practiced. However, bone loss during menopause transition is around 10–12% (may be higher in Asian ethnicity), and rapid loss happens in the initial 3–5 years after menopause [28, 30]. This can be effectively prevented by oestrogen and bisphosphonates [9].
  - Menopausal hormone therapy (MHT)
  - Selective oestrogen receptor modulators: agonists/antagonists
  - Tibolone
  - Anti-resorptive/anti-remodelling agents—bisphosphonates, denosumab

MHT (Menopausal Hormone Therapy) for Prevention of Osteoporosis [1, 9–11]

- Oestrogen alone or combined oestrogen-progestin therapy has been used in menopausal hormone therapy for women experiencing vasomotor, and genitourinary symptoms and in women with premature ovarian insufficiency. MHT is also beneficial in prevention of osteoporosis when used for these indications. However, MHT is not suggested solely for the purpose of prevention of osteoporosis.
- The FDA (Food and Drug Administration) stated oestrogen is approved solely for prevention of osteoporosis, for women with significant risk of osteoporosis and when non-oestrogen medications are considered inappropriate [31].
- NICE 2023 guidelines recommend use of MHT in reducing the fragility fracture risk. Guidelines state MHT benefits in terms of fewer fractures in women with current MHT users and women taking MHT for short term (less than 5 years). Data is currently not sufficient to support MHT for long duration, more than 5 years, to reduce fragility fracture [32].

- In Women's Health Initiative (WHI) study, oestrogen alone or combination of oestrogen-progestin therapy reduced risk of fractures by 34% (hip, vertebral, and total) compared to placebo in low risk population [33].
- The Danish Nurse Cohort Study, including 14,015 female nurses ≥50 years, taking MHT, concluded that hormone therapy reduced risk of hip fracture (hazard ratio 0.69) [34].
- The Danish Osteoporosis Prevention Study (DOPS)—women received MHT soon after menopause and followed up for 16 years, showed reduction in bone loss [35]. There was significant reduction in cardiovascular-related mortality in women receiving MHT.
- PERF study also enforced the short term use of MHT and effect on BMD. Women receiving MHT for 2–3 years had improved BMD up to 5 years after stopping MHT compared to placebo [36].
- MHT also prevents sarcopenia, improves muscle strength, improves balance, and reduces fall-related fractures.
- Benefits of MHT are reversed quickly on stoppage of MHT. It is essential to back up with bisphosphonate therapy on stopping.
- Women with osteopenia and who do not want to take or not fit for anti-resorptive medications within 10 years of menopause are ideal candidates for MHT osteoporosis prevention. Women more than 60 years or menopause attained more than 10 years are not ideal candidates for MHT as risks outweigh benefits. Women need to be involved in shared decision-making if MHT is required beyond 60 years.
- As MHT is not evaluated in women with osteoporosis, currently it is not recommended for treatment of osteoporosis.

Oestrogen Receptor Agonist/Antagonist [9, 10]

- Also called as selective estrogen receptor modulators (SERM)—exert weak oestrogenic effect on bone. Raloxifene and bazedoxifene are the SERMs used for bone health.
- Used in prevention and treatment of osteoporosis.
- Improvement in BMD by 1.6% at lumbar vertebra and 1.2% at femur neck was noted in clinical trial with raloxifene compared with placebo [37]. Beneficial effect is reversed on stoppage. Raloxifene has the advantage that it reduced risk of breast cancer in trials.
- Bazedoxifene is not yet approved as monotherapy for osteoporosis prevention or treatment. It is used in combination with conjugated oestrogens for the treatment of menopausal symptoms with osteopenia.

Tibolone, Synthetic Steroid

- Derived from Mexican yam, it releases metabolites of oestrogenic, pregestational and androgenic properties.
- Tibolone is approved for management of hot flushes, osteoporosis, and genitourinary symptoms.
- Reduction in risk of vertebral and non-vertebral fractures but increased risk of stroke is seen in studies [38].

Bisphosphonates

- Bisphosphonates interfere with osteoclast function and reduce bone resorption.
- Approved for prevention and treatment of osteoporosis.
- Alendronate and zoledronates are commonly used.
- Doses required for prevention are about 50% lesser compared to treatment dose.
- Considered for prevention of bone loss after stopping MHT or SERMs.
- Improvement in BMD from 3.1 to 6% in lumbar spine and from 1.8 to 4% in proximal femur is seen [39].
- BMD decreases slowly after stopping bisphosphonates.

Denosumab

- Denosumab is human monoclonal antibody. Acts by inhibiting RANK ligand and preventing bone resorption.
- It is studied in breast cancer survivors and found to prevent bone loss and reduce the risk of vertebral fractures in the first year by 50% [40].

Summary of pharmacotherapy used for prevention and dosage schedule are mentioned in Table 6.9.

Table 6.9 Drugs for prevention of postmenopausal osteoporosis [9]

Drug	Dosage
Conjugated oestrogen (equine or synthetic)	0.3 mg, 0.45 mg, 0.625 mg, 0.9 mg, 1.25 mg
Oestradiol	Oral, transdermal, vaginal rings
Oestradiol and norethindrone acetate	Oral 1 mg of oestradiol and 0.5 mg of norethindrone acetate 0.5 mg of oestradiol and 0.1 mg of norethindrone acetate
Ethinyl oestradiol and norethindrone acetate	2.5 mcg of ethinyl oestradiol and 0.5 mg norethindrone acetate 5 mcg of ethinyl oestradiol and 1 mg norethindrone acetate
Conjugated oestrogen and medroxyprogesterone acetate	0.625 mg of conjugated oestrogen and 2.5 mg of medroxyprogesterone acetate 0.625 mg of conjugated oestrogen and 5 mg of medroxyprogesterone acetate 0.45 mg of conjugated oestrogen and 1.5 mg of medroxyprogesterone acetate
Conjugated oestrogen and bazedoxifene	0.45 mg conjugated oestrogen and 20 mg bazedoxifene, orally daily
Tibolone	2.5 mg orally/day, daily
Raloxifene	60 mg daily, orally
Alendronate	35 mg/weekly, orally
Risedronate	35 mg/weekly or 150 mg/monthly, orally
Ibandronate	150 mg/monthly, orally
Zoledronate	Intravenous, every 2 years

- **Pharmacotherapy for Treatment of Postmenopausal Osteoporosis** [1, 26, 28, 9–11]
  - Anti-resorptive/anti-remodelling agents: Inhibitors of bone resorption: bisphosphonates, calcitonin and oestrogen receptor agonist/antagonist (SERM).
  - Osteo-anabolic drugs—stimulators of bone formation; parathyroid hormone analogues, anti-sclerostin monoclonal antibody (romosozumab).

6.6 Anti-resorptive/Anti-remodelling Drugs [9, 10, 26, 28]

These agents inhibit bone resorption by osteoclasts and thereby improving bone mineral density and reducing fracture risk. However, they cannot remodel microarchitecture of trabecular bone. Serum calcium should be corrected before starting these therapies. Effect on BMD and reduction of fractures is seen after using for 1 year.

These include:

- SERM—Raloxifene
- Bisphosphonates
- Denosumab
- Calcitonin-salmon

6.6.1 Raloxifene

- Is shown to effectively reduce the risk of vertebra fractures by 30–50% after 3 years of therapy [41]. Non-vertebral fracture reduction is not significant with raloxifene, with therapy up to 8 years.
- Raloxifene is associated with increase in risk of venous thromboembolism by three folds; hence risk should be started before initiating treatment.
- It is preferred in women with low risk of hip and non-vertebral fracture and high risk of breast cancer.

6.6.2 Bisphosphonates

- All bisphosphonates reduce the vertebral fracture risk by 41–70% in osteoporotic women at the end of 3 years of therapy. Alendronate, risedronate, and zoledronate have shown to reduce hip fracture by 28–50% and non-vertebral fracture by 20–38% in studies.
- Improvement in BMD plateaus after 5 years of use with no further benefit. Hence a *drug holiday* is recommended after 3–5 years of use, after assessing the fracture risk in women. If women are high-risk, they should be started on other group of drugs (anabolic agents). After 2 years of drug holiday, DXA scan is repeated, and bisphosphonates are restarted as indicated.

- If women are still high risk of developing fracture, they should be advised to start on Denosumab or anabolic drug.
- Fracture risk increases slowly after stopping bisphosphonates for 2 years.
- Alendronate and zoledronic acid are recommended for osteoporosis induced by steroid use.
- Adverse effects: Bone and muscle pain, gastrointestinal symptoms, and flu-like features in one third of patients on zoledronate. In women with impaired renal function, bisphosphonates should be used cautiously, and zoledronate is contraindicated as it is reported to cause renal failure in few cases. Osteonecrosis of jaw (ONJ) is a rare side effect of bisphosphonates reported as one in 10,000–1,00,000 patient years. In cancer case risk of ONJ is about 1–2%/year. Poor oral hygiene and invasive dental procedures are risk factors for osteonecrosis of jaw. ONJ is diagnosed by cone beam computerised tomography (CT) or MRI.

6.6.3 Denosumab

- Denosumab is a human monoclonal antibody. Acts by inhibiting RANK ligand and preventing bone resorption.
- Risk of vertebral fracture decreased by 68%, and hip fractures are reduced by 40% after 3 years of denosumab.
- Denosumab is used irrespective of renal function but hypocalcaemia is seen. Atypical femoral fracture osteonecrosis of jaw is reported as a rare effect after long-term use.
- Stopping treatment reverses effect in 1–2 years and bisphosphonates are recommended after stopping therapy with denosumab.
- Drug holiday is not recommended for denosumab.

6.6.4 Calcitonin-Salmon

- It is available as nasal spray, effective for bone pain after fracture. Improves ambulation rates during recovery following fracture.
- It is recommended in women who do not tolerate other treatment options.

6.7 Osteo-Anabolic Drugs: [9, 10, 26, 42]

- Drugs include:
  - Parathyroid hormone receptor agonists: Teriparatide, abaloparatide.
  - Romosozumab: Anti-sclerostin drug
- These drugs build bone and improve the microarchitecture and thickness of trabecular and cortical bone, respectively. More effective in improving BMD than anti-resorptive drugs.
- They are first choice therapy in women at very high risk of fracture.

- Treatment is restricted to 1–2 years as beneficial effect are plateaued after several months (anti-sclerostin agents) or after few years (PTH receptor agonists)

6.7.1 Parathyroid Hormone Receptor Agonists (PTH Agonists)

- Teriparatide and abaloparatide: Both are injectable preparations taken subcutaneously, similar to insulin injections.
- Act on parathyroid receptor and improve bone formation by activating the receptors.
- Improve microarchitecture of trabecular bone and endocortical thickness and increase BMD. Improvement in skeletal mass leads to reduced fracture risk, both vertebral and non-vertebral.
- Teriparatide decreased risk of vertebral fracture by 65% and non-vertebral fracture by 35% after treatment for 18–19 months. Available as metered dose injection pen device, for subcutaneous injection.
- Abaloparatide decreased risk of vertebral fracture by 86% and non-vertebral fracture by 43% after treatment for 18 months. Improved BMD benefits are maintained after switching to bisphosphonates for additional 2 years. Cost is 50% lesser than teriparatide.
- Orthostatic hypotension may be seen after initial injection. Hypocalcaemia is noted after use. Women should be calcium replete while using bisphosphonates. They are contraindicated in individuals with hypercalcemia, risk of osteosarcoma, or skeletal metastasis.
- Duration of use is restricted to 2 years of therapy. Teriparatide may be extended if fracture risk is still higher.
- *They are followed by bisphosphonate therapy to reduce bone resorption.*

6.7.2 Romosozumab

- Anti-sclerostin monoclonal antibody, which activates bone formation and inhibits bone resorption.
- Administered as subcutaneous injection on monthly basis (210 mg) or 2 monthly injections for 1 year.
- It is followed later by bisphosphonate therapy for 2 years.
- BMD increases by 13.3% in lumbar spine and 6.8% in total hip, and aggregate improvement after 2 years of bisphosphonate therapy is 14.9–18.1%.
- Romosozumab significantly reduced vertebral fracture risk by 73% and clinical fracture risk by 36% after 1 year of therapy compared to placebo.
- Injection site and hypersensitivity reactions are seen with romosozumab.
- Romosozumab is not used in women at high risk of cardiovascular disease especially who have experienced recent ischaemic heart disease or strokes.
- Drugs used for postmenopausal osteoporosis treatment and dosages are summarised in Table 6.10.
- Pharmacotherapy is stopped if no fractures and T score improves above −2.5.

Table 6.10 Pharmacotherapy for treatment of osteoporosis [9]

Drug	Route of administration	Dosage
Raloxifene	Oral	60 mg/day
Alendronate	Oral	70 mg/day
Risedronate	Oral	35 mg weekly or 150 mg monthly
Ibandronate	Oral, intravenous	150 mg/monthly or 3 mg intravenous
Zoledronate	Intravenous	5 mg, intravenous, yearly injection
Denosumab	Subcutaneous injection	60 mg/6 monthly injection
Teriparatide	Subcutaneous injection	20 mcg/daily
Abaloparatide	Subcutaneous injection	80 mcg/daily
Romosozumab	Subcutaneous injection	210 mg/monthly
Calcitonin	Nasal spray	200 units, daily

6.8 Summary

- Accelerated bone loss happens in the initial 3–5 years following menopause, about 10–12% of BMD decreases, may be higher in Asians.
- Age is an important predictor of bone density and bone loss. Many factors include peak bone mass, hormonal status, calcium and vitamin D intake, and parental fracture influence osteoporosis.
- Type 1 osteoporosis refers to postmenopausal osteoporosis; Type 2 is age related osteoporosis after 65 years in both genders.
- Osteoporosis is a progressive health condition that needs lifelong management to prevent fractures and improve quality of life.
- Osteopenia is usually asymptomatic and may have features like chronic backache, loss of balance, loss of height, and kyphosis. Sarcopenia is associated with osteopenia and present with reduced muscle mass, low speed of walking, and reduced strength in hand grip.
- Age more than 65 years is an indication for tests for assessment of BMD. Postmenopausal women are evaluated for risk factors for fractures.
- All postmenopausal women should be counselled regarding healthy lifestyle, sun exposure, physical activity, and nutrition rich in protein and calcium.
- If women have vasomotor or urogenital symptoms, menopausal hormone therapy is recommended, which prevents osteoporosis also.
- Bone mineral density is assessed by many tests, DXA is considered the gold-standard test. T score obtained by DXA is used to classify osteopenia and osteoporosis.
- T score ≤ -2.5 is considered osteoporosis. Fragility fracture irrespective of T score is considered as osteoporosis. T score between -1 and -2.5 with high fracture risk on FRAX is also to be considered for osteoporosis treatment.
- Clinical risk scoring for osteoporosis like FRAX scoring or simple OSTA scoring can be used to assess the risk of osteoporotic fractures. Fracture probability *risk more than 20% and hip fracture risk more than 3% over 10 years in FRAX* are taken as threshold for pharmacological treatment.

- Clinical stratification of women into low risk, high risk, and very high risk as proposed by the International Menopause Society based on T score and fracture risk helps in planning, guiding treatment for osteoporosis.
- Lifestyle modification consisting of diet with adequate amounts of protein, calcium (1200 mg/day), and vitamin D (600 IU/day) are essential for managing osteoporosis. All types of exercises are good in improving bone and muscle mass. Women with osteoporosis to practice simple muscle-strengthening and balance exercises. Measures to prevent fall are and important step in avoiding fractures.
- Take diet history regarding calcium-rich foods. Serum vitamin D (1,25-hydroxy vitamin D) is measured in women with osteoporosis, and supplements are given if deficiency.
- Counselling to stop smoking and alcohol.
- Menopausal hormone therapy is recommended as prevention for osteoporosis, which is used in women with low risk. Anti-resorptive agents including SERM, tibolone, bisphosphonates, and denosumab are recommended for high-risk women. Anabolic drugs are given for women under very high-risk category.
- Secondary causes of osteoporosis particularly drugs causing osteoporosis (corticosteroids, proton pump inhibitors) should be kept in mind while managing osteoporosis.
- Bone turnover markers may be used in the initial management and help patients in counselling regarding improvement after treatment. Increased markers suggest rapid bone loss and high fracture risk.
- Raloxifene and bisphosphonates are recommended as initial agents to prevent bone resorption. Bone-building agents (anabolic drugs) are given for high-risk women.

Key Points

- Assessment of BMD is vital in postmenopausal women.
- Menopausal hormone therapy should be considered in women at risk of osteoporosis with menopausal symptoms. MHT advantages are more, if initiated within 10 years of menopause or up to 60 years of age.
- Anti-resorptive drugs reduce bone turn over by inhibiting osteoclastic activity. Raloxifene, tibolone, bisphosphonates, and denosumab are effective anti-resorptive agents. Bisphosphonates are generally used for 3–5 years followed by drug holiday of 2–3 years. If fracture risk is high, then these are followed by anabolic drugs.
- Renal impairment is a contraindication for bisphosphonate therapy.
- Denosumab: No restriction on duration of use. No drug holiday for denosumab.
- Osteo-anabolic drugs recommended are PTH receptor agonists (teriparatide and abaloparatide), romosozumab (anti-sclerostin antibody) which increase bone formation by improvement in microarchitecture and cortical thickness of bones.
- Calcitonin nasal spray is used for reducing pain associated with fractures and decreases time for mobilisation after recent vertebral fracture.

- Anabolic drugs are given for 1–2 years followed again by anti-resorptive therapy to reduce bone loss. PTH receptor agonists are not used in hypercalcaemia, osteosarcoma, and skeletal metastasis. Romosozumab is not used in women at high risk for cardiovascular events like recent ischaemic heart disease and stroke.

References

1. WHO Scientific Group on the Prevention and Management of Osteoporosis (2000: Geneva, Switzerland). Prevention and management of osteoporosis: report of a WHO scientific group. World Health Organization; 2003. https://apps.who.int/iris/handle/10665/42841.
2. NIH Consensus Development Panel on Osteoporosis Prevention, Diagnosis, and Therapy. Osteoporosis prevention, diagnosis, and therapy. JAMA. 2001;285:785–95.
3. Wright NC, Looker AC, Saag KG, et al. The recent prevalence of osteoporosis and low bone mass in the United States based on bone mineral density at the femoral neck or lumbar spine. J Bone Miner Res. 2014;29:2520–6.
4. Singer A, Exuzides A, Spangler L, et al. Burden of illness for osteoporotic fractures compared with other serious diseases among postmenopausal women in the United States. Mayo Clin Proc. 2015;90:53–62.
5. Joshi VR, Mangat G, Balakrishnan C, Mittal G. Osteoporosis—Approach in Indian scenario. J Assoc Physicians India. 1998;46:965–7.
6. Krishna U, Mehta RU. Osteoporosis—Incidence and implications. J Obstet Gynecol India. 2000;50:150–6.
7. Adult official positions of the ISCD, updated in 2019. https://iscd.org/wp-content/uploads/2021/09/2019-Official-Positions-Adult-1.pdf. Accessed 4 June 2023.
8. Cooper C, Campion G, Melton LJ 3rd. Hip fractures in the elderly: a world-wide projection. Osteoporos Int. 1992;2:285–9.
9. Management of Osteoporosis in Postmenopausal Women: The 2021 Position Statement of The North American Menopause Society" Editorial Panel. Management of osteoporosis in postmenopausal women: the 2021 position statement of The North American Menopause Society. Menopause. 2021;28(9):973–997. https://doi.org/10.1097/GME.0000000000001831. PMID: 34448749.
10. Camacho PM, Petak SM, Binkley N, Diab DL, Eldeiry LS, Farooki A, Harris ST, Hurley DL, Kelly J, Lewiecki EM, Pessah-Pollack R, McClung M, Wimalawansa SJ, Watts NB. American Association of Clinical Endocrinologists/American College of Endocrinology clinical practice guidelines for the diagnosis and treatment of postmenopausal osteoporosis—2020 update. Endocr Pract. 2020;26(Suppl 1):1–46. https://doi.org/10.4158/GL-2020-0524SUPPL. PMID: 32427503.
11. Meeta M, Harinarayan CV, Marwah R, Sahay R, Kalra S, Babhulkar S. Clinical practice guidelines on postmenopausal osteoporosis: *an executive summary and recommendations—Update 2019–2020. J Midlife Health. 2020;11(2):96–112. https://doi.org/10.4103/jmh.JMH_143_20. Epub 2020 Aug 10. PMID: 33281419; PMCID: PMC7688018.
12. Cruz-Jentoft AJ, Bahat G, Bauer J, Boirie Y, Bruyère O, Writing Group for the European Working Group on Sarcopenia in Older People 2 (EWGSOP2), and the Extended Group for EWGSOP2. Sarcopenia: revised European consensus on definition and diagnosis. Age Ageing. 2019;48:16–31.
13. Al Saedi A, Stupka N, Duque G. Pathogenesis of osteoporosis. Handb Exp Pharmacol. 2020;115(12):3318–25.
14. Raisz LG. Pathogenesis of osteoporosis: concepts, conflicts, and prospects. J Clin Invest. 2005;115(12):3318–25.

15. Jilka RL, Hangoc G, Girasole G, Passeri G, Williams DC, Abrams JS, et al. Increased osteoclast development after estrogen loss: mediation by interleukin-6. Science. 1992;257(5066):88–91.
16. Manolagas SC, Jilka RL. Bone marrow, cytokines, and bone remodeling. Emerging insights into the pathophysiology of osteoporosis. N Engl J Med. 1995;332(5):305–11. https://doi.org/10.1056/NEJM199502023320506. PMID: 7816067.
17. Cummings SR, Browner WS, Bauer D, Stone K, Ensrud K, Jamal S, Ettinger B. Endogenous hormones and the risk of hip and vertebral fractures among older women. Study of Osteoporotic Fractures Research Group. N Engl J Med. 1998;339:733–8.
18. Tella SH, Gallagher JC. Prevention and treatment of postmenopausal osteoporosis. J Steroid Biochem Mol Biol. 2014;142:155–70. https://doi.org/10.1016/j.jsbmb.2013.09.008. Epub 2013 Oct 29. PMID: 24176761; PMCID: PMC4187361.
19. Greendale GA, Sowers MF, Han W, Huang M-H, Finkelstein JS, Crandall CJ, Lee JS, Karlamangla AS. Bone mineral density loss in relation to the final menstrual period in a multiethnic cohort: results from the Study of Women's Health Across the Nation (SWAN). J Bone Miner Res. 2012;27(1):111.
20. Reddy PG, Mithal A, Rao DS. Bone mineral density in healthy Asian Indian women: development of a reference database and implications for diagnosis of osteoporosis in Indian women living in the United States. J Bone Miner Res. 2002;17 Suppl 1:SA270.
21. Elam REW. In: Diamond HS, Chief Editor. Osteoporosis, practice essentials. Medscape. https://emedicine.medscape.com/article/330598-overview. Accessed 4 June 2023.
22. Muslim D, Mohd E, Sallehudin A, Tengku Muzaffar T, Ezane A. Performance of osteoporosis self-assessment tool for Asian (OSTA) for primary osteoporosis in post-menopausal Malay women. Malays Orthop J. 2012;6(1):35–9. https://doi.org/10.5704/MOJ.1203.011. PMID: 25279040; PMCID: PMC4093580.
23. Rubin KH, Friis-Holmberg T, Hermann AP, Abrahamsen B, Brixen K. Risk assessment tools to identify women with increased risk of osteoporotic fracture: complexity or simplicity? A systematic review. J Bone Miner Res. 2013;28(8):1701–17. https://doi.org/10.1002/jbmr.1956. PMID: 23592255.
24. Licata A, Binkley N, Petak SM, Camacho P. Consensus statement by the American Association of Clinical Endocrinologists and American College of Endocrinology on the quality of DXA scans and reports. Endocr Pract. 2018;24:220–9.
25. Lewiecki EM, Binkley N, Morgan SL, et al. Best practices for dual-energy X-ray absorptiometry measurement and reporting: International Society for Clinical Densitometry Guidance. J Clin Densitom. 2016;19:127–40.
26. de Villiers TJ, Goldstein SR. Update on bone health: the International Menopause Society white paper 2021. Climacteric. 2021;24(5):498–504. https://doi.org/10.1080/13697137.2021.1950967. PMID: 34498505.
27. Institute of Medicine (US) Committee to Review Dietary Reference Intakes for Vitamin D and Calcium. In: Ross AC, Taylor CL, Yaktine AL, Del Valle HB, editors. Dietary reference intakes for calcium and vitamin D. Washington: National Academies Press (US); 2011.
28. Eastell R, Rosen CJ, Black DM, Cheung AM, Murad MH, Shoback D. Pharmacological management of osteoporosis in postmenopausal women: an Endocrine Society* clinical practice guideline. J Clin Endocrinol Metab. 2019;104(5):1595–622. https://doi.org/10.1210/jc.2019-00221. PMID: 30907953.
29. Thanapluetiwong S, Chewcharat A, Takkavatakarn K, Praditpornsilpa K, Eiam-Ong S, Susantitaphong P. Vitamin D supplement on prevention of fall and fracture: a meta-analysis of randomized controlled trials. Medicine (Baltimore). 2020;99(34):e21506. https://doi.org/10.1097/MD.0000000000021506. PMID: 32846760; PMCID: PMC7447507.
30. Finkelstein JS, Brockwell SE, Mehta V, et al. Bone mineral density changes during the menopause transition in a multiethnic cohort of women. J Clin Endocrinol Metab. 2008;93:861–8.
31. Premarin (conjugated estrogens) tablets, USP for oral use [package insert]. Philadelphia: Wyeth Pharmaceuticals; 2014. [FDA].
32. National Institute for Health and Care Excellence. (2015, updated 2019). Menopause: diagnosis and management. (NICE guideline no. 23.) nice.org.uk/guidance/ng23.

33. Cauley JA, Robbins J, Chen Z, et al.; Women's Health Initiative Investigators. Effects of estrogen plus progestin on risk of fracture and bone mineral density: the Women's Health Initiative randomized trial. JAMA. 2003;290:1729–1738.
34. Hundrup YA, Ekholm O, Hoidrup S, Davidsen M, Obel EB. Risk factors for hip fracture and a possible effect modification by hormone replacement therapy. The Danish nurse cohort study. Eur J Epidemiol. 2005;20(10):871–7. https://doi.org/10.1007/s10654-005-2151-z. PMID: 16283478.
35. Mosekilde L, Hermann AP, Beck-Nielsen H, Charles P, Nielsen SP, Sørensen OH. The Danish Osteoporosis Prevention Study (DOPS): project design and inclusion of 2000 normal perimenopausal women. Maturitas. 1999;31(3):207–19. https://doi.org/10.1016/s0378-5122(99)00006-7. PMID: 10340280.
36. Bagger YZ, Tankó LB, Alexandersen P, Hansen HB, Møllgaard A, Ravn P, Qvist P, Kanis JA, Christiansen C. Two to three years of hormone replacement treatment in healthy women have long-term preventive effects on bone mass and osteoporotic fractures: the PERF study. Bone. 2004;34(4):728–35. https://doi.org/10.1016/j.bone.2003.12.021. PMID: 15050905.
37. Delmas PD, Bjarnason NH, Mitlak BH, et al. Effects of raloxifene on bone mineral density, serum cholesterol concentrations, and uterine endometrium in postmenopausal women. N Engl J Med. 1997;337:1641–7.
38. Cummings SR, Ettinger B, Delmas PD, et al.; LIFT Trial Investigators. The effects of tibolone in older postmenopausal women. N Engl J Med. 2008;359:697–708.
39. Grey A, Bolland MJ, Horne A, et al. Five years of anti-resorptive activity after a single dose of zoledronate—results from a randomized doubleblind placebo-controlled trial. Bone. 2012;50:1389–93.
40. Gnant M, Pfeiler G, Dubsky PC, et al.; Austrian Breast and Colorectal Cancer Study Group. Adjuvant denosumab in breast cancer (ABCSG-18): a multicentre, randomised, double-blind, placebo-controlled trial. Lancet. 2015;386:433–443.
41. Ettinger B, Black DM, Mitlack BH, et al. Reduction of vertebral fracture risk in postmenopausal women with osteoporosis treated with raloxifene: results from a 3-year randomized clinical trial. Multiple Outcomes of Raloxifene Evaluation (MORE) Investigators. JAMA. 1999;282:637–45.
42. Solling ASK, Harslof T, Langdahl B. Current status of bone-forming therapies for the management of osteoporosis. Drugs Aging. 2019;36:625–38.

Menopause and Oral Health

7

Sidhartha Sharma, Arunakshi Krishnan, Arnab Mukherjee, and Vijay Kumar

7.1 Introduction

Oral diseases are chronic and progressive conditions that compromise the oral and dental health. In recent years, it has been postulated that oral diseases have a bidirectional relationship with systemic health, in addition to their pronounced global prevalence and obvious public health concern [1, 2]. Several systemic diseases, including cardiovascular diseases, Alzheimer's disease, diabetes, rheumatoid arthritis, and some malignancies, have been associated with oral health status [3–6].

Similarly, the menopause has also been linked to significant orofacial alterations. Menopause is the irreversible cessation of menstruation as a result of the loss of ovarian follicular activity. A natural menopause is diagnosed retrospectively after 12 months of amenorrhoea with no pathological association [7]. It occurs between the ages of 45 and 55 (mean 50–52) [8]. "Perimenopause" (climacterium) is the period beginning when the first alterations in the menstrual cycle are observed and ending 1 year after the last period [7]. Numerous physiological changes occur in women nearing menopause, the majority of which are due to reduced oestrogen production. A deficiency in oestrogen can result in a variety of symptoms, including flushing, perspiration, osteoporosis, cardiovascular disease, cognitive disease, urogenital infections, and skin changes [3]. Although the systemic aspects of menopause are well-documented, oral discomfort as a component of menopausal complaints is still poorly understood. Healthcare practitioners must be familiar with the oral symptoms of menopausal women to properly diagnose and treat these patients. This chapter therefore aims to shed light on the oral manifestations of menopause.

S. Sharma (✉) · A. Krishnan · V. Kumar
Division of Conservative Dentistry and Endodontics, Centre for Dental Education and Research, All India Institute of Medical Sciences, New Delhi, India
e-mail: sid.aiims@aiims.edu

A. Mukherjee
Private Practitioner, Malda, West Bengal, India

R. Garg (ed.), *Management of Menopause*,
https://doi.org/10.1007/978-981-96-0239-1_7

7.2 Pathophysiology of Oestrogen Deficiency in the Oral Cavity

Oestrogen's function in cell growth and regulation is well-known, and it exerts its effects via oestrogen receptors (ERs) [9]. There are two subtypes of oestrogen receptors (ERs). ER-α is predominantly expressed in typical oestrogen-target tissues, such as mammary ducts and endometrium. ER-β is found in epithelial tissues including colonic, prostatic, and oral epithelium as well as acinar and ductal cells of the salivary gland. Except for the squamous cell layer, ER is found in all gingival and buccal mucosal epithelial layers. The distribution of ER differs from that of androgen receptors, which are largely limited to the basal epithelium. This distinction may reflect the reactivity of oral keratinocytes to oestrogens both early and late in the epithelial maturation process, as opposed to androgens, which appear to have an effect only during the early stage [10, 11].

ER-β serves a significant role in the maintenance and function of salivary glands. Immunopositivity for ER-β was found in mucous and serous acinar cells, as well as intercalated, striated, and excretory ductal cells, in varied degrees. The minor salivary glands were the most immunoreactive. The exact mechanism by which oestrogens mediate these actions remains unknown. It could be ascribed to the modulation of the expression of key growth factors (e.g. nerve growth factor) [10].

The other function of oestrogen includes the following [9]:

- Regulates bone turnover
- Antagonises resorption of periodontal tissues
- Collagen synthesis and maintenance
- Stimulates gingival fibroblast synthesis
- Increase of anti-inflammatory cytokines (interleukin (IL)-10, TGF-b)
- Decrease of pro-inflammatory cytokines (IL-1, IL-6, TNF-a)
- Reduction of B-cell apoptosis and alters its maturation
- Promotion of dendritic cell maturation
- Direct antioxidant effects

These findings may explain the sensitivity of oral tissues to oestrogens and the significance of hormone replacement therapy (HRT) in relieving postmenopausal symptoms [10].

7.3 Changes Occurring in the Oral Cavity of Menopausal Women

The effect of menopause on the oral cavity can broadly be divided into three headings:

1. **Effect on Saliva**

   Saliva is essential for maintaining the health of the oral tissues. Menopause may have the following effects:

(a) **Xerostomia and hyposalivation**: Hyposalivation is an objective reduction in the salivary flow rate, whereas xerostomia is defined as "a subjective sensation of dry mouth", which is typically correlated with hyposalivation [12]. A 40–50% reduction in salivary flow renders the patient symptomatic and susceptible to xerostomia [13]. Menopausal women have been shown to have a higher prevalence of xerostomia than premenopausal women [6]. However, its prevalence and severity may not be proportional to the rate of saliva secretion [12, 14, 15]. Salivary flow rate is commonly believed to be affected by oestrogen levels, with postmenopausal women having lower flow rates than menstruating women. Taga 2021 discovered that the volume of unstimulated saliva in perimenopausal women was substantially lower than in women without these conditions [16]. Kullander and Sonesson, as well as Laine and Virtanen, found that menopausal women secrete less saliva than menstruating women [17, 18]. Rukmini discovered a decrease in the pH and flow rate of saliva in healthy postmenopausal women compared to controls [19]. Postmenopausal women have decreased unstimulated and stimulated submandibular and sublingual salivary gland flow compared to premenopausal women, a finding unrelated to any medication effect [3, 20]. Studies on menopausal women have produced contradictory results regarding the reduction in salivary flow. Saluja et al. discovered that the salivary flow rate of menopausal women devoid of systemic and local disease was not significantly different [6]. Ship et al. and Ben Aryeh et al. found that the rate of salivary flow did not change significantly during menopause [14, 15].
(b) **Altered salivary composition**: The composition of saliva depends on the rate of secretion. It has been observed that menopausal women have significantly altered salivary composition. Low salivary flow rate decreases salivary pH as a result of decreased bicarbonate release [6]. Saluja et al. (2014) discovered that the salivary pH values of postmenopausal women were significantly lower and near the critical pH of 5.5, which could contribute to enamel demineralisation and the onset and progression of dental caries [6]. Compared to the control group, Yalcin et al. found decreased potassium concentration, substantially increased sodium concentration, and no difference in chlorine values in postmenopausal women [21]. Ben Aryeh et al. found no statistical difference between the sodium and potassium levels of healthy and menopausal women [15]. Multiple studies have confirmed that an increase in concentration of inorganic calcium in saliva which can accelerate the mineralisation of plaque and calculus formation [1, 22–24]. This is due to calcium-phosphate metabolism dysregulation, which results in increased calcium discharge into saliva [1, 25–29]. A decrease in salivary lysozyme concentration has been shown which prevents the antibacterial, antiviral, and antifungal activities of the saliva [28, 30–33].
(c) **Associated symptoms/disease**: Decreased salivary flow may increase the prevalence of oral dysesthesia, dysphagia, and taste alterations (dysgeusia) [3, 5, 34–38]. Reduced saliva leads to physical dryness and the loss of saliva's antibacterial properties, resulting in an increased incidence of dental

caries, periodontitis, halitosis, infections such as candida infection, tongue fissuring, depapillation, ulcers, oral mucositis, and lack of denture retention, all of which have a negative impact on the quality of life [12, 39].

(d) **Management**: The following management is suggested [1, 2, 4–6]:
- Ensure enough fluid intake of >1.5 L/day.
- Sucking ice cubes and sipping water frequently.
- In cases of xerostomia, artificial saliva (substitutes containing mucin or preparations containing carboxymethylcellulose) or saliva substitutes (hyaluronic acid or methylcellulose) must be prescribed.
- Salivary stimulants or sialagogues, such as sugar-free gum, lozenges, and xylitol tablets, can be prescribed to increase secretions.
- In severe cases, cholinergic parasympathomimetic compounds (e.g., pilocarpine or bromhexine) are used to alleviate the symptoms.
- Antifungal medications like clotrimazole and nystatin must be prescribed when fungal cultures are positive.
- Mouthwashes containing alcohol and toothpastes containing whitening agents and sodium lauryl sulphate are contraindicated because they exacerbate dry mouth and aggravate the oral mucosa.
- Avoidance of hard texture, spicy, and sweet foods as well as carbonated drinks.
- Local administration of natural moisturising and coating preparations, such as linseed oil, evening primrose oil, linseed, and mallow flower.
- Three to 6 months of dental follow-up appointments.

2. **Effect on Oral Mucosa**

The following effects can be seen:

(a) **Mucosal changes**: As a result of oestrogen's role in the maturation of the oral epithelium, menopausal women have mucosa that is thin, atrophic, folded, and less elastic. This, combined with mucosal dehydration, renders the oral mucosa vulnerable to local mechanical trauma, abrasions, and ulcerations, making it difficult to wear removable oral prosthesis. To avoid additional traumatisation of the oral mucosa, dentures should be made as smooth as feasible with an adequate fit [1, 25, 40]. Concurrent senile atrophic gingivitis develops in some women, resulting in an unnatural paleness of the gingival tissues. Others have menopausal gingivostomatitis, which is characterised by dry and shiny gingivae that bleed readily and range in colour from excessively pale to highly erythematous [41].

(b) **Burning mouth syndrome (BMS)**

BMS is defined as "burning pain in the tongue or other oral mucous membrane associated with normal signs and laboratory findings lasting at least 4–6 months" [42]. It is psychogenic or idiopathic in character, and the term BMS should only be used when a definite cause has not been found [35, 43, 44]. BMS is most common in middle-aged postmenopausal women in their fifth to seventh decade, with a prevalence of 10–40% [16, 43, 45, 46].

- **Aetiology**

- The specific cause of burning mouth syndrome is unknown [35, 47–50]. Reduced oestrogen levels can promote alterations in salivation causing peripheral neuropathic alterations in the oral mucosal membrane, which have been linked to BMS [48]. One of the most frequently accepted explanations is that loss of chorda tympani (facial) nerve function disinhibits the trigeminal nerve, resulting in pain along trigeminal pathways [45, 51]. Studies of tongue biopsy from BMS patients revealed reductions in the number of unmyelinated fibres associated with the taste papilla, as well as a reduction in the number of intraepithelial fibres and structural and functional abnormalities in the nervous system [52–54].
- **Clinical features**
- In the absence of noticeable lesions in the mucosa, the triad of symptoms comprises mouth pain, altered taste, and altered salivation [43, 48, 55, 56]. Pain is frequently described as a burning, scalding, stinging, or tingling sensation in the mouth, typically on the tongue (anterior two-thirds), lower lip, mucosa, and hard palate [43, 48, 50, 57]. The location of pain is not pathognomonic, as it frequently involves multiple sites [50]. Pain is exacerbated by hot and spicy foods, excessive speaking, and a stressful lifestyle and alleviated by cold foods, work, and distractions [43, 56–59]. Pain may be constant daily, develop gradually or spontaneously, and be associated with a precipitating event. The burning sensation is at its weakest upon awakening, reappears after the first meal, and increases in intensity throughout the day, reaching its peak in the evening [51, 60]. Patients have difficulty staying asleep, but do not typically awaken during the night [43, 48]. This occurs daily for more than 2 hours per day and for more than 3 months [2]. This results in psychological changes like irritability, anxiety, and depression, alterations in the sleep cycle, and overall quality of life [61]. Five clinical diagnostic criteria are suggested: (1) Daily reporting of deep and bilateral burning pain. (2) The duration of burning pain is at least 4–6 months. (3) Constant or increasing intensity throughout the day. (4) No deterioration but improvement on eating and drinking. (5) No disturbance in sleep. Taste disorder, xerostomia, sensory or chemosensory alterations, and mood or psychological disorders are additional criteria [47, 62].
- **Management**
- In the absence of a gold-standard treatment, management is empiric and centred on the symptom management [43, 47, 52]. It is recommended to rule out hyposalivation and candidiasis and to treat them if they are present [1, 3, 43, 47, 50, 57].
  - Topical

    Topical clonazepam 1 mg for 3 min, three times per day, for 2 weeks; Currently, topical clonazepam appears to be the most effective treatment, with nearly half of all patients showing improvement [63–65].

Low-level laser therapy (LLLT) stimulates the synthesis of serotonin and endorphins while reducing that of bradykinin, thereby easing burning sensations. LLLT inhibits the depolarisation of C fibres, which are accountable for the transmission of pain and thermal stimuli [66, 67].

0.15% benzydamine hydrochloride, administered thrice daily, has analgesic, anaesthetic, and anti-inflammatory effects, but the results are inconsistent [50, 68].

Capsaicin is an analgesic that functions as a desensitising agent on sensory afferent neurons to alleviate burning symptoms [47, 50, 69, 70].

70% aloe vera gel applied thrice daily reduces symptom [71].

– Systemic

Sun et al. discovered symptom alleviation after administration of vitamins BC, B12, folic acid, and minerals as a supplement [50, 72].

Systemic clonazepam (0.5 mg/day) and alprazolam (0.25 mg to 2 mg/day) are commonly used to treat BMS pain, and they likely work by disrupting the neuropathologic mechanism underlying the pain. It is an effective option for short-term therapy [73].

The use of the potent antioxidant and neuroprotective agent alpha lipoic acid (ALA 200 mg three times daily) in the management of BMS has conflicting results, as Femiano et al. discovered improvement in 96% of patients and Granot et al. confirmed this [74, 75], while Cavalcanti and Lopez-Jornet failed to discover a significant improvement in the tested patients [76, 77].

Use of tricyclic antidepressants such as amitriptyline, desipramine, imipramine, clomipramine, and nortriptyline (beginning dose of 5–10 mg/day and progressive increase to 50 mg/day), even though they exacerbate xerostomia symptoms [50, 78].

Selective serotonin reuptake inhibitors for 8 weeks and duloxetine at 30–60 mg/day, a dual action antidepressant that inhibits both serotonin and noradrenaline, result in a considerable improvement in oral burning sensation [50, 78].

Antipsychotic medications such as amisulpride and levosulpiride demonstrate good patient compliance in short-term interventions and have been shown to alleviate patients' burning symptoms and improve patient compliance [50].

Low doses of centrally acting medications such as benzodiazepines, tricyclic antidepressants, gabapentin, etc. are used to control pain [43]. A combination of drugs, such as clonazepam, gabapentin, and baclofen has been suggested (gabapentin 300 mg/day thrice daily or ALA 600 mg/day and gabapentin 300 mg/day for 2 months) [51].

Some patients may benefit from HRT; however, it cannot be guaranteed that HRT will be an effective treatment for all patients [79].

Psychological support and reassurance are needed. Combining cognitive behavioural therapy with alpha-lipoic acid and/or clonazepam appears to be highly promising [43, 80].

(c) **Autoimmune diseases**

Atrophic changes can lead to autoimmune changes such as oral lichen planus (OLP), pemphigus vulgaris or benign mucosal pemphigoid [1–3, 9]. An increased incidence of OLP has been reported in perimenopausal women than in premenopausal women (10.9% versus 0.5–2%) [1]. Lichen planus (LP) is an autoimmune inflammatory disorder affecting skin and mucous membrane. It manifests as papules and plaques that are pruritic, violaceous, and most prevalent on the wrists, lower back, and ankles. Wickham striae, a lattice-like network of white lines, overlies the lesions but is most readily observed on the buccal oral mucosa, where erosions may also be present [81]. It is more prevalent in women with excessive anxiety, depression, and psychological disorders [1, 2, 82]. Elimination of irritant factors (rough fillings, spicy foods, poor oral hygiene, and toothpaste containing sodium lauryl sulphate) constitutes the majority of treatment [2]. Topical corticosteroids (triamcinolone acetonide 0.1%; clobetasol propionate 0.05%; dexamethasone 0.05% for a month, two to four times daily) are the most effective first-line treatment for OLP, while topical calcineurin inhibitors (tacrolimus 0.1% or pimecrolimus 1% for two to four times daily) are promising as second-line medications for refractory cases [9, 83–86].

3. **Effect on Periodontal Health**

Periodontitis is a chronic inflammatory disease characterised by the progressive degradation of tooth-supporting tissues, including alveolar bone, which may result in tooth loss. Although periodontitis is undoubtedly caused by bacteria, the outcome and prognosis of the disease are ultimately determined by the host's inflammatory response and other risk factors [87]. Osteoporosis is a multifactorial chronic disease characterised by decreased bone mass owing to systemic and/or local bone resorption and deterioration of the microarchitecture of the skeleton [1, 3, 88, 89]. It has few risk factors in common with periodontitis. Menopause is characterised by a significant decrease in oestrogen, inhibition of calcium absorption, and decreased protection against bone resorption, which appears to be detrimental for both periodontitis and osteoporosis [87, 90]. Consequently, it is hypothesised that periodontal degradation may be influenced by systemic changes in bone mineral density (BMD) brought on by osteoporosis, particularly during menopause [3, 91–94]. Periodontitis is characterised by progressive and irreversible bone and periodontal ligament attachment loss. Symptoms include red, swollen gums, persistent bad odour, pus discharge, and loose or separating teeth. This can eventually result in tooth loss [95]. The rate of bone loss in postmenopausal women is predictive of tooth loss; the risk of tooth loss quadruples for every 1% annual decrease in bone mineral density of the entire body [92, 95]. In addition, women with severe osteoporosis are three times more likely to be edentulous than healthy, age-matched controls [96].

- **Etiopathogenesis**

- A lack of oestrogen can result in both diminished resistance and increased action. The osteoporosis-related systemic bone resorption may lead to osteoporotic mandible changes and alveolar bone loss [96–100]. The reduction of the mandibular cortical width and the thinning of the trabecular maxillary bone result in a "weakened resistance" of the periodontium to infection, thereby exacerbating alveolar bone loss in periodontitis [1]. On the other hand, elevated levels of pro-inflammatory mediators such as IL-1, IL-6, IL-8, RANKL, GCSF, GM CSF, and TNF have been detected in oestrogen deficiency, and they may play crucial roles in the promoting the activity of osteoclasts via nuclear factor-kappa B signalling. Aside from that, these mediators may act locally to impair the tissue response to periodontitis, thereby exacerbating the inflammatory response and accelerating systemic bone resorption by modulating the host response [101]. Changes in oral microcirculation, antioxidant defence, and the growth and differentiation of periodontal fibroblast may also contribute to the increased risk of periodontitis that occurs during menopause [4, 21, 84, 102, 103]. The risk is also affected by a higher concentration of ionised calcium in saliva, which accelerates the mineralisation of dental plaque and promotes calculus formation [1, 26–29]. In addition, menopausal women with higher depressive mood scores may practice poor oral hygiene, thereby increasing their risk of periodontitis [104–106].
- **Relationship between osteoporosis and loss of alveolar bone**
- As osteoporosis is characterised by the generalised thinning of trabecular and cortical bone, it has been hypothesised that the alveolar bone encircling the teeth in osteoporotic patients is more prone to periodontal bone loss. Growing evidence strongly supports a correlation between systemic and alveolar bone loss (ABL). All ten clinical investigations published between 1996 and 2020 examining the relationship between systemic bone loss and ABL revealed an inverse correlation between systemic BMD and ABL [87].
- **Relationship between osteoporosis and loss of clinical attachment**
- Evidence is only moderately suggestive of a correlation between systemic BMD and clinical attachment loss (CAL). CAL reflects the cumulative experience of periodontal disease and is a crucial outcome measure for periodontitis diagnosis and staging. Seventeen of the 23 studies published between 1995 and 2020 revealed a correlation between CAL and osteoporosis. In severe periodontitis, the loss of clinical attachment results in the deterioration of supporting alveolar bone support and loss of teeth. Eleven of the 16 studies that evaluated the relationship between tooth loss and systemic BMD found a positive correlation, while 5 studies found conflicting results. When confounding factors such as age and smoking were accounted for, a large multicentre study revealed a significant link between tooth loss and systemic BMD [87].
- **Management**
- Plaque accumulation is essential for the advent of periodontal attachment loss in postmenopausal women. Menopause may not pose a threat to the periodontium in such women with good oral health. To prevent periodontitis in suscep-

tible women, it is essential to remove bacterial plaque biofilm with good oral hygiene, to schedule regular dental visits, and to manage osteoporosis [95, 99].

4. **Dental implants and menopause**

   In ovariectomised animals (without functional occlusion), the volume of surrounding trabecular bone volume and the contact between the placed dental implant and new trabecular bone are significantly reduced compared to the results for non-ovariectomised animals. However, neither the cortical bone volume nor the contact with the implant changed around the implant [3, 107, 108]. August et al. discovered that maxillary implants of postmenopausal women without HRT showed unsuccessful integration with bone significantly more frequently (13.8%) than the ones placed in premenopausal women (6.3%) and postmenopausal women receiving HRT (8.1%). This indicates that oestrogen deficiency may be a risk factor for maxillary implant failure [109].

5. **Hormone replacement therapy**

   Clinicians usually prescribe hormone replacement therapy (HRT) to alleviate menopausal transition symptoms or to prevent chronic diseases that are thought to occur at this time, partly because of long-term oestrogen deficiency [3]. The use of HRT for the prevention of diseases other than menopause-related symptoms may not be justified [110–113]. Nonetheless, it is evident that many women benefit from HRT, which may also have oral implications [3, 110]. Oral discomfort may be caused by steroid hormone withdrawal in only a subset of postmenopausal women, and HRT may ameliorate the clinical symptoms and cytologic characteristics of this patient population [114, 115]. HRT exerts its effects via a variety of mechanisms and pathways. Its anti-inflammatory mechanism includes inhibition of matrix metalloproteinase, prostaglandin, or osteoclast and stimulation of osteoblast [110, 116, 117]. HRT reduces the synthesis of proinflammatory cytokines (IL-1, tumour necrosis factor-α and IL-6) by mononuclear cells, T-cell–mediated inflammation and leukocyte formation in bone marrow [3, 118, 119]. Allen et al. conducted a systematic review of the health and economic effects of HRT in postmenopausal women for dental care and found that the HRT group consistently had better dental outcomes than the non-HRT group [120]. However, the majority of the included studies were single-arm trials or observational, and there was a dearth of large, randomised trials [9, 114, 120]. The role of HRT in relieving oral symptoms and signs is controversial as the effect is highly individual so that some women with menopausal symptoms benefit from HRT while others do not. Future gene profiling may identify women benefiting or not from the use of HRT [121].

   - **HRT in periodontitis**
   - Multiple studies have found that hormone replacement therapy improves periodontal health and tooth retention in women. Haas et al. (2009) reported that the prevalence of periodontitis in postmenopausal women who did not use HRT was substantially higher than in premenopausal women [122]. Taguchi et al. (2004) found in a study of 330 postmenopausal Japanese women that oestrogen may increase tooth retention by reinforcing the peri-

odontal attachment surrounding teeth, but not by affecting the bone porosity [123]. In an epidemiological study involving 4290 participants in Germany, Meisel et al. (2008) discovered that postmenopausal women using oestrogen had more teeth than males of the same age. In addition, women without HRT in this study had fewer teeth than other women [124]. This finding is consistent with the Women's Health Study from the United States, in which current HRT users had a 24% reduced risk of tooth loss than non-users among 42,171 postmenopausal women [125]. Nonetheless, few studies have produced contradictory findings. Lopez-Marcos et al. (2005) discovered no significant effect on periodontal status in 210 women who received or did not receive HRT [126]. The association between HRT and periodontal disease was more pronounced in women with menopause younger than 45 years [90].

- **HRT and saliva**
- Several studies have reported that women receiving HRT experience less oral discomfort, resulting in an improvement in quality of life. This may be attributed to an increase in saliva secretion [3, 18, 127, 128]. Thus, HRT may enhance both the quality and quantity of saliva in postmenopausal women [18]. In their study of 43 healthy premenopausal and postmenopausal females in the United States, however, Ship et al. (1991a) found no changes in salivary volume, indicating that menopause or HRT do not substantially affect salivary gland function among healthy women [14]. Since the evidence on the impact of menopause on saliva is based on a small number of patients and there are no randomised controlled trials on the effect of HRT on saliva, these partially contradictory results need to be confirmed in larger studies [121, 128].
- **HRT and BMS**
- It was discovered that HRT can alleviate oral burning symptoms and enhance cytologic characteristics, particularly in perimenopausal and postmenopausal women. In postmenopausal women, Volpe et al. discovered that 12 out of 22 patients with oral symptoms improved after treatment with estradiol [79]. Lopez-Jornet et al. discovered that women with burning symptoms and oestrogen receptors in the oral mucosa respond to hormone replacement, whereas patients without these receptors do not; however, there is no certainty that HRT will be a successful treatment [61].

7.4 Conclusion

Numerous physical and psychological symptoms of menopause negatively impact oral health. Oral health specialists, gynaecologists, endocrinologists, and physicians must be aware of the challenges associated with menopause and provide these women with a comprehensive health plan that includes oral health care. To obtain the best possible outcome, dentists must collaborate closely with gynaecologists by referring postmenopausal women with oral symptoms, if necessary, for medical intervention.

References

1. Ciesielska A, Kusiak A, Ossowska A, Grzybowska ME. Changes in the oral cavity in menopausal women—A narrative review. Int J Environ Res Public Health. 2021;19(1):253.
2. Bruckmann C. "Oral menopause"—Do you know this phenomenon? Womens Health Sci J. 2018;2:106.
3. Friedlander AH. The physiology, medical management and oral implications of menopause. J Am Dent Assoc. 2002;133(1):73–81.
4. Sen S, Sen S, Dutta A, Abhinandan, Kumar V, Singh AK. Oral manifestation and its management in postmenopausal women: an integrated review. Prz Menopauzalny. 2020;19(2):101–3.
5. Mutneja P, Dhawan P, Raina A, Sharma G. Menopause and the oral cavity. Indian J Endocrinol Metab. 2012;16(4):548–51.
6. Saluja P, Shetty V, Dave A, Arora M, Hans V, Madan A. Comparative evaluation of the effect of menstruation, pregnancy and menopause on salivary flow rate, pH and gustatory function. J Clin Diagn Res. 2014;8(10):ZC81–5.
7. Research on the menopause in the 1990s. Report of a WHO Scientific Group. World Health Organ Tech Rep Ser. 1996;866:1–107.
8. McKinlay SM, Brambilla DJ, Posner JG. The normal menopause transition. Maturitas. 1992;14(2):103–15.
9. Ashraf M, Kamp E, Musbahi E, DeGiovanni C. Menopause, skin and common dermatoses. Part 4: oral disorders. Clin Exp Dermatol. 2022;47(12):2130–5.
10. Välimaa H, Savolainen S, Soukka T, Silvoniemi P, Mäkelä S, Kujari H, et al. Estrogen receptor-beta is the predominant estrogen receptor subtype in human oral epithelium and salivary glands. J Endocrinol. 2004;180(1):55–62.
11. Ojanotko-Harri A, Forssell H, Laine M, Hurttia H, Bläuer M, Tuohimaa P. Immunohistochemical detection of androgen receptors in human oral mucosa. Arch Oral Biol. 1992;37(6):511–4.
12. Niklander S, Veas L, Barrera C, Fuentes F, Chiappini G, Marshall M. Risk factors, hyposalivation and impact of xerostomia on oral health-related quality of life. Braz Oral Res. 2017;31:e14.
13. Minicucci EM, Pires RBC, Vieira RA, Miot HA, Sposto MR. Assessing the impact of menopause on salivary flow and xerostomia. Aust Dent J. 2013;58(2):230–4.
14. Ship JA, Patton LL, Tylenda CA. An assessment of salivary function in healthy premenopausal and postmenopausal females. J Gerontol. 1991;46(1):M11–5.
15. Ben Aryeh H, Gottlieb I, Ish-Shalom S, David A, Szargel H, Laufer D. Oral complaints related to menopause. Maturitas. 1996;24(3):185–9.
16. Taga T, Ito K, Takamatsu K, Ogawa M, Funayama S, Inoue M. Menopausal symptoms are associated with oral sensory complaints in perimenopausal women: an observational study. BMC Womens Health. 2021;21:262.
17. Kullander S, Sonesson B. Studies on saliva in menstruating, pregnant and post-menopausal women. Acta Endocrinol (Copenh). 1965;48:329–36.
18. Laine M, Leimola-Virtanen R. Effect of hormone replacement therapy on salivary flow rate, buffer effect and pH on perimenopausal and postmenopausal women. Arch Oral Biol. 1996;41(1):91–6.
19. Rukmini JN, Sachan R, Sibi N, Meghana A, Malar CI. Effect of menopause on saliva and dental health. J Int Soc Prev Community Dent. 2018;8(6):529–33.
20. Streckfus CF, Baur U, Brown LJ, Bacal C, Metter J, Nick T. Effects of estrogen status and aging on salivary flow rates in healthy Caucasian women. Gerontology. 1998;44(1):32–9.
21. Yalcin F, Gurgan S, Gul G. Oral health in postmenopausal Turkish women. Oral Health Prev Dent. 2006;4(4):227–33.
22. Rajesh KS, Zareena, Hegde S, Arun Kumar MS. Assessment of salivary calcium, phosphate, magnesium, pH, and flow rate in healthy subjects, periodontitis, and dental caries. Contemp Clin Dent. 2015;6(4):461–5.
23. Fiyaz M, Ramesh A, Ramalingam K, Thomas B, Shetty S, Prakash P. Association of salivary calcium, phosphate, pH and flow rate on oral health: a study on 90 subjects. J Indian Soc Periodontol. 2013;17(4):454–60.

24. Sinor MZ. Association between salivary parameters and periodontal disease. Int Med J (1994). 2013;20:1–5.
25. Srebrzyńska-Witek A, Koszowski R. Effect of menopause on salivary glands and oral mucosa. Menopausal Rev. 2013;5:418–22.
26. Agha-Hosseini F, Mirzaii-Dizgah I, Moghaddam PP, Akrad ZT. Stimulated whole salivary flow rate and composition in menopausal women with oral dryness feeling. Oral Dis. 2007;13(3):320–3.
27. Sewón LA, Karjalainen SM, Söderling E, Lapinleimu H, Simell O. Associations between salivary calcium and oral health. J Clin Periodontol. 1998;25(11 Pt 1):915–9.
28. Cydejko A, Kusiak A, Grzybowska ME, Kochańska B, Ochocińska J, Maj A, et al. Selected physicochemical properties of saliva in menopausal women—A pilot study. Int J Environ Res Public Health. 2020;17(7):2604.
29. Soundarya B, Massillamani F, Kailasam S, Jayashree G, Narmadha N, Sornaa N. Salivary menopausal markers and oral health status—A hidden hook up. J Midlife Health. 2022;13(2):157–62.
30. Pink R, Simek J, Vondrakova J, Faber E, Michl P, Pazdera J, et al. Saliva as a diagnostic medium. Biomed Pap Med Fac Univ Palacky Olomouc Czech Repub. 2009;153(2):103–10.
31. Lynge Pedersen AM, Belstrøm D. The role of natural salivary defences in maintaining a healthy oral microbiota. J Dent. 2019;80(Suppl 1):S3–12.
32. Fábián TK, Hermann P, Beck A, Fejérdy P, Fábián G. Salivary defense proteins: their network and role in innate and acquired oral immunity. Int J Mol Sci. 2012;13(4):4295–320.
33. Yeh CK, Dodds MW, Zuo P, Johnson DA. A population-based study of salivary lysozyme concentrations and candidal counts. Arch Oral Biol. 1997;42(1):25–31.
34. Mott AE, Grushka M, Sessle BJ. Diagnosis and management of taste disorders and burning mouth syndrome. Dent Clin North Am. 1993;37(1):33–71.
35. Zakrzewska J, Buchanan JAG. Burning mouth syndrome. BMJ Clin Evid. 2016;2016:1301.
36. Frutos R, Rodríguez S, Miralles-Jorda L, Machuca G. Oral manifestations and dental treatment in menopause. Med Oral. 2002;7(1):26–30, 31–5.
37. Samsioe G. The menopause revisited. Int J Gynaecol Obstet. 1995;51(1):1–13.
38. Chaveli B, Pérez MG, Jimenez Y. Dental considerations in pregnancy and menopause. J Clin Exp Dent. 2011;3:e135–44.
39. Wolff A, Fox PC, Ship JA, Atkinson JC, Macynski AA, Baum BJ. Oral mucosal status and major salivary gland function. Oral Surg Oral Med Oral Pathol. 1990;70(1):49–54.
40. Petkowicz B, Piotrkowicz J, Szeszko Ł, Banakiewicz K, Zieliński P. Selected aspects of oral cavity diseases in menopausal women. Menopausal Rev. 2013;4:352–7.
41. Talo Yildirim T, Kaya F. The effects of menopause on periodontal tissue. Int Dent Res. 2011;1:81.
42. Merskey H. Classification of chronic pain: descriptions of chronic pain syndromes and definitions of pain terms. Pain. 1986;Suppl 3:226.
43. Dahiya P, Kamal R, Kumar M, Niti, Gupta R, Chaudhary K. Burning mouth syndrome and menopause. Int J Prev Med. 2013;4(1):15–20.
44. ADA Division of Communications; Journal of the American Dental Association. For the dental patient. Burning mouth syndrome. J Am Dent Assoc. 2005;136(8):1191.
45. Bergdahl M, Bergdahl J. Burning mouth syndrome: prevalence and associated factors. J Oral Pathol Med. 1999;28(8):350–4.
46. Ślebioda Z, Szponar E. Burning mouth syndrome—a common dental problem in perimenopausal women. Prz Menopauzalny. 2014;13(3):198–202.
47. Bookout GP, Ladd M, Short RE. Burning mouth syndrome. In: StatPearls [Internet]. Treasure Island: StatPearls Publishing; 2023 [cited 2023 Jul 31]. http://www.ncbi.nlm.nih.gov/books/NBK519529/.
48. Lee YH, Chon S. Burning mouth syndrome in postmenopausal women with self-reported sleep problems. Cranio. 2020;38(4):221–32.

49. Payano Sosa JS, Da Silva JT, Burrowes SAB, Yoo SY, Keaser ML, Meiller TF, et al. Time of day influences psychophysical measures in women with burning mouth syndrome. Front Neurosci. 2021;15:698164.
50. Aravindhan R, Vidyalakshmi S, Kumar MS, Satheesh C, Balasubramanium AM, Prasad VS. Burning mouth syndrome: a review on its diagnostic and therapeutic approach. J Pharm Bioallied Sci. 2014;6(Suppl 1):S21–5.
51. Grushka M, Epstein JB, Gorsky M. Burning mouth syndrome. Am Fam Physician. 2002;65(4):615–20.
52. Vaidya R. Burning mouth syndrome at menopause: elusive etiology. J Midlife Health. 2012;3(1):3–4.
53. Lauria G, Majorana A, Borgna M, Lombardi R, Penza P, Padovani A, et al. Trigeminal small-fiber sensory neuropathy causes burning mouth syndrome. Pain. 2005;115(3):332–7.
54. Yilmaz Z, Renton T, Yiangou Y, Zakrzewska J, Chessell IP, Bountra C, et al. Burning mouth syndrome as a trigeminal small fibre neuropathy: increased heat and capsaicin receptor TRPV1 in nerve fibres correlates with pain score. J Clin Neurosci. 2007;14(9):864–71.
55. Taichman LS, Havens AM, Van Poznak CH. Potential implications of adjuvant endocrine therapy for the oral health of postmenopausal women with breast cancer. Breast Cancer Res Treat. 2013;137(1):23–32.
56. Cerchiari DP, de Moricz RD, Sanjar FA, Rapoport PB, Moretti G, Guerra MM. Burning mouth syndrome: etiology. Braz J Otorhinolaryngol. 2006;72(3):419–23.
57. Burning mouth syndrome|National Institute of Dental and Craniofacial Research [Internet]. [cited 2023 Jul 31]. https://www.nidcr.nih.gov/health-info/burning-mouth.
58. Ozasa K, Noma N, Kobayashi M, Takizawa K, Young A, Eliav E, et al. Association between anxiety and descending pain modulation of thermal stimuli in patients with burning mouth syndrome: a cross-sectional study. J Oral Facial Pain Headache. 2022;36(1):67–77.
59. Ozasa K, Noma N, Young A, Korczeniewska OA, Eliav E, Imamura Y. Potential differences in somatosensory function during premenopause and early and late postmenopause in patients with burning mouth syndrome: an observational case-control study. J Dent Sci. 2022;17(1):399–406.
60. Grinspan D, Fernández Blanco G, Allevato MA, Stengel FM. Burning mouth syndrome. Int J Dermatol. 1995;34(7):483–7.
61. López-Jornet P, Camacho-Alonso F, Andujar-Mateos P, Sánchez-Siles M, Gómez-Garcia F. Burning mouth syndrome: an update. Med Oral Patol Oral Cir Bucal. 2010;15(4):e562–8.
62. Scala A, Checchi L, Montevecchi M, Marini I, Giamberardino MA. Update on burning mouth syndrome: overview and patient management. Crit Rev Oral Biol Med. 2003;14(4):275–91.
63. Gremeau-Richard C, Woda A, Navez ML, Attal N, Bouhassira D, Gagnieu MC, et al. Topical clonazepam in stomatodynia: a randomised placebo-controlled study. Pain. 2004;108(1–2):51–7.
64. Mínguez Serra MP, Salort Llorca C, Silvestre Donat FJ. Pharmacological treatment of burning mouth syndrome: a review and update. Med Oral Patol Oral Cir Bucal. 2007;12(4):E299–304.
65. Cui Y, Xu H, Chen FM, Liu JL, Jiang L, Zhou Y, et al. Efficacy evaluation of clonazepam for symptom remission in burning mouth syndrome: a meta-analysis. Oral Dis. 2016;22(6):503–11.
66. Matsuoka H, Chiba I, Sakano Y, Toyofuku A, Abiko Y. Cognitive behavioral therapy for psychosomatic problems in dental settings. Biopsychosoc Med. 2017;11:18.
67. Al-Maweri SA, Javed F, Kalakonda B, AlAizari NA, Al-Soneidar W, Al-Akwa A. Efficacy of low level laser therapy in the treatment of burning mouth syndrome: a systematic review. Photodiagn Photodyn Ther. 2017;17:188–93.
68. Buchanan JA, Zakrzewska JM. Burning mouth syndrome. BMJ Clin Evid. 2010;2010:1301.
69. Spanemberg JC, Cherubini K, de Figueiredo MAZ, Yurgel LS, Salum FG. Aetiology and therapeutics of burning mouth syndrome: an update. Gerodontology. 2012;29(2):84–9.
70. Kisely S, Forbes M, Sawyer E, Black E, Lalloo R. A systematic review of randomized trials for the treatment of burning mouth syndrome. J Psychosom Res. 2016;86:39–46.

71. López-Jornet P, Camacho-Alonso F, Molino-Pagan D. Prospective, randomized, double-blind, clinical evaluation of Aloe vera Barbadensis, applied in combination with a tongue protector to treat burning mouth syndrome. J Oral Pathol Med. 2013;42(4):295–301.
72. Sun A, Wu KM, Wang YP, Lin HP, Chen HM, Chiang CP. Burning mouth syndrome: a review and update. J Oral Pathol Med. 2013;42(9):649–55.
73. Nagler RM, Hershkovich O. Sialochemical and gustatory analysis in patients with oral sensory complaints. J Pain. 2004;5(1):56–63.
74. Femiano F. Burning mouth syndrome (BMS): an open trial of comparative efficacy of alpha-lipoic acid (thioctic acid) with other therapies. Minerva Stomatol. 2002;51(9):405–9.
75. Granot M, Nagler RM. Association between regional idiopathic neuropathy and salivary involvement as the possible mechanism for oral sensory complaints. J Pain. 2005;6(9):581–7.
76. Cavalcanti DR, da Silveira FRX. Alpha lipoic acid in burning mouth syndrome—a randomized double-blind placebo-controlled trial. J Oral Pathol Med. 2009;38(3):254–61.
77. López-Jornet P, Camacho-Alonso F, Leon-Espinosa S. Efficacy of alpha lipoic acid in burning mouth syndrome: a randomized, placebo-treatment study. J Oral Rehabil. 2009;36(1):52–7.
78. Van Houdenhove B, Joostens P. Burning mouth syndrome. Successful treatment with combined psychotherapy and psychopharmacotherapy. Gen Hosp Psychiatry. 1995;17(5):385–8.
79. Volpe A, Lucenti V, Forabosco A, Boselli F, Latessa AM, Pozzo P, et al. Oral discomfort and hormone replacement therapy in the post-menopause. Maturitas. 1991;13(1):1–5.
80. Bergdahl J, Anneroth G, Perris H. Cognitive therapy in the treatment of patients with resistant burning mouth syndrome: a controlled study. J Oral Pathol Med. 1995;24(5):213–5.
81. Arnold DL, Krishnamurthy K. Lichen Planus. In: StatPearls [Internet]. Treasure Island: StatPearls Publishing; 2023 [cited 2023 Jul 31]. http://www.ncbi.nlm.nih.gov/books/NBK526126/.
82. Dvorak G, Monshi B, Hof M, Bernhart T, Bruckmann C, Rappersberger K. Gender aspects in oral health-related quality of life of oral lichen planus patients. Int J Stomatol Occlusion Med. 2015;8:33–40.
83. Oberti L, Alberta L, Massimo P, Francesco C, Dorina L. Clinical management of oral lichen planus: a systematic review. Mini Rev Med Chem. 2019;19(13):1049–59.
84. Scardina GA, Messina P. Oral microcirculation in post-menopause: a possible correlation with periodontitis. Gerodontology. 2012;29(2):e1045–51.
85. Petruzzi M, Lucchese A, Lajolo C, Campus G, Lauritano D, Serpico R. Topical retinoids in oral lichen planus treatment: an overview. Dermatology. 2013;226(1):61–7.
86. Gupta S, Ghosh S, Gupta S. Interventions for the management of oral lichen planus: a review of the conventional and novel therapies. Oral Dis. 2017;23(8):1029–42.
87. Yu B, Wang CY. Osteoporosis and periodontal diseases—An update on their association and mechanistic links. Periodontol 2000. 2022;89(1):99–113.
88. Lenell C, Peña-Chávez R, Burdick RJ, Rogus-Pulia N. The relationship between menopause and dysphagia: a scoping review. Womens Health Rep (New Rochelle). 2022;3(1):990–7.
89. Hernández-Vigueras S, Martínez-Garriga B, Sánchez MC, Sanz M, Estrugo-Devesa A, Vinuesa T, et al. Oral microbiota, periodontal status, and osteoporosis in postmenopausal females. J Periodontol. 2016;87(2):124–33.
90. Lee Y, Kim I, Song J, Hwang KG, Choi B, Hwang SS. The relationship between hormone replacement therapy and periodontal disease in postmenopausal women: a cross-sectional study the Korea National Health and Nutrition Examination Survey from 2007 to 2012. BMC Oral Health. 2019;19(1):151.
91. Jeffcoat MK, Chesnut CH. Systemic osteoporosis and oral bone loss: evidence shows increased risk factors. J Am Dent Assoc. 1993;124(11):49–56.
92. Krall EA, Dawson-Hughes B, Papas A, Garcia RI. Tooth loss and skeletal bone density in healthy postmenopausal women. Osteoporos Int. 1994;4(2):104–9.
93. Genco RJ, Grossi SG. Is estrogen deficiency a risk factor for periodontal disease? Compend Contin Educ Dent Suppl. 1998;(22):S23–S29.
94. Klemetti E, Collin HL, Forss H, Markkanen H, Lassila V. Mineral status of skeleton and advanced periodontal disease. J Clin Periodontol. 1994;21(3):184–8.

95. Buencamino MCA, Palomo L, Thacker HL. How menopause affects oral health, and what we can do about it. Cleve Clin J Med. 2009;76(8):467–75.
96. Kribbs PJ. Comparison of mandibular bone in normal and osteoporotic women. J Prosthet Dent. 1990;63(2):218–22.
97. von Wowern N, Klausen B, Kollerup G. Osteoporosis: a risk factor in periodontal disease. J Periodontol. 1994;65(12):1134–8.
98. Ronderos M, Jacobs DR, Himes JH, Pihlstrom BL. Associations of periodontal disease with femoral bone mineral density and estrogen replacement therapy: cross-sectional evaluation of US adults from NHANES III. J Clin Periodontol. 2000;27(10):778–86.
99. Zenk JK. The ADA council on access, prevention, and interprofessional relations. Northwest Dent. 2016;95(3):7–8.
100. Jeffcoat MK, Lewis CE, Reddy MS, Wang CY, Redford M. Post-menopausal bone loss and its relationship to oral bone loss. Periodontol 2000. 2000;(23):94–102.
101. Peng J, Chen J, Liu Y, Lyu J, Zhang B. Association between periodontitis and osteoporosis in United States adults from the National Health and Nutrition Examination Survey: a cross-sectional analysis. BMC Oral Health. 2023;23(1):254.
102. Baltacioğlu E, Akalin FA, Alver A, Balaban F, Unsal M, Karabulut E. Total antioxidant capacity and superoxide dismutase activity levels in serum and gingival crevicular fluid in post-menopausal women with chronic periodontitis. J Clin Periodontol. 2006;33(6):385–92.
103. Mascarenhas P, Gapski R, Al-Shammari K, Wang HL. Influence of sex hormones on the periodontium. J Clin Periodontol. 2003;30(8):671–81.
104. Yakar N, Türedi A, Emingil G, Şahin Ç, Köse T, Silbereisen A, et al. Oral health and emotional well-being in premenopausal and postmenopausal women: a cross-sectional cohort study. BMC Womens Health. 2021;21(1):338.
105. Zeleke BM, Bell RJ, Billah B, Davis SR. Vasomotor symptoms are associated with depressive symptoms in community-dwelling older women. Menopause. 2017;24(12):1365–71.
106. Yoshida N, Sugimoto K, Suzuki S, Kudo H. Change in oral health status associated with menopause in Japanese dental hygienists. Int J Dent Hyg. 2018;16(1):157–64.
107. Motohashi M, Shirota T, Tokugawa Y, Ohno K, Michi K, Yamaguchi A. Bone reactions around hydroxyapatite-coated implants in ovariectomized rats. Oral Surg Oral Med Oral Pathol Oral Radiol Endod. 1999;87(2):145–52.
108. Yamazaki M, Shirota T, Tokugawa Y, Motohashi M, Ohno K, Michi K, et al. Bone reactions to titanium screw implants in ovariectomized animals. Oral Surg Oral Med Oral Pathol Oral Radiol Endod. 1999;87(4):411–8.
109. August M, Chung K, Chang Y, Glowacki J. Influence of estrogen status on endosseous implant osseointegration. J Oral Maxillofac Surg. 2001;59(11):1285–9; discussion 1290–1291.
110. Tarkkila L, Furuholm J, Tiitinen A, Meurman JH. Oral health in perimenopausal and early postmenopausal women from baseline to 2 years of follow-up with reference to hormone replacement therapy. Clin Oral Investig. 2008;12(3):271–7.
111. Cherry N, Gilmour K, Hannaford P, Heagerty A, Khan MA, Kitchener H, et al. Oestrogen therapy for prevention of reinfarction in postmenopausal women: a randomised placebo controlled trial. Lancet. 2002;360(9350):2001–8.
112. Herrington DM, Reboussin DM, Brosnihan KB, Sharp PC, Shumaker SA, Snyder TE, et al. Effects of estrogen replacement on the progression of coronary-artery atherosclerosis. N Engl J Med. 2000;343(8):522–9.
113. Rossouw JE, Anderson GL, Prentice RL, LaCroix AZ, Kooperberg C, Stefanick ML, et al. Risks and benefits of estrogen plus progestin in healthy postmenopausal women: principal results from the Women's Health Initiative randomized controlled trial. JAMA. 2002;288(3):321–33.
114. Suri V, Suri V. Menopause and oral health. J Midlife Health. 2014;5(3):115–20.
115. Forabosco A, Criscuolo M, Coukos G, Uccelli E, Weinstein R, Spinato S, et al. Efficacy of hormone replacement therapy in postmenopausal women with oral discomfort. Oral Surg Oral Med Oral Pathol. 1992;73(5):570–4.
116. Mariotti A. Sex steroid hormones and cell dynamics in the periodontium. Crit Rev Oral Biol Med. 1994;5(1):27–53.

117. Soory M. Targets for steroid hormone mediated actions of periodontal pathogens, cytokines and therapeutic agents: some implications on tissue turnover in the periodontium. Curr Drug Targets. 2000;1(4):309–25.
118. Norderyd OM, Grossi SG, Machtei EE, Zambon JJ, Hausmann E, Dunford RG, et al. Periodontal status of women taking postmenopausal estrogen supplementation. J Periodontol. 1993;64(10):957–62.
119. Reinhardt RA, Payne JB, Maze CA, Patil KD, Gallagher SJ, Mattson JS. Influence of estrogen and osteopenia/osteoporosis on clinical periodontitis in postmenopausal women. J Periodontol. 1999;70(8):823–8.
120. Allen IE, Monroe M, Connelly J, Cintron R, Ross SD. Effect of postmenopausal hormone replacement therapy on dental outcomes: systematic review of the literature and pharmacoeconomic analysis. Manag Care Interface. 2000;13(4):93–9.
121. Meurman JH, Tarkkila L, Tiitinen A. The menopause and oral health. Maturitas. 2009;63(1):56–62.
122. Haas AN, Rösing CK, Oppermann RV, Albandar JM, Susin C. Association among menopause, hormone replacement therapy, and periodontal attachment loss in southern Brazilian women. J Periodontol. 2009;80(9):1380–7.
123. Taguchi A, Sanada M, Suei Y, Ohtsuka M, Nakamoto T, Lee K, et al. Effect of estrogen use on tooth retention, oral bone height, and oral bone porosity in Japanese postmenopausal women. Menopause. 2004;11(5):556–62.
124. Meisel P, Reifenberger J, Haase R, Nauck M, Bandt C, Kocher T. Women are periodontally healthier than men, but why don't they have more teeth than men? Menopause. 2008;15(2):270–5.
125. Grodstein F, Colditz GA, Stampfer MJ. Tooth loss and hormone use in postmenopausal women. Compend Contin Educ Dent Suppl. 1998;(22):S9–16.
126. López-Marcos JF, García-Valle S, García-Iglesias AA. Periodontal aspects in menopausal women undergoing hormone replacement therapy. Med Oral Patol Oral Cir Bucal. 2005;10(2):132–41.
127. Leimola-Virtanen R, Helenius H, Laine M. Hormone replacement therapy and some salivary antimicrobial factors in post- and perimenopausal women. Maturitas. 1997;27(2):145–51.
128. Eliasson L, Carlén A, Laine M, Birkhed D. Minor gland and whole saliva in postmenopausal women using a low potency oestrogen (oestriol). Arch Oral Biol. 2003;48(7):511–7.

Menopause and Eye Health

8

Ritu Sharma and Pinky Mishra

8.1 Overview

Increased life expectancy has led to increased encounters with age-related ocular diseases among women. According to the World Health Organisation (WHO), over the last one decade, there has been 22% increase in the number of postmenopausal women, with further expectation that women aged 60 years could survive for another 21 years. Elderly women are at high risk for developing various ocular disorders with gender-specific predilection for women. The deteriorated eye health will ultimately compromise the quality of life and make women more susceptible to psychological issues—depression, anxiety, etc. Hence menopause offers an important opportunity to address the ocular health of these women.

8.2 Pathophysiology of Various Ocular Diseases Encountered in Menopause

Various epidemiological, genetic, and clinical factors have emerged as potential risk factors. Role of oestrogen and androgens in ocular disorders has been extensively studied. Oestrogen receptors, ER-α and ER-β, are abundantly expressed throughout the ocular surfaces. Selective ER modulators (SERMs, tamoxifen) and aromatase inhibitors (anastrozole) reduce oestrogen and cause visual side effects. Oestrogen via oestrogen receptors exerts anti-inflammatory effect, reduces intraocular pressure (IOP), prevents retinal ganglion cell loss, and maintains ocular perfusion and haemostasis, thus protects against age-related diseases like glaucoma, cataract, and age-related macular degeneration (AMD). The time of hormone replacement therapy (HRT) administration is also an important factor to be considered.

R. Sharma (✉) · P. Mishra
Government Institute of Medical Sciences, Greater Noida, UP, India

R. Garg (ed.), *Management of Menopause*,
https://doi.org/10.1007/978-981-96-0239-1_8

The menopausal effects on eyes include alteration in the quantity and quality of tear film, corneal changes in shape and thickness, retinal perfusion changes, changes in lens transparency, and inflammation in vitreous humour resulting in dry eyes, refractive errors, open angle glaucoma, age-related macular degeneration, Leber's hereditary optic neuropathy, and progression of cataract. Women may be asymptomatic or present with spectrum of symptoms which affect quality of life (Box 8.1).

Box 8.1 Various Symptoms in Ocular Disorders Among Postmenopausal Women

Asymptomatic

Dryness, itching, burning

Discomfort, pain, redness

Watering, crusting

Blurring of vision, double vision, halos, reduced night vision

Reduced contrast sensitivity, faded colours

Floaters (cobweb like patterns seen due to debris floating in the liquified vitreous humour)

Scintillating scotoma (flashing lights or blind spots due to reduced retinal perfusion, reduced collagen causing vitreous detachment)

8.2.1 Menopause and Dry Eye Syndrome/Keratoconjunctivitis Sicca [1]

It is a tear film disorder resulting subsequent to either increased deficiency of tears or increased evaporation of tears, with reported prevalence of 32% in one of the Indian studies [2].

The tear film consists of three layers: outermost layer, oil; middle, aqueous; and innermost, mucin. The meibomian glands secrete oils (consisting of lipids and proteins) which have antibacterial and lubricating action, and also inhibit evaporation. The lacrimal glands secrete aqueous which has antibacterial action due to the presence of lysozyme and lactoferrin. The mucin is secreted by goblet cells and protects against debris, friction, and antigens (due to presence of IgA) [3]. Hence dysfunction of meibomian glands and/or lacrimal glands can result in dry eye syndrome with the former being the major contributor. The tear film also contains epidermal growth factor EGF, omega-3 fatty acids which repair ocular epithelium, and transforming growth factor-beta TGF-β which has anti-inflammatory activity.

Both lacrimal and meibomian glands have oestrogen and androgen receptors. Testosterone stimulates lipid production and has anti-inflammatory action; hence reduced testosterone levels in menopausal women cause meibomian gland as well as lacrimal gland dysfunction. Oestradiol downregulates the enzymes responsible for exocrine gland tissue lysis, stimulates tumour necrosis factor-alpha (TNF-α), and has pro-inflammatory action. It is suggested that it is the altered oestrogen/androgen balance secondary to alteration of receptors in menopausal females which is important in pathophysiology of dry eye syndrome. Loss of oestrogen receptors make hormone replacement therapy (HRT) ineffective in dry eye syndrome; rather it has been reported to worsen the symptoms [4, 5].

The *aetiology* is multifactorial, and the risk factors include menopause, advanced age, type 2 diabetes (by accelerating decline of the meibomian gland), thyroid disorders, autoimmune diseases like Sjogren's syndrome (affect exocrine glands), history of laser eye surgery (destroy corneal epithelial cells), neurological disorders like Bell's palsy and stroke, and certain medications like beta blockers, diuretics, anticholinergics, antihistamines (reduce tear production and increase intraocular pressure), HRT especially unopposed oestrogen therapy, etc. Environmental factors such as air pollution (cause ocular inflammation), low humidity, excessive wind or cold or hot weather (increase tear evaporation), and increased screen time have also been identified as risk factors for dry eye syndrome [5, 6].

The **symptoms** include dryness, burning, gritting sensation, redness, crusting, light sensitivity/photophobia, eye fatigue, reflex watering, etc. The damage to ocular surfaces predisposes the patients to infections (bacterial keratitis, blepharitis); loss of aqueous layer predisposes to visual refractory disturbances and post-operative complications following eye surgeries; neurosensory damage due to loss of corneal oestrogen receptors leads to decreased blinking and tear reflex.

8.3 Investigations to Diagnose Dry Eye Syndrome

- **Tear film osmolarity testing**: to measure the number of concentrated electrolytes on the ocular surface or osmotic strength of tear film. Dry eye syndrome is diagnosed when the osmolarity is >300 mOsm/L and an inter-eye difference of >8 mOsm/L.
- **Schirmer test**: to assess tear volume and the amount of ocular film breakdown. Dry eye syndrome is diagnosed when tear production less than 14 mm after 5 min.
- **Meibography**: to determine the lacrimal duct patency.
- Ocular surface staining.

Good history, examination, and investigations will determine whether dry eye is due to evaporative cause or aqueous deficiency, and the management is then decided accordingly. The dry eye syndrome can be managed by educating women regarding various simple but effective lifestyle modifications targeting various risk factors.

8.3.1 Menopause and Glaucoma [7]

Glaucoma is the most important cause for irreversible blindness subsequent to the slow progressive neurodegeneration of retinal ganglion cells (RGCs) in optic nerve. About 80 million people worldwide are suffering from glaucoma.

There are different types of glaucoma: primary open-angle glaucoma (POAG), acute angle closure glaucoma, secondary glaucoma, congenital glaucoma, and normal tension glaucoma, with primary open-angle glaucoma being the most common and age-related.

The risk factors associated with POAG include advanced age, positive family history, late menarche, early menopause (2.6-fold increased risk), short duration between menarche to menopause, longer duration of oral contraceptive pill (OCP) use (25% increased risk with >5 years use) and bilateral oophorectomy, associated medical disorders like diabetes, hypertension, corneal thinning, prolonged corticosteroids use, eye injuries, smoking, alcohol, etc. History of far-sightedness is a risk factor for closed-angle glaucoma [8].

The oestradiol levels are inversely proportional to intraocular pressure. Menopause results in increased intraocular pressure by 1–3 mmHg; further women undergoing menopause at an early age are at higher risk of developing POAG [9]. It has been proposed that POAG may result either due to retinal ganglion cell (RGC) damage secondary to raised intraocular pressure (**mechanical theory**), or due to neurodegeneration secondary to reduced perfusion to the optic nerve (**vascular theory**); and oestrogen plays role in both. Oestrogen, via oestrogen receptors ER-α and ER-β, increases optic nerve perfusion by upregulating the vasodilator nitric oxide synthase from ocular endothelium, regulating smooth muscle tone and vascular resistance. Oestrogen also affects IOP by affecting the synthesis and outflow of tears. To find whether oestrogen action is mediated through the outflow pathway or through alteration of tissue biomechanical properties, a case control study conducted on Brown Norway rats reported that in ovariectomised rats compared with sham controls, there was 34% decrease in outflow facility ($P = 0.011$) and 19% increase in ocular compliance, respectively ($P = 0.019$), hence concluding that oestrogen act via multifactorial pathways [10].

HRT (oestrogen alone) has been reported to have beneficial effects—reducing IOP, improving quality and quantity of tears, and improving ocular perfusion, hence reducing the risk of open angle glaucoma [11]. However, there are studies where the results are inconclusive or contradictory. The "critical period hypothesis" may explain the inconsistencies, which states that time of HRT administration is important—in perimenopausal period HRT is beneficial, whereas in postmenopausal women if administered after prolonged period of oestrogen deprivation, it may be detrimental [12].

The **symptoms** include gradual peripheral visual loss, blind spots, blurring, halos, pain, fatigue, redness, reduced contrast sensitivity, headaches, nausea, vomiting, etc.

Investigations to diagnose glaucoma include the following:

Gonioscopy: examination of eye angle to find out whether angle is blocked or open

Tonometry: to measure the intraocular pressure IOP, which if >22 mmHg diagnose glaucoma and normal IOP is 12–21 mmHg.

Pachymetry: to measure corneal thickness.

Ophthalmoscopy/dilated eye examination: for detailed examination of optic nerve.

Visual field test/perimetry: to assess peripheral vision loss.

Optical coherence tomography (OCT): is a noninvasive test where images of the retina/optic nerve are studied.

Slit lamp examination: for optical nerve assessment.

Ultrasound eye: to examine various dimensions and blood flow.

There is no cure for glaucoma and the damage is permanent. However, the progression can be delayed by medication/procedures targeted to reduce intraocular pressure.

8.3.2 Menopause and Age-Related Macular Degeneration (AMD) [13, 14]

The macula, small area in the centre of the retina, is responsible for central vision, the clearest and sharpest vision. Macula contains rods and cones and macular pigment (carotenoids—lutein, zeaxanthin, and meso-zeaxanthin). The macular pigment protects the retina from oxidative stress and absorbs harmful blue light.

Age-related macular degeneration (AMD), an important cause of progressive central vision loss in elderly population, is the most common cause of adult blindness >55 years of age in developed countries with expected 288 million people suffering from AMD by 2040. There are **two types of AMD**—neovascular/exudative or wet form (10–15%, abnormal leaky blood vessel grows with rapid visual loss) and atrophic/dry form (85–90%, gradual loss of photoreceptor cells occurs due to tiny yellow protein deposits called drusen, with progressive visual loss).

AMD is the result of the interplay between environmental and genetic risk factors—advanced age, smoking, diabetes, cardiovascular diseases, complement factor abnormalities, positive family history, poor nutrition, prolonged UV light exposure, etc.

In retinal pigment epithelium (RPE), the expression of ER-α, ER-β, and genes regulated by oestrogen suggests link between oestrogen status and AMD. Oestrogen containing HRT and OCP lowers the risk of AMD, especially neovascular AMD. Long-term OCP usage, however, is reported to be associated with structural changes in the posterior segment—the macula, the retinal nerve fibre layer, and choroidal thickness. In a recent study, age and diabetes mellitus emerged as independent risk factors for developing age-related macular degeneration, regardless of menopause [15]. Owing to limited understanding of the association between menopause and AMD, the pathophysiology of AMD remains unclear and still needs further investigation.

Leber's hereditary optic neuropathy (LHON), a retinal disease, is caused by mutations in the mitochondrial genes encoding the subunits of NADH dehydrogenase. It results in optic atrophy and central vision loss. Oestrogen is again said to have role in its pathogenesis.

The **symptoms** include reduced night vision (first symptom), blurring, distorted images, straight lines appearing wavy, difficulty recognising faces, and blank/dark areas in the centre of vision.

Investigations for diagnosing AMD include the following:

Dilated eye examination: for thorough examination.

Amsler grid test: Amsler grid has straight lines with lots of dots in the centre which to a woman with AMD may look distorted—blurry, wavy, or broken. It is used to diagnose AMD and to monitor its progress.

Fluorescein angiography: may reveal leaking blood vessels at the macula.

Optical coherence tomography (OCT): is a noninvasive test where images of retina or macula are studied.

Optical coherence tomography angiography (OCTA): instead of fluorescein dye, laser reflection is used; and OCT scan provides 3D images of ocular blood flow.

There is no cure for AMD and only the progression can be delayed by medication. Atrophic AMD management include lifestyle changes, and age-related eye disease study-2 supplements (AREDS-2 supplements—lutein, zeaxanthin, vitamins C, E, zinc), while neoplastic AMD management includes anti-VEGF injections (anti-vascular endothelial growth factors) or laser surgery.

8.3.3 Menopause and Cataract [16]

Cataract involves opacification of the lens due to clumping of lens proteins, thus interfering with light transmission and vision. Cataract is an important and major cause of visual impairment especially in the elderly population worldwide. Its incidence is directly proportional to the age and is more prevalent in postmenopausal **women** compared with age-matched men.

Cataract can be classified into various kind, namely, **posterior, subcapsular, cortical, nuclear, and mixed variety**. In postmenopausal women, there is increased prevalence of cortical cataract. On the other hand, early menarche and late menopause are associated with reduced incidence of cataract formation (especially cortical cataract), while late menarche is associated with increased risk of nuclear cataract [17]. Various epidemiological studies have shown a protective effect of HRT among postmenopausal users (current users/ever-users) as compared to non-users on nuclear cataract formation. The duration of HRT is reported to be inversely related to the prevalence of cataract. Another study has shown that endogenous oestrogen exposure of more than 32 years and prolonged HRT use >3 years were reported to have protective effect on age-related cataract development [18, 19]. Oestrogen protects against **transforming growth factor**-beta (TGF-β) which is responsible for inducing **lenticular opacities**. **Antioxidant** properties of oestrogen preserves mitochondrial function and ATP levels in lens, preventing cataract progress. Hence, the evidence available suggests a possible protective role of oestrogen in delaying cataract formation.

Apart from advanced age and menopause, smoking, diabetes, genetic factors, excessive sunlight exposure, and injury are other risk factors for cataract. Tamoxifen, an oestrogen antagonist, accelerates the development of cataract.

Symptoms include blurred vision, reduced night vision, double vision, halos, frequent change of prescription, fading of colours, increased sensitivity to glare, etc.

Investigations for diagnosing cataract include the following:

Visual acuity test: to evaluate vision clarity.

Slit lamp examination: to examine the lens opacities.

Dilated eye examination: for detailed examination.

Tonometry: to measure the intraocular pressure to rule out other causes of reduced vision.

Colour vision test, contrast sensitivity test, visual field test: to assess the extent of cataract and field of vision.

8.4 Maintaining Eye Health in Menopause

Since the ocular changes in menopause are usually irreversible, periodic eye check-ups are important. A validated eye questionnaire should be administered to assess the quality of eye health. Emphasis should be on improving awareness about the symptoms of eye problems among menopausal women, optimising the control of underlying health issues—diabetes and hypertension—and educating women regarding the various simple lifestyle management options available. Adopting healthy diet and regular exercise are absolutely essential in maintaining eye health.

8.5 Comprehensive Eye Examination [20]

Regular eye examinations help in early detection and management of cataract, glaucoma, AMD, dry eyes, etc., thereby preventing vision loss. Comprehensive eye examination in low-risk women is recommended as below:

- At 40 years—baseline comprehensive eye evaluation
- 40–54 years—every 2–4 years
- 55–64 years—every 1–3 years
- >65 years—every 1–2 years

In high-risk women, a comprehensive eye examination is recommended more frequently, e.g. in people at high risk for glaucoma development, the schedule is as follows:

- 40–54 years—every 1–3 years
- 55–64 years—every 1–2 years
- >65 years—every 6–12 months

8.6 Management of Ocular Disorders in Menopause [1, 7, 13, 16]

Investigations required will depend on the provisional diagnosis made on the basis of history and ophthalmological examination. Management include lifestyle management options and specific management depending on the diagnosis made.

8.7 Nutrition and Hydration

Hormonal imbalance in menopause results in oxidative stress. Air pollution and UV rays also generate reactive oxygen species which leads to dry eye symptoms. Oxidative stress increases the risk of dry eye syndrome, AMD, and cataract.

Omega-3 fatty acids: Omega-3 fatty acids (especially eicosapentaenoic acid, docosahexaenoic acid) and omega-6 fatty acids help in lipid synthesis, reduce tear osmolarity, improve tear film stability, and have anti-inflammatory action. Lipid mediators formed protect goblet cells and reduce barrier disruption, hence enhancing ocular surface homeostasis. They prevent dry eyes and AMD. The rich sources of omega-3 and omega-6 fatty acids include vegetable oils, spinach, almonds, flaxseeds, chia seeds, eggs, fish oils, walnuts, and canola oil.

Vitamins and minerals: Vitamins C and D promote the production of lactoferrin, an antioxidant, hence have protective role. Vitamin C also regenerates collagen and other antioxidants and inhibits glycation and hence advanced glycation end products AGEs in lens responsible for cataract. Vitamin E (alpha tocopherol) helps to maintain integrity of cell membranes in retina and to maintain meibomian gland function. Vitamin A is required in the synthesis of rhodopsin in rods responsible for night vision and in synthesis of mucin. Green tea contains antioxidants like catechins and polyphenols and is helpful to maintain eye health. Carotenoids, lutein, and zeaxanthin reduce glare by filtering blue light and protect against AMD. So antioxidants prevent age-related eye problems like dry eye syndrome, AMD, and cataract.

Antioxidant-rich diet includes green leafy vegetables, broccoli, bell pepper, corn, eggs, citrus fruits, etc. Maqui berry is a super fruit with antioxidant properties, rich in vitamins C and E and omega-3 and omega-6 fatty acids.

Phyto-oestrogen-rich diet (e.g. flax and soy) and HRT improve visual sensitivity.

Zinc is a component of antioxidant enzyme superoxide dismutase and helps to metabolise vitamin A into its active form. Zinc absorption decreases in menopause increasing susceptibility to AMD and cataract; hence its supplementation is required.

Adequate hydration is essential in synthesis and maintaining the tear film. Drinking eight to ten glasses of water per day is therefore recommended; however, intake depends on activity, climate, and age.

8.8 Topical Eye Drops

Artificial tears: Osmolarity-lowering topical, lipid-based artificial tears containing ingredients like hyaluronic acid, polyethylene glycol, and propylene glycol are prescribed in dry eyes. They protect ocular surface epithelium and promote the repair of the damaged corneal epithelium. The artificial tears are supportive only and not therapeutic. The frequency of use may be increased in dry weather and in digital work. The preservatives in these preparations can cause allergy or irritation; hence preservative-free formulations are preferred.

Corticosteroids: Prescribed in dry eyes by ophthalmologist only. They have anti-inflammatory action by inhibiting cytokines and leukocytes, hence helpful in immunological disorders like Sjogren's syndrome. However, they should be used under supervision for short-term period only, as long-term use is associated with glaucoma, cataract, eye infections, and corneal thinning.

Immunomodulatory agents: Prescribed in dry eyes by ophthalmologist only. Cyclosporin exerts anti-inflammatory action by inhibiting interleukin 2.

IOP-lowering eye drops: Prescribed in glaucoma and may contain beta blockers (reduce tear production, e.g. timolol), alpha-adrenergic agonists (reduce tear production and improve outflow as well, e.g. apraclonidine), prostaglandin analogues (improve tear outflow, e.g. latanoprost), carbonic anhydrase inhibitors (reduce tear production, e.g. dorzolamide), or cholinergic agents (improve tear outflow, e.g. pilocarpine).

8.9 Systemic Medications

They are prescribed if topical preparations are ineffective.

Beta blockers, carbonic anhydrase: Are prescribed in glaucoma as oral tablets.

Anti-VEGF (anti-vascular endothelial growth factor) injections: given intravitreally to inhibit neovascularisation in wet AMD, e.g. aflibercept, bevacizumab, and ranibizumab.

8.10 Other Strategies

- ***Maintain optimal temperature and humidity***: Air conditioner and heater can reduce humidity in the air. Humidifier can be of help to maintain optimal humidity and reduce tear evaporation. Clean humidifier regularly.
- ***Reduce exposure*** to dust and allergens.
- ***UV-protective sunglasses*** reduce oxidative damage to ocular structures.
- ***Switch contact lenses*** to silicone hydrogel soft lenses, or moisturising lenses with regular contact lens breaks to avoid dry eye symptoms.
- ***Suitable eyeglasses*** may be helpful to improve vision.
- ***Minimise screen time*** as prolonged screen time reduces blinking and cause eye strain. Follow 20-20-20 rule, i.e. break every 20 min, and look at something

20 feet away for 20 seconds. Adjust brightness and contrast and position screen so that screen top is at level with the eyes; this will reduce tear evaporation by avoiding the need to open eyes wide.

- ***Regular blinking*** helps to evenly distribute tear film. For blinking practice close eyes gently, hold for 2 s, and open eyes widely; repeat for 2–3 min. The blinking practice is recommended several times a day. Apart from this conscious blinking, efforts are also promoted.
- ***Warm, moist compresses***: These emulsify the solidified fluid in the meibomian glands at the eyelashes base, maintain eyelid hygiene, and promote tear secretion.
- ***Control underlying medical disorders***: optimise blood sugar levels and blood pressure to prevent progression of AMD, glaucoma, cataract, etc.
- ***Stop smoking and alcohol*** as it can accelerate dry eye, AMD, and cataract. Helpful in management of non-communicable diseases (NCD) also.
- ***Regular exercise***: Thirty minutes of moderate exercise 5 days a week helps to improve the blood perfusion, stimulates the antioxidant and anti-inflammatory response, and helps to manage diabetes and blood pressure, hence reduce the risk of glaucoma, AMD, diabetic, and hypertensive retinopathy.
- ***Adequate sleep***: Hormonal changes in menopause causes sleep deprivation which decreases parasympathetic activity essential for tear production and secretion. Women are, therefore, advised to have 7–9 h of sleep. Relaxation techniques and avoiding caffeine and digital devices help to improve sleep quality.
- ***Relieve stress***: Stress causes ocular inflammation. Relaxation techniques like deep breathing, meditation, and yoga are helpful to relieve stress.
- ***Acupuncture***: It has been reported to stimulate the tears synthesis in the lacrimal gland and hence may prove useful in dry eyes.

8.11 Hormone Replacement Therapy (HRT)

Oestrogen plays a significant role in eye health. HRT has a protective role against cataract, AMD, and raised IOP. However, as there are concerns related to the associated side effects, HRT is to be prescribed only when the benefits outweigh the possible risks and should be used under supervision only. Phyto-oestrogen-rich diet (e.g. flax and soy) improves visual sensitivity.

8.12 Surgery

It is the definitive option in some cases, while is opted as the last resort in others.

- Surgery is the definitive treatment in cataract which involves lensectomy and IOL implantation. In the case of secondary cataract/posterior capsule opacification, YAG capsulotomy is recommended.
- In dry eyes, punctal plugs may be inserted to decrease drainage and evaporation of tears.

- Surgery is the last resort in glaucoma management when other options prove ineffective. Trabeculectomy is done to facilitate drainage of aqueous humour either by shunt surgery or with help of laser.
- Laser peripheral iridotomy may be required in emergency in acute angle closure glaucoma.
- Laser surgery or photodynamic therapy (injectable light activated drug) may be required in neovascular AMD for abnormal vessel destruction.

8.13 Other Supportive Measures

Women with AMD may use voice activated technology (Siri, Alexa) and audiobooks, large fonts, and magnifying glass. They may join support groups for AMD to get emotional support.

8.14 Conclusion

Menopause can negatively affect the eye health of women by predisposing them to a spectrum of ocular disorders, thereby adversely affecting the overall quality of life. Oestrogen has a definitive role to play. Given the potential risks associated with HRT, it should be used cautiously. A holistic and pragmatic approach to menopausal eye health focussing on healthy lifestyle and regular comprehensive eye examinations with ophthalmologist are recommended.

Key Points

- The role of oestrogen and androgens in ocular disorders has been well established.
- There is sufficient evidence available to support the association of menopause with development of age-related ocular disorders, the most important being dry eye syndrome, glaucoma, age-related macular degeneration, and cataract.
- Ocular damage and subsequent visual loss are irreversible in glaucoma and AMD. In glaucoma there is peripheral vision loss, while in AMD there is central vision loss.
- Regular comprehensive eye examination is recommended.
- Control underlying medical disorders that will slow the progression of ocular changes.
- Maintain eye hygiene, use sunglasses, minimise screen time, and follow the 20-20-20 rule. Do regular exercise, take adequate rest, and stop smoking.
- Take diet rich in omega-3 fatty acids; vitamin C, E, and zinc; carotenoids; phytoestrogens; and maintain adequate hydration.
- Usually topical preparations like artificial tears and IOP-lowering eye drops are prescribed, reserving the systemic preparations for nonresponsive cases.
- Surgery is the definitive option in cataract, while is opted as the last resort in glaucoma.

- HRT has a protective role against cataract, AMD, and raised IOP. However, HRT should be used cautiously as due to scarcity of large-scale and longitudinal studies, direct causal link between oestrogen deficiency and various ocular disorders remains inconclusive.

References

1. American Academy of Ophthalmology. Menopause and dry eye syndrome. 2019. https://www.aao.org/eye-health/tips-prevention/menopause-dry-eye-syndrome.
2. Agarwal R, Singh P, Rajpal T, et al. Hospital based study of prevalence of dry eye in post-menopausal women. Indian J Clin Exp Ophthalmol. 2016;2(1):57–62.
3. Stern ME, Schaumburg CS, Pflugfelder SC. Dry eye as a mucosal autoimmune disease. Int Rev Immunol. 2013;32:19–41. https://doi.org/10.3109/08830185.2012.748052.
4. Shen G, Ma X. High levels of 17b-estradiol are associated with increased matrix metalloproteinase-2 and metalloproteinase-9 activity in tears of postmenopausal women with dry eye. J Ophthalmol. 2016;2016:2415867. https://doi.org/10.1155/2016/2415867.
5. Villatoro AJ, Fernández V, Claros S, et al. Regenerative therapies in dry eye disease: from growth factors to cell therapy. Int J Mol Sci. 2017;18(11):2264. https://doi.org/10.3390/ijms18112264. PMID: 29143779; PMCID: PMC5713234.
6. Singh M, Digumarti L, Agarwal N, Vaze N, Shah R, Malik S. Clinical practice guidelines on menopause: *an executive summary and recommendations: Indian Menopause Society 2019–2020. J Midlife Health. 2020;11(2):55. https://doi.org/10.4103/jmh.JMH_137_20.
7. American Academy of Ophthalmology. What is glaucoma? Symptoms, causes, diagnosis, treatment. 2021. https://www.aao.org/eye-health/diseases/what-is-glaucoma.
8. Madjedi KM, Stuart KV, Chua SYL, et al. The association of female reproductive factors with glaucoma and related traits: a systematic review. Ophthalmol Glaucoma. 2022;5(6):628–47. https://doi.org/10.1016/j.ogla.2022.06.003. Epub 2022 Jun 9. PMID: 35691565; PMCID: PMC10051419.
9. Panchami SR, Shenoy JP, Shivakumar J, Kole SB. Postmenopausal intraocular pressure changes in South Indian females. J Clin Diagn Res. 2013;7:1322–4.
10. Feola AJ, Sherwood JM, Pardue MT, et al. Age and menopause effects on ocular compliance and aqueous outflow. Invest Ophthalmol Vis Sci. 2020;61(5):16. https://doi.org/10.1167/iovs.61.5.16.
11. Vajaranant TS, Maki PM, Pasquale LR, et al. Effects of hormone therapy on intraocular pressure: the Women's Health Initiative-Sight Exam study. Am J Ophthalmol. 2016;165:115–24.
12. Scott E, Zhang QG, Wang R, Vadlamudi R, Brann D. Estrogen neuroprotection and the critical period hypothesis. Front Neuroendocrinol. 2012;33(1):85–104.
13. American Academy of Ophthalmology. What is macular degeneration? 2019. https://www.aao.org/eye-health/diseases/amd-macular-degeneration.
14. Cleveland Clinic. Macular degeneration. 2023. https://my.clevelandclinic.org/health/diseases/15246-macular-degeneration.
15. Yuk J-S, Hwang JH. Menopause and the risk of developing age-related macular degeneration in Korean women. J Clin Med. 2022;11(7):1899. https://doi.org/10.3390/jcm11071899.
16. American Academy of Ophthalmology (AAO). What are cataracts? 2021. https://www.aao.org/eye-health/diseases/what-are-cataracts.
17. Kanthan GL, Wang JJ, Burlutsky G, et al. Exogenous oestrogen exposure, female reproductive factors and the long-term incidence of cataract: the Blue Mountains Eye Study. Acta Ophthalmol. 2010;88:773–8. https://doi.org/10.1111/j.1755-3768.2009.01565.x. PubMed: 19489760.

18. Lai K, Cui J, Ni S, Zhang Y, He J, et al. The effects of postmenopausal hormone use on cataract: a meta-analysis. PLoS One. 2013;8(10):e78647. https://doi.org/10.1371/journal.pone.0078647.
19. Noran NH, Salleh N, Zahari M. Relationship between reproductive exposures and age-related cataract in women. Asia Pac J Public Health. 2007;19:23–8. https://doi.org/10.1177/10105395070190020501. PubMed: 18050560.
20. Eye exam frequency. American Academy of Ophthalmology. https://www.aao.org/education/clinical-statement/frequency-of-ocular-examination.

Menopause and Sexual Health

9

Soniya Dhiman and Oishika Chakraborty

9.1 Introduction

Menopause is a natural event associated with several physical and psychological changes that herald a complex period in life for women. While these women commonly seek medical attention for physical discomfort or ailments, they are reluctant to discuss their sexual health. Human sexuality is a complex phenomenon and an integral part of a healthy life and should not abruptly come to an end with the onset of menopause [1]. As defined by the World Health Organization (WHO) [2] "Sexual health is a state of physical, emotional, mental and social wellbeing related to sexuality; not merely the absence of dysfunction or infirmity". It has been recognized by the WHO as an important component of women's health [2].

9.2 Prevalence

Its prevalence is still unclear. In premenopausal women's age group, its prevalence ranged between 22.7 and 72.2%; in perimenopausal-aged women, it was 37.3–78.2%; and in postmenopausal-aged women, it was extremely reported a wide variety of prevalence ranges and was estimated between 8.7 and 89.01% [3].

9.3 Sexual Dysfunction

Earlier sexual dysfunctions are defined as chronic problems (minimum of 3 months), which occur in 75% of sexual events and are associated with personal distress [4]. DSM-5 [5] defines female sexual dysfunction (FSD) as a condition lasting at least

S. Dhiman (✉) · O. Chakraborty
AIIMS, New Delhi, India

R. Garg (ed.), *Management of Menopause*,
https://doi.org/10.1007/978-981-96-0239-1_9

6 months for at least 75% of sexual encounters and causing significant distress to the individual and not explained by any non-sexual mental illness, drugs or substance abuse, stressor, medical condition, or a consequence of severe relationship distress.

These can broadly be classified into disorders of persistent lack of arousal [6, 7], disorders of orgasm, dysfunction of pelvic floor musculature, or disorders of pelvic pain-related penetration [8].

9.4 Risk Factors of Female Sexual Dysfunction [9]

1. **Poor Physical Health**: Due to advanced age, any medical condition has an adverse effect on sexual health.
2. **Poor Mental Health**: Mental-emotional issues like depression and anxiety, intensity of menopausal emotional symptoms, feelings about the sexual partner, level of self-confidence and self-esteem, body image, and feelings of sexual attraction all have a direct impact on sexual function.
3. **Genitourinary Problems**: Duration and type of menopause either surgical or natural have its impact on genitourinary tissue, which adversely affects sexual health.
4. **Poor Partner's Health**: The age of the partner and any medical condition of the partner have a direct impact on sexual experience of the woman.
5. **Social Factors**: The following social factors have a direct or indirect impact on the sexual experience of the woman:
   (a) Education level and occupation of a woman and her partner
   (b) Access to a sexual partner and change in sexual partner
   (c) Duration of relationship, frequency of sexual intercourse, and quality of relationship
   (d) Socioeconomic status, cultural background, and religious beliefs
   (e) Sexual knowledge, perceived health status, lifestyle, previous sexual activity, and social expectations
   (f) Access to healthcare
   (g) History of previous divorce or death of a spouse and racial and ethnic differences
   (h) Substance abuse (tobacco, alcohol, etc.)
   (i) History of sexual abuse or conflict with partner

9.5 Pathophysiology

9.5.1 Hormones

Changes that occur during the menopausal transition result from reduced ovarian reserve. Cycles in this stage are characterized by increased follicle-stimulating hormone (FSH), decreased inhibin B, and irregular cycle lengths [10]. By the time of the last menstrual cycle, women enter a persistent state of hypergonadotropism as a result of decreased oestradiol [11, 12]. Serum androgen levels, on the other hand, demonstrate a less steep decline [13, 14]. A decrease in sex hormone-binding globulin also observed during menopause. This indicates a complex interplay between estrogen and androgens during menopausal transition [15].

9.5.2 Chronic Diseases

Diseases like hypertension, diabetes, depression, neurological diseases, urinary incontinence, and osteoarthritis commonly impact sexual function [16–18]. Vascular disease reduces vulvovaginal vasodilation and thus sexual arousal [19]. Reduced physical function in obese women and women with osteoarthritis may also adversely affect sexual activity. Additionally, sexual dysfunction observed in women with diabetes is attributed to reduced energy, altered body image, and suboptimal vaginal engorgement during orgasm [17].

9.5.3 Pelvic Organ Prolapse

Pelvic organ prolapse is associated with dyspareunia, chronic pelvic pain, and modified self-image.

9.5.4 Vulvovaginal Atrophy

Decreased levels of oestrogen leading to decreased lactobacilli and altered vaginal flora are associated with vulvovaginal atrophy, characterized by thin, pale, and dry vaginal and vulvar surfaces. Symptomatic vulvovaginal atrophy affects as many as 45% of postmenopausal women affected [20]. It is often accompanied by diminished secretions from sebaceous glands and reduced vaginal lubrication during sexual stimulation [21]. This may lead to pain with intercourse further causing decreased interest and frank avoidance of sexual activity [22].

9.6 Hypoactive Sexual Desire Disorder

Hypoactive sexual desire disorder (HSDD) occurs when there is a persistent or recurrent absence of sexual fantasies or desire for sexual activity that results in personal distress without any organic or iatrogenic cause [23]. DSM-V has grouped HSDD with female sexual arousal disorder (FSAD) under the category of female sexual interest/arousal disorders as described above [24]. HSDD correlates with low feelings of physical and emotional satisfaction, poor self-image, and unhappiness [20].

9.7 Medications

Medications associated with sexual dysfunction are given in Box 9.1 [17, 18]:

Box 9.1

1. Antidepressants/mood stabilizers like SSRIs, tricyclic antidepressants, MAO inhibitors, benzodiazepines, lithium
2. Antipsychotics
3. Cardiovascular medications like Beta-blockers, digoxin, statins, spironolactone
4. Hormonal preparations like oral contraceptives, GnRH agonists, anti-androgens
5. Neuroleptic medications
6. Steroids
7. Antiepileptics
8. Antihistamines
9. Anticholinergics

9.8 Approach to a Postmenopausal Woman with Sexual Dysfunction

9.8.1 History

Proper history should be taken. In addition to sexual health complaints, history must be elicited for other problems associated with menopause (Box 9.2).

Box 9.2

History:

- Time since menopause
- Age at which menopause was acquired
- Type of menopause (medical vs surgical)
- Whether the menopausal transition was smooth or associated with abnormal uterine bleeding (AUB)
- Any urinary symptoms like frequency, urgency, urinary incontinence
- Any personal or family history of cardiovascular event
- Any history of recent fractures/ shortening of height
- Any history of spotting/bleeding
- Any history of vaginal dryness
- History of sexual problems. Menopausal women seeking healthcare can be screened using preformed, validated questionnaires (Box 9.3)

Box 9.3 Validated Tests
1. Decreased Sexual Desire Screener [25]
2. Brief Sexual Symptom Checklist [26]
3. Female Sexual Function Index [27]
4. Revised Female Sexual Distress Scale [28]
5. Pelvic Organ Prolapse/Urinary Incontinence Sexual Questionnaire [29]

In addition to these screening questionnaires, a thorough history should be taken about chronic illnesses, use of any medications, any urinary complaints, etc.

Examination: A thorough examination has to be carried out in all symptomatic patients. The following points need to be considered.

General physical examination	To rule out chronic illnesses like hypertension, obesity
Gynaecological examination	
Local examination	• Hair may be grey and sparse • Look for any loss of fat from labia majora • Any discolouration or hypopigmentation of vulva must be looked for • Any mass has to be seen
Per speculum examination	• Vagina may be pale and dry with loss of rugosities • Cervix may be small • Patient may be asked to cough to look for uterocervical descent, cystocele, rectocele, stress urinary incontinence
Per vaginal examination	• Cervix may be flushed with fornices • Size of uterus should be commented upon. Uterus may be small and atrophic • One should do a bimanual palpation to rule out forniceal masses
Pap smear should be taken if not taken before	
All organic causes of sexual dysfunction must be ruled out on physical examination:	Vulvovaginal atrophy Pelvic organ prolapse Urinary incontinence Lichen sclerosus Clitoral phimosis

9.9 Available Treatment

9.9.1 Psychological

Psychological counselling may be used alone or in conjunction with directed medical therapies. Alternatives to counselling include psychotherapy, cognitive behavioural therapy, mindfulness and sexual skills training, and individual, couple, or group sexual counselling [30].

9.9.2 Oestrogen

Local vaginal oestrogen therapy is recommended as the preferred treatment for symptomatic vulvovaginal atrophy [31]. It increases vaginal lubrication and reduces dyspareunia [20]. Low dose vaginal oestrogen formulations come in vaginal creams, tablets, and rings. Systemic absorption is low for these preparations, and they are not effective for the relief of vasomotor symptoms [21].

9.9.2.1 Androgen

While transdermal testosterone can be used for HSDD, oral and intramuscular preparations are not recommended. Side effects are dyslipidaemia, acne, and hirsutism. Contraindications to testosterone therapy include pregnancy, severe acne, hirsutism, androgenic alopecia, and high baseline free testosterone levels. Serum levels should be monitored, with assessment at baseline, 3–6 weeks after initiation, and every 6 months thereafter. It should not be more than that in young women (2.8 nmol/L) [32]. Positive effects may not be felt until 3 months after beginning therapy. It is not a Food and Drug Administration (FDA)-approved drug therapy for the treatment of female sexual interest and arousal disorders.

9.10 Recent Advances

Flibanserin is a serotonin agonist-antagonist that has been approved by the Food and Drug Administration (FDA) for the treatment of HSDD in premenopausal women without depression, although one study (the SNOWDROP trial) has also shown efficacy in postmenopausal women [33]. The most common side effects are dizziness, insomnia, nausea, and headache.

Bremelanotide, a melanocortin 4-receptor agonist, recently approved in the USA as the first on-demand, injectable medication to increase sexual desire [34].

9.11 Newer Modalities

Lorexys (combination of bupropion and trazodone) is a potential medication for HSDD. It is an oral, nonhormonal medication that works by balancing the neurotransmitters that regulate sexual inhibition and excitation [32].

9.12 Management

9.12.1 Painful Sex

Vulvovaginal atrophy and pain can affect the sexuality of both partners, resulting in avoidance of sex. Low-dose local oestrogen, lubricants and moisturizers, vaginal ovules of dehydroepiandrosterone (DHEA), or oral ospemifene can be used [35]. Pelvic floor muscular hypertonicity alone or in combination with bowel and bladder dysfunction may require a multidisciplinary approach involving pelvic floor physiotherapy, vaginal dilators, mindfulness, and yoga [36, 37]. Onabotulinum toxin as a treatment for pelvic floor muscle hypertonicity is under trial [38]. Lastly, affected couples can be counselled for sexual interactions that do not involve penetration.

9.12.2 HSDD/Low Libido

Reversible medical causes (e.g. hypothyroidism, use of selective serotonin reuptake inhibitors [SSRIs] or oral contraceptive pills) or psychosocial factors are to be addressed. Transdermal testosterone improves sexual function in postmenopausal women, increasing sexual desire, arousal, orgasm, pleasure, and sexual responsiveness [39, 40]. The suggested off-label dosage is one-half pump of 1% androgen gel, preferably on the posterior calf (one-tenth the male dosage). Bremelanotide is an on-demand injection that is FDA-approved.

9.12.3 Arousal Disorders

There is a lack of subjective arousal from any physical or non-physical stimuli characterized by decreased pelvic blood flow and lubrication. In women without reversible medical or psychosocial causes, phosphodiesterase inhibitors (low-dose sildenafil) can be used [30]. Cognitive behavioural sex therapy, particularly mindfulness and mechanical devices like clitoral suction devices and sex toys, are also under investigation [41, 42].

9.12.4 Anorgasmia

There are no approved, on-label treatments for anorgasmia. Primary anorgasmia (lifelong inability to achieve orgasm) is hard to treat. Secondary anorgasmia (anorgasmia in an individual who has achieved orgasm before) may occur due to psychosocial reasons like a change in partner or the nature of the relationship or can be secondary to medications like SSRIs. In such cases, the dose of SSRIs may be titrated, or alternate treatment with bupropion may be considered [16]. In both cases, physical lesions like clitoral phimosis or lichen sclerosis must be ruled out and, if present, treated [4]. Where no organic cause is found, psychoeducation, mindfulness, directed masturbation, sensate focus techniques, or vibrators may help individuals who have never achieved an orgasm [16].

9.13 Summary

Disorders of sexual health in menopausal women are a common problem, yet often neglected. It is due to either hesitation on the part of the woman to express or the physician to enquire. Given the significant distress it causes to these women, physicians should not omit sexual history taking and pelvic floor examination in these women. Where behavioural and lifestyle changes are helpful, they should be encouraged. Those without any identifiable causes can be offered pharmacotherapy to improve their quality of life.

References

1. Caruso S, Rapisarda A, Cianci S. Sexuality in menopausal women. Curr Opin Psychiatry. 2016;29:323–30.
2. Defining sexual health [Internet]. [cited 2023 Jul 11]. https://www.who.int/teams/sexual-and-reproductive-health-and-research/key-areas-of-work/sexual-health/defining-sexual-health.
3. Khani S, Azizi M, Elyasi F, Kamali M, Moosazadeh M. The prevalence of sexual dysfunction in the different menopausal stages: a systematic review and meta-analysis. Int J Sex Health. 2021;33:439. https://doi.org/10.1080/19317611.2021.1926039.
4. Simon JA, Lukas VA. Distressing sexual function at midlife: unmet needs, practical diagnoses, and available treatments. Obstet Gynecol. 2017;130(4):889–905.
5. American Psychiatric Association. Diagnostic and statistical manual of mental disorders, 5th ed. Text Revision (DSM-5-TR). Washington: American Psychiatric Association; 2022.
6. Faubion SS, Rullo JE. Sexual dysfunction in women: a practical approach. Am Fam Physician. 2015;92(4):281–8.
7. Clayton AH, Valladares Juarez EM. Female sexual dysfunction. Med Clin North Am. 2019;103(4):681–98.
8. American Psychiatric Association. Diagnostic and statistical manual of mental disorders: DSM-5. 5th ed. Arlington: American Psychiatric Association Publishing; 2013.
9. McCool-Myers M, Theurich M, Zuelke A, Knuettel H, Apfelbacher C. Predictors of female sexual dysfunction: a systematic review and qualitative analysis through gender inequality paradigms. BMC Womens Health. 2018;18(1):108. https://doi.org/10.1186/s12905-018-0602-4. PMID: 29929499; PMCID: PMC6013982.
10. Santoro N, Chervenak JL. The menopause transition. Endocrinol Metab Clin North Am. 2004;33(4):627–36.
11. Burger HG, Hale GE, Dennerstein L, Robertson DM. Cycle and hormone changes during perimenopause: the key role of ovarian function. Menopause. 2008;15(4 Pt 1):603–12.
12. Santoro N, Brown JR, Adel T, Skurnick JH. Characterization of reproductive hormonal dynamics in the perimenopause. J Clin Endocrinol Metab. 1996;81(4):1495–501.
13. Dennerstein L, Randolph J, Taffe J, Dudley E, Burger H. Hormones, mood, sexuality, and the menopausal transition. Fertil Steril. 2002;77(Suppl 4):S42–8.
14. Rothman MS, Carlson NE, Xu M, Wang C, Swerdloff R, Lee P, et al. Reexamination of testosterone, dihydrotestosterone, estradiol and estrone levels across the menstrual cycle and in postmenopausal women measured by liquid chromatography-tandem mass spectrometry. Steroids. 2011;76(1–2):177–82.
15. Burger HG, Dudley EC, Cui J, Dennerstein L, Hopper JL. A prospective longitudinal study of serum testosterone, dehydroepiandrosterone sulfate, and sex hormone-binding globulin levels through the menopause transition. J Clin Endocrinol Metab. 2000;85(8):2832–8.
16. Kingsberg SA, Rezaee RL. Hypoactive sexual desire in women. Menopause. 2013;20(12):1284–300.
17. Ambler DR, Bieber EJ, Diamond MP. Sexual function in elderly women: a review of current literature. Rev Obstet Gynecol. 2012;5(1):16–27.
18. Buster JE. Managing female sexual dysfunction. Fertil Steril. 2013;100(4):905–15.
19. Nascimento ER, Maia ACO, Pereira V, Soares-Filho G, Nardi AE, Silva AC. Sexual dysfunction and cardiovascular diseases: a systematic review of prevalence. Clinics (Sao Paulo). 2013;68(11):1462–8.

20. Nappi RE, Wawra K, Schmitt S. Hypoactive sexual desire disorder in postmenopausal women. Gynecol Endocrinol. 2006;22(6):318–23.
21. Management of symptomatic vulvovaginal atrophy: 2013 position statement of The North American Menopause Society. Menopause. 2013;20(9):888–902; quiz 903–4.
22. Tan O, Bradshaw K, Carr BR. Management of vulvovaginal atrophy-related sexual dysfunction in postmenopausal women: an up-to-date review. Menopause. 2012;19(1):109–17.
23. Brotto LA. The DSM diagnostic criteria for hypoactive sexual desire disorder in women. Arch Sex Behav. 2010;39(2):221–39.
24. Vahia VN. Diagnostic and statistical manual of mental disorders 5: a quick glance. Indian J Psychiatry. 2013;55(3):220–3.
25. Clayton AH, Goldfischer ER, Goldstein I, Derogatis L, Lewis-D'Agostino DJ, Pyke R. Validation of the decreased sexual desire screener (DSDS): a brief diagnostic instrument for generalized acquired female hypoactive sexual desire disorder (HSDD). J Sex Med. 2009;6(3):730–8.
26. Hatzichristou D, Kirana PS, Banner L, Althof SE, Lonnee-Hoffmann RAM, Dennerstein L, et al. Diagnosing sexual dysfunction in men and women: sexual history taking and the role of symptom scales and questionnaires. J Sex Med. 2016;13(8):1166–82.
27. Rosen R, Brown C, Heiman J, Leiblum S, Meston C, Shabsigh R, et al. The female sexual function index (FSFI): a multidimensional self-report instrument for the assessment of female sexual function. J Sex Marital Ther. 2000;26(2):191–208.
28. Derogatis L, Clayton A, Lewis-D'Agostino D, Wunderlich G, Fu Y. Validation of the female sexual distress scale-revised for assessing distress in women with hypoactive sexual desire disorder. J Sex Med. 2008;5(2):357–64.
29. Rogers RG, Coates KW, Kammerer-Doak D, Khalsa S, Qualls C. A short form of the pelvic organ prolapse/urinary incontinence sexual questionnaire (PISQ-12). Int Urogynecol J Pelvic Floor Dysfunct. 2003;14(3):164–8; discussion 168.
30. American College of Obstetricians and Gynecologists' Committee on Practice Bulletins—Gynecology. Female sexual dysfunction: ACOG practice bulletin clinical management guidelines for obstetrician-gynecologists, number 213. Obstet Gynecol. 2019;134(1):e1–18.
31. Gass MLS, Cochrane BB, Larson JC, Manson JE, Barnabei VM, Brzyski RG, et al. Patterns and predictors of sexual activity among women in the hormone therapy trials of the Women's Health Initiative. Menopause. 2011;18(11):1160–71.
32. Davis SR, Davison SL, Donath S, Bell RJ. Circulating androgen levels and self-reported sexual function in women. JAMA. 2005;294(1):91–6.
33. Simon JA, Kingsberg SA, Shumel B, Hanes V, Garcia M, Sand M. Efficacy and safety of flibanserin in postmenopausal women with hypoactive sexual desire disorder: results of the SNOWDROP trial. Menopause. 2014;21(6):633–40.
34. Dhillon S, Keam SJ. Bremelanotide: first approval. Drugs. 2019;79(14):1599–606.
35. Johnston S, Bouchard C, Fortier M, Wolfman W. Guideline no. 422b: menopause and genitourinary health. J Obstet Gynaecol Can. 2021;43(11):1301–1307.e1.
36. Morin M, Carroll MS, Bergeron S. Systematic review of the effectiveness of physical therapy modalities in women with provoked vestibulodynia. Sex Med Rev. 2017;5(3):295–322.
37. Orr N, Wahl K, Joannou A, Hartmann D, Valle L, Yong P; International Society for the Study of Women's Sexual Health's (ISSWSH) Special Interest Group on Sexual Pain. Deep dyspareunia: review of pathophysiology and proposed future research priorities. Sex Med Rev [Internet]. 2020 [cited 2023 Aug 4];8(1):3–17. https://pubmed.ncbi.nlm.nih.gov/30928249/.
38. Pacik PT, Geletta S. Vaginismus treatment: clinical trials follow up 241 patients. Sex Med. 2017;5(2):e114–23.
39. Somboonporn W, Davis S, Seif MW, Bell R. Testosterone for peri- and postmenopausal women. Cochrane Database Syst Rev. 2005;(4):CD004509.
40. Islam RM, Bell RJ, Green S, Page MJ, Davis SR. Safety and efficacy of testosterone for women: a systematic review and meta-analysis of randomised controlled trial data. Lancet Diabetes Endocrinol. 2019;7(10):754–66.

41. Kingsberg SA, Althof S, Simon JA, Bradford A, Bitzer J, Carvalho J, et al. Female sexual dysfunction-medical and psychological treatments, committee 14. J Sex Med. 2017;14(12):1463–91.
42. Alexander M, Bashir K, Alexander C, Marson L, Rosen R. Randomized trial of clitoral vacuum suction versus vibratory stimulation in neurogenic female orgasmic dysfunction. Arch Phys Med Rehabil. 2018;99(2):299–305.

10 Urinary Problems at Menopause

Richa Vatsa, Soniya Dhiman, and Prabhat Agrawal

10.1 Introduction

The estimated mean age of menopause in India is 46 years [1], earlier than the western world, being 51 years in the USA [2]. Life expectancy in India for females was 68.2 years in 2011 sample registration system data and expected to increase to 74.7 years by 2035 [3]. On an average a woman spends one third of her life after menopause. Almost half of postmenopausal women experience genitourinary syndrome of menopause (GSM) which includes vulval, vaginal, and urinary discomfort [4, 5]. The pelvic floor disorders (PFDs) include urinary incontinence (UI) that can be stress, urge, or mixed, fecal incontinence, and pelvic organ prolapse. Pelvic floor disorders (PFDs) are a major hindrance to this healthy life in postmenopausal women. The PFDs occurs due to weakness of pelvic muscles after menopause. Other than menopause, there are various risk factors for PFDs like prior hysterectomy, vaginal birth, obesity, smoking, and inheriting a connective tissue disorder [6].

10.2 Prevalence and Disease Burden

The urinary symptoms after menopause, which is a part of spectrum of genitourinary syndrome of menopause, are a major handicap. It significantly decreases quality of life (QOL), has a major impact on sexual life, and can lead to social isolation and depression [7, 8]. Treating them improves QOL and sexual satisfaction [6]. The PFDs are often underreported by females; the reason being that they consider it as a normal part of aging and incurable. Also, these symptoms might lead to

R. Vatsa (✉) · S. Dhiman
Department of Obstetrics and Gynecology, AIIMS, New Delhi, India

P. Agrawal
PG Department of Medicine, SN Medical College, Agra, India

R. Garg (ed.), *Management of Menopause*,
https://doi.org/10.1007/978-981-96-0239-1_10

stigmatization and social isolation, which can be a contributory factor in delay or not seeking treatment. Incontinence might affect social and work life of females resulting in her independence being affected [9]. Furthermore, PFDs and huge economic burden and healthcare burden and have been expected to increase more in the future due to increase in proportion of the aging population. The PFDs affect women of all age groups, but older ones are affected more. The prevalence increase from 6% in women aged 20–29 to 53% in women older than 80 years [10]. Almost 44–57% of middle-aged and postmenopausal women [11] experience some involuntary urine loss which increases to the tune of 75% in older women [12]. Epidemiological studies have shown the spike in prevalence of UI around time of menopause, and almost 70% women date their onset of UI symptoms at final menstrual period [13]. There is a difference in incontinence experienced by old age and young age. Younger females experience more of stress urinary incontinence (SUI) resulting from pelvic floor trauma, whereas older women experience more of mixed or urger urinary incontinence (UUI) due to overactive bladder with or without contribution from sphincter dysfunction [14, 15].

10.3 Urinary Problems at Menopause and Their Etiology

Lower urinary tract epithelium is related embryologically to genital epithelium both of which originate from primitive urogenital sinus, so both are sensitive to effect of steroid hormones [16]. The hormone estrogen has a proliferative effect of the urogenital tract, and menopause has adverse effect on urogenital system also.

10.3.1 Menopause and Lower Urinary Tract Symptoms

Loss of estrogen at menopause leads to molecular and functional changes in lower urinary tract. These are mucosal thinning of the urethra and bladder resulting in characteristic lower urinary tracts symptoms (LUTS) of menopause which includes urethritis, urge incontinence, and urinary frequency. Nocturia is also a bothering symptom in these females. Estrogen has trophic effect on collagen, and menopause results in loss of collagen in the urogenital system also. This weakens the bladder neck muscles, causing symptoms of stress incontinence. The bladder compliance decreases and urethral sphincter becomes less contractile. A study done by Yoshida et al. showed that estrogen deficiency due to ovariectomy in mouse leads to increase in acetylcholine release from cholinergic nerves and increases detrusor contractility [17]. The incontinence seen in postmenopausal women is mixed type with predominant component being UUI [18]. Reduced estrogen leads to alkaline vaginal pH resulting in altered vaginal flora and increases susceptibility to infection by urogenital and fecal pathogen. This results in ascending infection causing urethritis, cystitis, and urinary tract infection (UTI). The main symptoms are vaginal dryness, superficial dyspareunia, urinary frequency, urgency, and recurrent UTI (rUTI). The main urinary symptom of menopause is urinary urgency seen in almost 10% postmenopausal women but can also present as rUTI [19, 20]. The effects of menopause on genitourinary problems have been questioned by some studies. Quiroz et al. in their study found that age was the risk factor for PFDs and menopausal status was not associated with increased odds of reporting symptoms [21]. And some studies have even found that loss of estrogen at menopause is not a significant risk factor for PFDs [22]. Contrary to that, a study on animal models to see the response to low estrogen, uncoupled from aging, has found that low estrogen develops changes similar to those seen in genitourinary tract of menopausal women [23]. Certain association like childbirth, tissue loss, and comorbidities are inherent with aging, all of which can be contributing to these PFDs. Nevertheless, the association between loss of estrogen and occurrence PFDs seems logical as both genital tract and lower urinary tract contain estrogen receptors [24]. There must be other contributory factors also because all postmenopausal women do not have these symptoms. This controversy is difficult to resolve as it is difficult to do studies to see the effect of menopause exclusively, due to complexity to separate menopausal status from aging and other comorbidities. Vaginal microbiota and inflammatory markers have not been found to be associated with symptom severity [25]. Age is a risk factor of urinary incontinence. Obesity is a major contributory factor, and obesity increases the risk of incontinence around three times from non-obese women [26]. Though pregnancy and vaginal delivery are a risk factor for UI, studies have shown that all aspects of UI are seen in nulliparous women [26]. The women who delivered their babies by vaginal delivery have more chances of UI than by caesarean section [27]. There are many other risk factors like caffeine intake, smoking, diabetes, depression, constipation, cognitive impairment, and functional impairment. Studies have also been done on urinary microbiome and urinary symptoms. It is different from vaginal and gut microbiome. The urobiome has less bacterial diversity and low overall bacterial number. The alteration in urobiome has been associated with pathologies, best described till date being UUI, a significant LUTS in postmenopausal women. Pearce et al., classified urinary bacteria in urine collected by transurethral catheter, using 16S rRNA gene sequencing to classify bacterial DNA and expanded quantitative urine culture (EQUC) techniques to isolate live bacteria from women with UUI and compared it to a cohort without UUI [28]. The study found significant difference in type and amount of bacteria present between the two groups. Studies have found that estrogen use and high body mass index (BMI) are associated with increased urobiome diversity [29]. This can be the possible explanation of decrease in symptoms of UUI in postmenopausal women with estrogen supplementation. Topical estrogen treatment can improve urobiome as seen with vaginal microbiome, and good-quality studies will answer this question.

10.3.2 Menopause and Recurrent Urinary Tract Infection

Incidence of rUTI increases with advancing age and is an important cause of morbidity in postmenopausal females. The incidence increase with age, occurring in up to 15% of women over 60 which increases to 20% for women aged >65 years [30]. Females are anyways more prone to development of UTI because of short urethra than males, and menopause increases this further. Normal lactobacilli-dominant flora maintains acidic pH of vagina and prevents pathogen growing in the vagina. The potential uropathogen in the gut flora is thought to be responsible for rUTI. The postmenopausal lactobacilli-deficient vagina is more prone to be colonized by these gut pathogens resulting in rUTI. Estrogen has proliferative effect on bladder urothelium [31]; it increases the expression of tight junction proteins (E cadherin) in bladder epithelial cell thus strengthening the urothelial barrier [32]. Further expression of antimicrobial peptide by bladder epithelial cells increased, namely, hBD1–3, ribonuclease 7, and psoriasin [32]. These peptides are present more in premenopausal urine, and treatment with estrogen increases their secretion in urine. Further, topical estrogen cream changes vaginal flora and makes it more physiological. These can be the explanation of effect of estrogen in prevention of rUTI as seen in studies [33]. Acting on the etiology of rUTI, i.e., alteration of vaginal flora and vaginal probiotic supplementation have been tried for r UTI in postmenopausal women. A recent study on prevention of rUTI with *Lactobacillus crispatus*-containing vaginal suppositories has found that vaginal microbiota of postmenopausal women with rUTI is differed from healthy controls and their lack of *Lactobacillus* and relatively dominant of *Enterobacteriaceae*. Authors found that vaginal *Lactobacillus*-containing suppositories can prevent RC by stabilizing vaginal dysbiosis [34].

10.4 Assessing Urinary Incontinence

10.4.1 History Taking and Physical Examination

By careful history taking, women's UI can be categorized either as stress UI, urge UI, or mixed type with or without one being predominant. This is important as treatment depends on this categorization and directed to treat predominant symptom in mixed UI [35]. Aggravating and relieving factors for the symptom should be asked to guide for additional investigation. Clinician should use a validated urinary incontinence-specific symptom and quality-of-life questionnaire as it will be helpful in evaluation of therapies [35]. Detailed history should involve asking about condition which itself can cause symptoms of urinary incontinence like diabetes, multiple sclerosis, thyroid disease, prior cerebrovascular injury, prior spinal cord injury, back pain, prior back injuries, etc. Certain drugs also interfere with bladder function like muscle relaxants and alpha-blocking agents, and antihypertensive drugs (calcium-channel blockers and methyldopa) may exacerbate urethral smooth and skeletal muscle relaxation, causing stress urinary incontinence (SUI).

A detailed genitourinary, pelvic, and perineal examination should be done:

- Inspection of vagina and urethra to look for atrophy and ulceration
- Any visible perineal tear
- Any urinary leakage on cough or straining
- Genital prolapse

- Strength of perineal muscles
- Per vaginal examination to palpate the uterus, cervix, and adnexa

For evaluation of women with symptoms of urinary incontinence, bladder diary should be used. The bladder diary should cover minimum of 3 days of usual activity, both are working, and leisure days [36]. Performing Q-tip, Bonney, Marshall, and Fluid-Bridge tests in the assessment of women with urinary incontinence is not recommended. There are few points in history and examination when referral to a specialist service is indicated:

- Persisting bladder or urethral pain
- Palpable bladder on bimanual or abdominal examination after voiding
- Clinically benign pelvic masses
- Associated fecal incontinence
- Suspected neurological disease
- Symptoms of voiding difficulty
- Suspected urogenital fistulae
- Previous continence surgery
- Previous pelvic cancer surgery
- Previous pelvic radiation therapy

10.4.2 Investigations for Urinary Incontinence

Urinary tract infection needs to be ruled out before diagnosis of UI, urine dipstick, microscopy, and depending on the result, culture and antibiotic sensitivity should be ordered (Table 10.1). Investigations depend on the detailed history findings, given in Table 10.2.

Table 10.1 Interpretation of urine report [35]

Symptom of UTI	Urine test for leucocyte and nitrites	Action
Yes	Positive for both	Send a midstream urine specimen for culture and antibiotic sensitivity Prescribe an appropriate course of antibiotic treatment pending culture results
Yes	Negative for either	Send a midstream urine specimen for culture and analysis of antibiotic sensitivities. Consider the prescription of antibiotics pending culture results
No	Positive for either	Do not offer antibiotic without result of midstream urine culture
No	Negative for either	Do not send sample for midstream urine culture

Table 10.2 Investigations for urinary symptoms

Urine routine/microscopy ± midstream urine specimen for culture antibiotic sensitivities	To rule out UTI as cause of symptom
Ultrasonography for postvoid residual urine	Symptom suggestive of voiding dysfunction or recurrent UTI
Multichannel filling and voiding cystometry	Filed to respond to medical management in cases of OAB Before surgery for stress urinary incontinence in women who have any of the following: • Urge predominant mixed urinary incontinence or urinary incontinence in which the type is unclear • Symptoms suggestive of voiding dysfunction • Anterior or apical prolapse • A history of previous surgery for stress urinary incontinence
Cystoscopy	Not recommended for incontinence alone
Imaging (MRI, CT)	If pelvic or uterine mass suspected

10.4.3 Treatment for Urinary Incontinence

Urinary incontinence is underrecognized and undertreated in women. Timely identification will result in timely treatment, which can prevent complications of urinary incontinence like urinary tract infection and perineal ulceration [35]. History should be able to identify the predominant type of incontinence. Treatment depends on type and severity of incontinence. Treatment options are non-pharmacological which includes lifestyle modifications, pharmacological and surgical.

10.4.3.1 Non-pharmacological Management

These are the first-line treatment for urinary incontinence. These include lifestyle changes like weight loss, appropriate amount and type of fluid intake, and pelvic floor exercises. Obesity is a major risk factor for UI, and weight loss is beneficial in women whose BMI > 30 in all urinary incontinence [37]. Cutting down on alcohol intake is also useful. Due to feat of urinary frequency, old-age females tend to reduce the water intake, and that can lead to urinary tract infection. Fluid intake should be around 1.5–2 liters a day. It should neither be too large or too small a volume. A trial of caffeine intake reduction should be given to women with overactive bladder (OAB). Bladder training should be given for at least 6 weeks as first line for women with UUI and MUI as it is beneficial for all types of UI [37].

If this is not effective, OAB medicines should be added. Absorbent containment products, handheld urinals, or toileting aids to treat urinary incontinence should be offered for long-term management of UI as aid to others treatments or after other management options have failed.

Pelvic floor exercises improve the SUI; it is the first-line treatment for this condition, and women should be advised at least 3 months of pelvic floor muscle training (PFMT) [38]. This training programs should comprise at least eight contractions performed three times per day, and this should be continued if found beneficial. Perineometry or pelvic floor electromyography as biofeedback should not be used as a routine part of pelvic floor muscle training. Rather biofeedback should be considered for women who cannot actively contract pelvic floor muscles to aid motivation and adherence to therapy.

Incontinence pessaries have also been tried for SUI, but evidence does not support its use [39]. Though, NICE guidelines recommends its use for occasional SUI [38].

10.4.3.2 Medical Management for Overactive Bladder and Urge Incontinence

When 6 weeks trial of non-pharmacological treatment fails for UUI, switch to pharmacological treatment. After starting medication, review should be done at the fourth week. Continue medication if improvement is optimal. Change dose or medication when response is suboptimal or side effect is intolerable. Once on stable long-term treatment, women should be reviewed every 12 months or every 6 months if age is more than 75 years.

Antimuscarinic Agents

This class of drugs includes oxybutynin, tolterodine, and solifenacin, which are the mainstay of treatment of OAB and UUI. These drugs block muscarinic M2 and M3 receptors, thus reducing bladder contractility. A recently published Cochrane review has evaluated the oral anticholinergic drug verses placebo or no treatment for managing OAB [40]. It covered studies in all age group not exclusively postmenopausal age. The review found that anticholinergic drugs have modest but important improvement in overactive bladder syndrome symptoms compared with placebo treatment. Recent studies suggest that this is generally associated with only modest improvement in quality of life. All anticholinergics had high incidence of adverse effects which led to withdrawals in all anticholinergics except tolterodine. The benefit of long-term anticholinergics treatment or after treatment stops was not known [41].

Side-effect profile seen with these class of drugs are due to blockage of M2 and M3 receptors in other parts of body like the salivary gland (dry mouth), tear glands (dry eye and blurred vision), brain (dementia, cognitive impairment), and bowel smooth muscles (constipation). They have a side effect of constipation and dry mouth, and it is a major cause of discontinuation of drug in the long term. Counselling the patients that these side effects means that drug has started taking its action might give some positive effect on her psychology. The medicine doesn't have immediate onset of action; which might take at least 4 weeks. For long term compliance the patient needs to be counselled regarding expected side effects and ways to mitigate them like increasing fiber intake in food to prevent constipation. While prescribing anticholinergic to women, comorbidities should be kept in mind, and she must take care of the drugs she has been taking as there can be drug interactions. Anticholinergics can have cognitive impairment and one should be careful while prescribing these drugs especially oxybutynin, in old-age postmenopausal females.

ß-3 agonist: ß adrenoreceptors are seen in urothelium detrusor muscles. Subtypes of this receptors are ß 1, 2, and 3 with the ß 3 being most abundantly expressed in the urinary bladder [41, 42]. Adrenoreceptors causes bladder smooth muscle relaxation during the filling phase of micturition cycle, improving compliance in filling phase. Mirabegron is the first commercially available ß-3 adrenoceptor agonist for the treatment of OAB. Mirabegron has been tried with and without anticholinergics and various trials and found effective. One of the most common adverse effects of mirabegron is hypertension. A recent systemic review of 21 studies done on female patients with OAB has found that mirabegron has efficacy similar to anticholinergics in relieving all symptoms of OAB but with fewer side-effect profile [43]. Though the side effect was lesser, treatment continuation rates of both the drugs were similar: 54% and 55% in mirabegron and anticholinergic groups, respectively. The authors concluded that there is paucity of high-quality randomized controlled trials (RCTs) with large sample size and long-term follow-up to compare mirabegron with other drugs, sexual life, and effect on quality of life. Further hypertensive women were excluded from all the studies of this meta-analysis, so safety profile and efficacy of mirabegron in this group of patient remain unknown. The dose tried in different studies for OAB was 25 and 50 mg, with or without solifenacin 5 mg [44–47]. The combination therapy of mirabegron with solifenacin has been found to be more effective than either monotherapy and well tolerated [46, 47]. Studies have also found the cardiovascular favorable safety profile of long-term treatment with mirabegron in combination with antimuscarinics [48].

Desmopressin: Nocturia significantly affects quality of life by compromising sleep. In population studies, frequency of nocturia was found to be about 50% in women, increasing with age [49]. In the EPIC study, the frequency of nocturia was 43.9% in women aged 39 or younger and reached 70.8% for women aged >60 years [50]. Nocturia can be due to nocturnal polyuresis, low nocturnal bladder capacity, or a combination of both. The first one is responsible for almost 70% of cases [51]. Other causes of nocturia like diuretic intake, congestive heart failure, diabetes mellitus, and pituitary disorders should be ruled out before giving this treatment. Conservative treatment should be considered before starting pharmacological treatment, conservative treatment should be considered, which involves limiting the amount of fluid intake in the evening hours ideally 4–6 h before sleep; avoiding fluid which irritates bladder like alcohol, coffee, tea etc.; emptying the bladder every time possible before bedtime; treatment of constipation; and for patients on diuretic, changing the time of drug from evening to morning who take diuretics in the evening. Time of at least 1–3 months should be given for these measures to be effective. Treatment of nocturia relies mostly on medical treatment of OAB, but this intervention has low success rate to treat the nocturia [52]. Desmopressin has shown promising results especially in nocturia due to nocturnal polyuresis. Mun et al., evaluated 60 women of more than 60 years age who failed to respond to conservative treatment for nocturia, all were given desmopressin 0.1 mg oral at bedtime for 12 weeks.

Authors found desmopressin an effective treatment for nocturnal polyuria in females, and it also improved sleep quality [53]. Furthermore in a systemic review of five studies (378 women) done on effect of desmopressin on female patients with OAB and nocturia, the drug was found efficacious in significantly reducing night-time urine production, episodes of nocturia, and urgency episodes and improves quality and duration of sleep. The efficacy of combination therapy of desmopressin and anticholinergic was very high with least side effects [54]. The efficacy of combination therapy of tolterodine and desmopressin has been proven in randomized controlled trial also [55]. The dose used in studies ranges from lowest dose of 0.2 mg to highest dose of 0.4 mg, 1 h before going to sleep sublingual; there is no need to take water with the drug. The dose titration is over 1–3 weeks. The treatment takes at least 7 days to start its action, so evaluation of treatment should be done at least after 3 weeks and ideally after 3 months [56, 57]. The reported adverse effect of the drug are hyponatremia, facial puffiness, headache, dizziness, diarrhea, and oliguria, hyponatremia being most worrisome. Desmopressin should be avoided in women over 65 years with hypertension or cardiovascular diseases. Females are more prone to develop hyponatremia than men. Treatment should be started only when baseline serum sodium is within the normal range (i.e., 135–145 mmol/L). The test should be repeated at 4–8 days, 1 month after start of treatment and then every 3–6 months depending on the risk.

Failed Medical Management for UUI

Another treatment which can be tried is bladder wall injection with Botulinum toxin A. Women choosing to have this treatment should be explained about the risk of UTI and urinary retention. In the event of urinary retention, patient might need intermittent self-catheterization as long as needed. If patient can't do intermittent self-catheterization, she should be willing to accept temporary indwelling catheter. Initial dose used is 100 units of Botulinum toxin A. First review after treatment should be within 12 weeks, and if there is inadequate response, increase dose to 200 units. For women not responding or not willing to take injection of Botulinum toxin A, percutaneous sacral nerve stimulation can be offered.

Augmentation cystoplasty and urinary diversion are the last resort for women with OAB who are not responding to other treatments. Women need lifelong follow-up after these surgeries.

10.4.3.3 Second-Line Treatment for Stress Urinary Incontinence

Surgical Management

When pelvic floor exercises doesn't work, surgical option should be offered. Various options are there like colposuspension (open or laparoscopic) *or* an autologous rectus fascial sling, retropubic mid-urethral sling. For all the surgical procedures, evidence of benefit is there, but long-term safety evidence is not available especially for mesh procedures. For mesh procedures, type 1 macroporous polypropylene mesh should be used. Trans-obturator approach for mid-urethral mesh placement should not be done.

Medical management: Duloxetine should not be offered routinely as second-line treatment for SUI, only when women prefer pharmacological treatment over surgical treatment or not suitable for surgical treatment, this drug can be offered as second-line treatment.

Urethral bulking agents: These are less invasive surgical options. These can be tried when surgical options have failed or women want to avoid invasive surgery or want to avoid mesh placement [36]. Various bulking agents have been tried like polyacrylamide hydrogel, silicon particles, carbon beads, calcium hydroxyapatite, and cross-linked vinyl dimethyl-polydimethylsiloxane [36]. Though these are permanent materials, effect might reduce over time, and repeat injection might be needed to achieve optimum effect. Again evidence on long-term effectiveness and adverse events is not available.

10.4.4 Estrogen Treatment for LUTS

Estrogen is essential for urogenital health and function. Estrogen receptors are found in the female squamous epithelium of the proximal and distal urethra, vagina, and trigone of the bladder and in the squamous epithelium of the anal canal [58]. Furthermore, they are expressed in the paraurethral tissues, urethral sphincter, uterosacral ligaments, and pelvic floor musculature [58]. When estrogen was supplemented in ovariectomized mice, there was a decrease in both acetylcholine release and detrusor contractility [6]. This might be the likely explanation of decrease in LUTS in postmenopausal women after estrogen supplementation, and studies have found efficacy of this intervention similar to anticholinergic treatment for OAB symptoms. Ellington et al., compared tolterodine with intavaginal estrogen for OAB in 58 postmenopausal women in a randomized controlled trial and found that both interventions were equally effective at 12 weeks for OAB symptoms [59]. All the participants were given combined therapy after 12 weeks, and improvement was better at 24 and 52 weeks compared to single therapy at 12 weeks, but authors concluded that need of combined therapy for OAB needs further evaluation [59]. Nelken et al., randomised 58 postmenopausal women with OAB to receive either intravaginal estrogen ring or oxybutynin. Authors found that there was a significant improvement in Urogenital Distress Inventory and Incontinence Impact Questionnaire scores in both groups, with benefit being equivalent in both the groups [60]. Available literature doesn't support benefit of estrogen supplementation in UI unanimously. The result is conflicting; some studies supporting the drug [61], but others do not find this intervention useful for UI [62, 63]. Cochrane review on estrogen treatment for UI in postmenopausal women concluded that local estrogen therapy is not useful in the long term, and systemic estrogen therapy worsens the symptoms of UI when compared to placebo [64]. This Cochrane review included 35 studies; out of that 6 trials were there on systemic estrogen treatment. The systemic estrogen worsened the symptoms of UI both in hysterectomized (estrogen-only HRT) and non-hysterectomized (estrogen and progesterone HRT) postmenopausal women. Normal urination is controlled by a small region in brainstem called Barrington's nucleus (Bar). A recent study have found the presence of ER α+ in Bar nucleus, the main function of which is to relax of muscles of urethral sphincter and facilitate [65]. This can be the explanation of systemic estrogen worsening the UI by acting on pontine center to cause urethral relaxation and urine release.

Local estrogen: Local estrogen preparations are more effective in relieving these symptoms than systemic HRT. So, in women with predominantly these symptoms, vaginal treatment should be given along with systemic HRT [66]. Local estrogen can be provided in the form of cream, ring, pessary, and tablets. Estrogen deficiency adds to loss of pelvic muscle strength resulting in stress urinary incontinence. Many times systemic HRT is contraindicated, local estrogen can be given in these cases also after consultation with menopause treatment specialists [67].

Duration of treatment: The systemic absorption of vaginal estrogen is very low. It is not needed to add progesterone for endometrial protection in women taking vaginal estrogen. But safety beyond 1 year of use has not been proven. So, advised is to take the lowest effective dose needed for symptom control. The problems reoccur after discontinuation of treatment. So vaginal estrogen can be used for as long as needed by the patient [67]. Routine monitoring of endometrial thickness is not needed in women on vaginal estrogen for urogenital atrophy, but women should be counselled to report if they experience unscheduled vaginal bleeding [67].

Systemic estrogen: Collagen decreases after menopause. Treatment with estrogen reduces collagen turnover and improves collagen quality [68, 69]. The results of studies done to see the effect estrogen urinary incontinence are mixed; some found it beneficial, but others have not. The landmark studies done on HRT, the Heart and Estrogen-Progestin Replacement Study (HERS) randomized trial and Nurses' Health Study reported increase of incontinence in hormone users [70, 71]. Some studies found improvement in SUI due to effect on urethral epithelium. A meta-analysis found improvement only in non-randomized studies. Some lubricants are also effective in this regard but not as effective as estrogen.

10.5 Summary

A significant part of females' life is spent after menopause. So, menopausal health and QOL are important. Estrogen deficiency is significant but not a necessary contributor to menopausal symptoms. The LUTS are a major obstacle to good QOL in menopausal females. Combination of anticholinergic and ß-3 agonist has shown promising results. Use of this combination in hypertensive females needs further study. Local estrogen also relieves symptoms of LUTS.

References

1. Singh M. Early age of natural menopause in India, a biological marker for early preventive health programs. Climacteric. 2012;15:581–6.

2. Schoenaker DA, Jackson CA, Rowlands JV, Mishra GD. Socioeconomic position, lifestyle factors and age at natural menopause: a systematic review and meta-analyses of studies across six continents. Int J Epidemiol. 2014;43:1542–62.
3. Government of India: Ministry of Home Affairs 2011. Office of the Registrar General & Census Commissioner, India; 2011. http://censusindia.gov.in. Accessed 2 Oct 2023.
4. Huang AJ, Moore EE, Boyko EJ, et al. Vaginal symptoms in postmenopausal women: self-reported severity, natural history, and risk factors. Menopause. 2010;17(1):121–6.
5. Santoro N, Komi J. Prevalence and impact of vaginal symptoms among postmenopausal women. J Sex Med. 2009;6(8):2133–42.
6. Good MM, Solomon ER. Pelvic floor disorders. Obstet Gynecol Clin North Am. 2019;46:527–40.
7. Huang AJ, Gregorich SE, Kuppermann M, et al. Day-to-day impact of vaginal aging questionnaire: a multidimensional measure of the impact of vaginal symptoms on functioning and well-being in postmenopausal women. Menopause. 2015;22(2):144–54.
8. Pinkerton JV, Bushmakin AG, Komm BS, Abraham L. Relationship between changes in vulvar- vaginal atrophy and changes in sexual functioning. Maturitas. 2017;100:57–63.
9. Nygaard I, Barber MD, Burgio KL, Kenton K, Meikle S, Schaffer J, Spino C, Whitehead WE, Wu J, Brody DJ, Pelvic Floor Disorders Network. Prevalence of symptomatic pelvic floor disorders in US women. JAMA. 2008;300(11):1311–6.
10. Wu JM, Vaughan CP, Goode PS, et al. Prevalence and trends of symptomatic pelvic floor disorders in U.S. women. Obstet Gynecol. 2014;123:141–8.
11. Carls C. The prevalence of stress urinary incontinence in high school and college-age female athletes in the midwest: implications for education and prevention. Urol Nurs. 2007;27(1):21–4, 39.
12. Boyington JE, Howard DL, Carter-Edwards L, Gooden KM, Erdem N, Jallah Y, Busby-Whitehead J. Differences in resident characteristics and prevalence of urinary incontinence in nursing homes in the southeastern United States. Nurs Res. 2007;56(2):97–107.
13. Robinson D, Cardozo L. Estrogens and the lower urinary tract. Neurourol Urodyn. 2011;30(5):754–7. https://doi.org/10.1002/nau.21106. PMID: 21661025.
14. Shamliyan T, Wyman J, Bliss DZ, Kane RL, Wilt TJ. Prevention of urinary and fecal incontinence in adults. Evid Rep Technol Assess (Full Rep). 2007;(161):1–379.
15. Committee 1 Epidemiology of urinary (UI) and fecal (FI) incontinence and pelvic organ prolapse (POP). Incontinence: 4th International Consultation on Incontinence; 2008 July 5–8, 2008; Paris. Health Publications Ltd.
16. Robinson D, Toozs-Hobson P, Cardozo L. The effect of hormones on the lower urinary tract. Menopause Int. 2013;19:155. https://doi.org/10.1177/1754045313511398.
17. Yoshida J, Aikawa K, Yoshimura Y, Shishido K, Yanagida T, Yamaguchi O. The effects of ovariectomy and estrogen replacement on acetylcholine release from nerve fibres and passive stretch-induced acetylcholine release in female rat bladder. Neurourol Urodyn. 2007;26(7):1050–5. https://doi.org/10.1002/nau.20438. PMID: 17480029.
18. Taylor HS, Pal L, Seil E. Chapter 17. Menopause transition and menopause hormone therapy. In: Speroff's clinical gynecological endocrinology and infertility. 9th ed. New Delhi: Wolters Kluver; 2019. p. 601.
19. Meeta M, Digumarti L, Agarwal N, Vaze N, Shah R, Malik S. Clinical practice guidelines on menopause: *an executive summary and recommendations: Indian menopause society 2019–2020. J Midlife Health. 2020;11:55–95.
20. Anglim B, Phillips C, Shynlova O, Alarab M. The effect of local estrogen therapy on the urinary microbiome composition of postmenopausal women with and without recurrent urinary tract infections. Int Urogynecol J. 2022;33(8):2107–17.
21. Quiroz LH, White DE, Juarez D, Shobeiri SA. Age effects on pelvic floor symptoms in a cohort of nulliparous patients. Female Pelvic Med Reconstr Surg. 2012;18:325–8.
22. Quiroz LH, White DE, Juarez D, Shobeiri SA. Age effects on pelvic floor symptoms in a cohort of nulliparous patients. Female Pelvic Med Reconstr Surg. 2012;18(6):325–8.

23. Miyagawa S, Iguchi T. Epithelial estrogen receptor 1 intrinsically mediates squamous differentiation in the mouse vagina. Proc Natl Acad Sci U S A. 2015;112:12986–91.
24. Blakeman PJ, Hilton P, Bulmer JN. Oestrogen and progesterone receptor expression in the female lower urinary tract, with reference to oestrogen status. BJU Int. 2000;86(1):32–8.
25. Mitchell CM, Ma N, Mitchell AJ, Wu MC, Valint DJ, Proll S, Reed SD, Guthrie KA, Lacroix AZ, Larson JC, Pepin R, Raftery D, Fredricks DN, Srinivasan S. Association between postmenopausal vulvovaginal discomfort, vaginal microbiota and mucosal inflammation. Am J Obstet Gynecol. 2021;225(2):159.e1–159.e15.
26. Al-Mukhtar Othman J, Åkervall S, Milsom I, Gyhagen M. Urinary incontinence in nulliparous women aged 25-64 years: a national survey. Am J Obstet Gynecol. 2017;216(2):149.e1–149.e11.
27. Lukacz ES, Lawrence JM, Contreras R, Nager CW, Luber KM. Parity, mode of delivery, and pelvic floor disorders. Obstet Gynecol. 2006;107(6):1253–60.
28. Pearce MM, Hilt EE, Rosenfeld AB, Zilliox MJ, Thomas-White K, Fok C, Kliethermes S, Schreckenberger PC, Brubaker L, Gai X, Wolfe AJ. The female urinary microbiome: a comparison of women with and without urgency urinary incontinence. mBio. 2014;5(4):e01283–14.
29. Thomas-White KJ, Kliethermes S, Rickey L, Lukacz ES, Richter HE, Moalli P, Zimmern P, Norton P, Kusek JW, Wolfe AJ, Brubaker L, National Institute of Diabetes and Digestive and Kidney Diseases Urinary Incontinence Treatment Network. Evaluation of the urinary microbiota of women with uncomplicated stress urinary incontinence. Am J Obstet Gynecol. 2017;216(1):55.e1–55.e16.
30. Keating KN, Perfetto EM, Subedi P. Economic burden of uncomplicated urinary tract infections: direct, indirect and intangible costs. Expert Rev Pharmacoecon Outcomes Res. 2005;5:457–66.
31. Blakeman PJ, Hilton P, Bulmer JN. Cellular proliferation in the female lower urinary tract with reference to oestrogen status. BJOG. 2001;108:813–6.
32. Lüthje P, Brauner H, Ramos NL, et al. Estrogen supports urothelial defense mechanisms. Sci Transl Med. 2013;5:190–80.
33. Raz R, Stamm WE. A controlled trial of intravaginal estriol in postmenopausal women with recurrent urinary tract infections. N Engl J Med. 1993;329(11):753–6.
34. Sekito T, Wada K, Ishii A, Iwata T, Matsubara T, Tomida S, Watanabe M, Araki M, Sadahira T. Etiology of recurrent cystitis in postmenopausal women based on vaginal microbiota and the role of *Lactobacillus* vaginal suppository. Front Microbiol. 2023;14:1187479.
35. Rosenberg MT, Dmochowski RR. Overactive bladder: evaluation and management in primary care. Cleve Clin J Med. 2005;72(2):149–56.
36. McGowan S, Campbell P, Dolan L. The use of urethral bulking agents in the treatment of stress urinary incontinence. Obstet Gynaecol. 2020;22:137–46. https://doi.org/10.1111/tog.12647.
37. Todhunter-Brown A, Hazelton C, Campbell P, Elders A, Hagen S, McClurg D. Conservative interventions for treating urinary incontinence in women: an overview of Cochrane systematic reviews. Cochrane Database Syst Rev. 2022;9(9):CD012337. https://doi.org/10.1002/14651858.CD012337.
38. National Institute for Health and Care Excellence (NICE). Urinary incontinence and pelvic organ prolapse in women: management. NICE guideline (NG123). London: NICE; 2019. https://www.nice.org.uk/guidance/ng123.
39. Lipp A, Shaw C, Glavind K. Mechanical devices for urinary incontinence in women. Cochrane Database Syst Rev. 2014;(12):CD001756.
40. Stoniute A, Madhuvrata P, Still M, Barron-Millar E, Nabi G, Omar MI. Oral anticholinergic drugs versus placebo or no treatment for managing overactive bladder syndrome in adults. Cochrane Database Syst Rev. 2023;5(5):CD003781.
41. Andersson KE, Arner A. Urinary bladder contraction and relaxation: physiology and pathophysiology. Physiol Rev. 2004;84(3):935–86. https://doi.org/10.1152/physrev.00038.2003.
42. Otsuka A, Shinbo H, Matsumoto R, Kurita Y, Ozono S. Expression and functional role of beta-adrenoceptors in the human urinary bladder urothelium. Naunyn Schmiedebergs Arch Pharmacol. 2008;377(4–6):473–81.

43. Hicks A, McCafferty GP, Riedel E, et al. GW427353 (solabegron), a novel, selective beta3-adrenergic receptor agonist, evokes bladder relaxation and increases micturition reflex threshold in the dog. J Pharmacol Exp Ther. 2007;323(1):202–9.
44. Athanasiou S, Pitsouni E, Grigoriadis T, Zacharakis D, Salvatore S, Serati M. Mirabegron in female patients with overactive bladder syndrome: what's new? A systematic review and meta-analysis. Eur J Obstet Gynecol Reprod Biol. 2020;251:73–82.
45. Abrams P, Kelleher C, Staskin D, et al. Combination treatment with mirabegron and solifenacin in patients with overactive bladder: exploratory responder analyses of efficacy and evaluation of patient-reported outcomes from a randomized, double-blind, factorial, dose-ranging, phase II study (SYMPHONY). World J Urol. 2017;35(5):827–38.
46. Mueller ER, van Maanen R, Chapple C, et al. Long-term treatment of older patients with overactive bladder using a combination of mirabegron and solifenacin: a prespecified analysis from the randomized, phase III SYNERGY II study. Neurourol Urodyn. 2019;38(2):779–92.
47. Katoh T, Igawa Y, Yamaguchi O, Kato D, Hamada T, Kuroishi K. Cardiovascular safety of antimuscarinic add-on therapy in patients with overactive bladder who had a suboptimal response to mirabegron monotherapy: a post hoc analysis from the Japanese MILAI II study. Low Urin Tract Symptoms. 2020;12(1):68–80.
48. Gratzke C, van Maanen R, Chapple C, Abrams P, Herschorn S, Robinson D, Ridder A, Stoelzel M, Paireddy A, Yoon SJ, Al-Shukri S, Rechberger T, Mueller ER. Long-term safety and efficacy of mirabegron and solifenacin in combination compared with monotherapy in patients with overactive bladder: a randomised, multicentre phase 3 study (SYNERGY II). Eur Urol. 2018;74(4):501–9.
49. Coyne KS, Sexton CC, Thompson CL, et al. The prevalence of lower urinary tract symptoms (LUTS) in the USA, the UK and Sweden: results from the Epidemiology of LUTS (EpiLUTS) study. BJU Int. 2009;104:352–60.
50. Irwin DE, Milsom I, Hunskaar S, Reilly K, Kopp Z, Herschorn S, Coyne K, Kelleher C, Hampel C, Artibani W, Abrams P. Population-based survey of urinary incontinence, overactive bladder, and other lower urinary tract symptoms in five countries: results of the EPIC study. Eur Urol. 2006;50(6):1306–14.
51. Chang SC, Lin AT, Chen KK, et al. Multifactorial nature of male nocturia. Urology. 2006;67:541–4. https://doi.org/10.1016/j.urology.2005.09.037.
52. Drangsholt S, Peyronnet B, Arcila-Ruiz M, Sussman RD, Palmerola R, Pape DR, Rosenblum N, Nitti VW, Brucker BM. Nocturia in female patients: current clinical features, treatment patterns and outcomes at a tertiary referral centre. Arab J Urol. 2019;17(1):82–6.
53. Mun JH, Kim SO, Yu HS, Chung HS, Kwon D. Effects of desmopressin for the treatment of nocturnal polyuria in elderly women: impact on related sleep quality. Can Urol Assoc J. 2015;9(11–12):E770–4.
54. Barakat B, Franke K, May M, Gauger U, Vögeli TA. Efficacy and safety of desmopressin on frequency and urgency in female patients with overactive bladder and nocturia, current clinical features and outcomes: a systematic review. Asian J Urol. 2022;9(1):27–34.
55. Rovner ES, Raymond K, Andruczyk E, Juul KV. Low-dose desmopressin and tolterodine combination therapy for treating nocturia in women with overactive bladder: a double-blind, randomized, controlled study. Low Urin Tract Symptoms. 2018;10(3):221–30.
56. Weiss JP, Herschorn S, Albei CD, van der Meulen EA. Efficacy and safety of low dose desmopressin orally disintegrating tablet in men with nocturia: results of a multicenter, randomized, double-blind, placebo controlled, parallel group study. J Urol. 2013;190:965–72.
57. Juul KV, Malmberg A, van der Meulen E, Walle JV, Norgaard JP. Low-dose desmopressin combined with serum sodium monitoring can prevent clinically significant hyponatraemia in patients treated for nocturia. BJU Int. 2017;119:776–84.
58. Panay N, Hamoda H, Arya R, Savvas M, on behalf of The British Menopause Society and Women's Health Concern. The 2013 British Menopause Society & Women's Health Concern recommendations on hormone replacement therapy. Menopause Int. 2013;19(2):59–68. https://doi.org/10.1177/1754045313489645.
59. Menopause: diagnosis and management. NICE guideline 2015. nice.org.uk/guidance/ng23.

60. Robinson D, Cardozo LD. The role of estrogens in female lower urinary tract dysfunction. Urology. 2003;62(4 Suppl 1):45–51.
61. Ellington DR, Szychowski JM, Malek JM, Gerten KA, Burgio KL, Richter HE. Combined Tolterodine and vaginal estradiol cream for overactive bladder symptoms after randomized single-therapy treatment. Female Pelvic Med Reconstr Surg. 2016;22(4):254–60. https://doi.org/10.1097/SPV.0000000000000256. PMID: 26945271; PMCID: PMC4919279.
62. Nelken RS, Ozel BZ, Leegant AR, Felix JC, Mishell DR Jr. Randomized trial of estradiol vaginal ring versus oral oxybutynin for the treatment of overactive bladder. Menopause. 2011;18(9):962–6. https://doi.org/10.1097/gme.0b013e3182104977. PMID: 21532512.
63. Fantl JA, Cardozo L, McClish DK. Estrogen therapy in the management of urinary incontinence in postmenopausal women: a meta-analysis. First report of the Hormones and Urogenital Therapy Committee. Obstet Gynecol. 1994;83:12–8.
64. Grady D, Brown JS, Vittinghoff E, Applegate W, Varner E, Snyder T, HERS Research Group. Postmenopausal hormones and incontinence: the Heart and Estrogen/Progestin Replacement Study. Obstet Gynecol. 2001;97:116–20.
65. Hendrix SL, Cochrane BB, Nygaard IE, et al. Effects of estrogen with and without progestin on urinary incontinence. JAMA. 2005;293:935–48.
66. Steinauer JE, Waetjen LE, Vittinghoff E, Subak LL, Hulley SB, Grady D, Lin F, Brown JS, for the Heart and Estrogen/Progestin Replacement Study Research Group, Postmenopausal hormone therapy. Does it cause incontinence? Obstet Gynecol. 2005;106:940.
67. Townsend MK, Curhan GC, Resnick NM, Grodstein F. Postmenopausal hormone therapy and incident urinary incontinence in middle-aged women. Am J Obstet Gynecol. 2009;200:86.e1.
68. Cody JD, Jacobs ML, Richardson K, Moehrer B, Hextall A. Oestrogen therapy for urinary incontinence in post-menopausal women. Cochrane Database Syst Rev. 2012;10:CD001405.
69. Keller JA, Chen J, Simpson S, Wang EH, Lilascharoen V, George O, Lim BK, Stowers L. Voluntary urination control by brainstem neurons that relax the urethral sphincter. Nat Neurosci. 2018;21(9):1229–38. https://doi.org/10.1038/s41593-018-0204-3. Epub 2018 Aug 13. PMID: 30104734; PMCID: PMC6119086.
70. Holland EFN, Studd JWW, Mansell JP, Leather AT, Bailey AJ. Changes in collagen composition and cross-links in bone and skin of osteoporotic post-menopausal women treated with percutaneous estradiol implants. Obstet Gynecol. 1994;83:180.
71. Castelo-Branco C, Pons F, Gratacos E, Fortuny A, Vanrell JA, Gonzalez-Merlo J. Relationship between skin collagen and bone changes during aging. Maturitas. 1994;18:199.

Menopause and Weight Management

11

Aryan Kashyap, Saloni Kamboj, and Prabhat Agrawal

11.1 Introduction

One of the hallmark events in a woman's life, which not only marks the end of her reproductive era but also brings with it a plethora of changes to which she must adapt, is menopause. Menopause has classically been defined as cessation of menstruation for 12 months since the last menstrual period, as a consequence of depletion of ovarian follicular reserve. While among the Caucasian women, the average age of menopause is 51.3 years, Indian women tend to attain menopause earlier than their western contemporaries, at an average of 46.6 years [1]. Thus, ovaries in Indian women tend to age earlier than their Caucasian counterparts, with a 6-year difference in favour of Caucasians [2].

Hypo-oestrogenemia in menopause, which occurs due to diminished follicular reserve, has been implicated in a variety of symptoms that include hot flashes, mood disorders, sleep disturbances, and urogenital tract problems that can be very distressing for a patient [3]. The risk of developing metabolic syndrome (MS), type 2 diabetes, osteoporosis, and cardiovascular diseases is also increased by metabolic derangements that appear at this time; the effects of oestrogen shortage include an increase in body weight, insulin resistance, osteogenic remodelling, and altered glucose and lipid metabolism. As demonstrated by the Framingham study, a 2.6-fold increase of cardiovascular events was found in postmenopausal women when compared to age-matched premenopausal controls [4].

A. Kashyap
CIMAR, Kochi, India

S. Kamboj (✉)
Departmental of Obstetrics and Gynaecology, AIIMS, Delhi, India

P. Agrawal
PG Department of Medicine, SN Medical College, Agra, India

R. Garg (ed.), *Management of Menopause*,
https://doi.org/10.1007/978-981-96-0239-1_11

The primary cause of metabolic irregularities in postmenopausal women is obesity, which is defined by the World Health Organization (WHO) as an abnormal or excessive fat buildup that may be harmful to one's health. The worldwide prevalence of obesity nearly tripled between 1975 and 2016 [5]. Obesity is one of the most important adverse events associated with the menopause, which not only is the progenitor of various endocrinological and gynaecological afflictions but is also a social problem and an economic burden. Prevalence of metabolic syndrome (MS) after menopause, closely associated with obesity, is estimated at the level of 31–55% [3]. The need of the hour is to promote weight management strategies based on lifestyle modification techniques which are in concordance with a woman's cultural and social practices, thus making such techniques more acceptable and palatable for our patients.

In this review, we will understand the pathophysiology of menopausal weight gain, the risk factors and wider implications of obesity among postmenopausal women, and strategies to prevent and manage obesity in menopausal patients.

11.2 Pathophysiology of Menopausal Weight Gain and Obesity

Even though the reason for central adiposity in menopausal women remains elusive, hypo-oestrogenism, along with genetic and exogenous factors plays a crucial role in menopausal weight gain and obesity (Fig. 11.1).

Adrenergic receptors, both the β adrenergic and the α2A adrenergic receptors, regulate lipid metabolism in adipocytes. Activation of β receptors increases

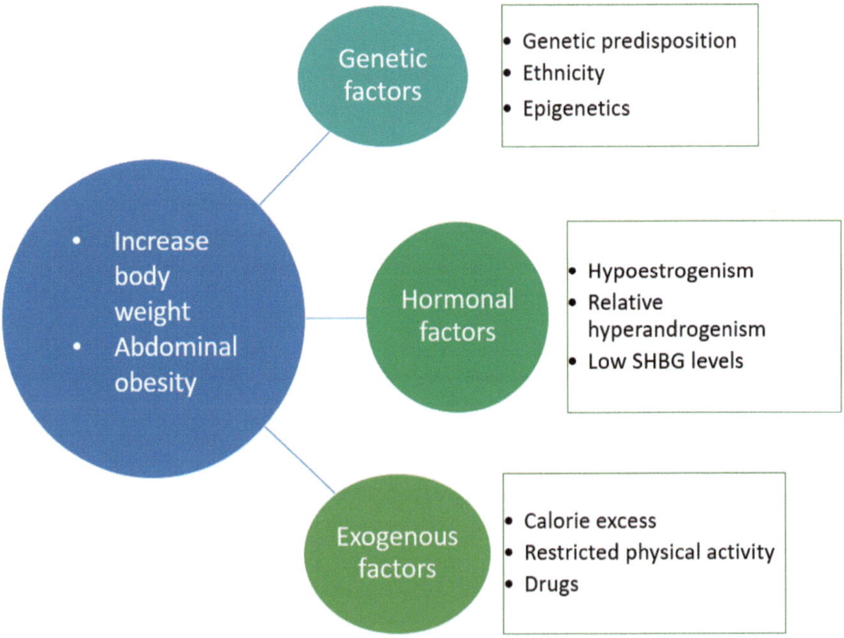

Fig. 11.1 Factors contributing to obesity and menopausal weight gain

lipolysis, while the stimulation of α2A receptors results in an anti-lipolytic action and promotes accumulation of fat [6]. Oestrogen by binding to its nuclear receptors—the ERα and the ERβ receptors—regulates the expression of adrenergic receptors in adipose tissues. Oestrogen upregulates the expression of α2A adrenergic receptors in the subcutaneous fat tissue, with no effect on the visceral fat. Erα receptor activation also stimulates β adrenergic action in visceral adipocytes which helps in reducing abdominal fat mass. This explains the reason for a gynaecoid distribution of fat in a premenopausal woman, which is commonly referred to as a 'pear-shaped' figure [7]. Moreover, oestrogen has also been shown to increase fat oxidation in skeletal muscles and at the same time inhibit hepatic and muscle lipogenesis [8].

Oestrogen also plays a cardinal role in the regulation of various adipokines and cytokines which are secreted from adipose tissues. Oestrogen upregulates the expression and sensitivity of leptin receptors in the hypothalamus, thereby potentiating the action of leptin as a centrally acting appetite suppressant [9]. Adiponectin, a cytokine with actions opposite to leptin, which has been implicated in the pathogenesis of insulin resistance, has been shown to have a negative correlation with oestrogen levels [10]. Moreover, the inhibitory effect of oestrogen on proinflammatory cytokines such as interleukin-6 (IL-6) and tumour necrosis factor-α (TNF-α) confers cardioprotective effect to oestrogen.

During menopause, low levels of oestrogen decrease the hepatic synthesis of sex hormone-binding globulin (SHBG). Since SHBG is important for binding testosterone, low SHBG levels in menopause lead to an increase in the pool of bioavailable testosterone, leading to a relative hyperandrogenic state.

Together with low oestrogen levels and a relative hyperandrogenic state, menopause is heralded by an unfavourable fat redistribution, with increased abdominal and visceral adiposity—which means that a menopausal woman changes from a 'pear-shape' to an 'apple-shape' (Fig. 11.2).

11.2.1 Oestrogen and Central Regulation of Appetite

The central control on appetite is exerted by the hypothalamus—particularly by the arcuate, ventromedial and the paraventricular nucleus. Stimulation of various

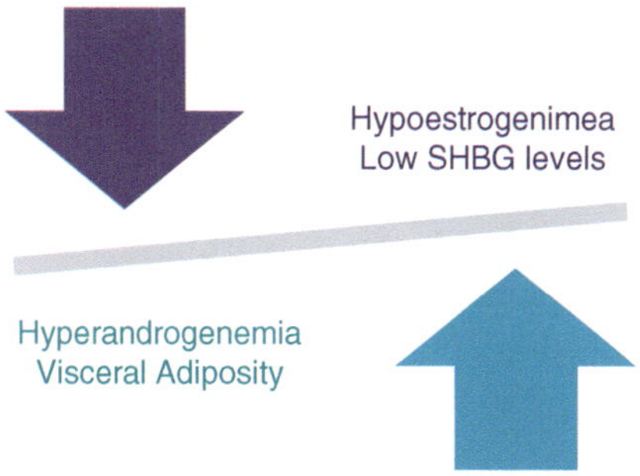

Fig. 11.2 Low SHBG levels in menopause due to low oestrogen levels cause a relative increase in bioavailable testosterone, which leads to an increase in visceral fat deposition

neurons in this region exerts a regulatory action on appetite: which can either be an orexigenic (stimulating hunger) or an anorexigenic (reducing hunger) effect.

In experimental studies done in mammals, expression and activation of Erα receptor in the hypothalamic proopiomelanocortin (POMC) neurons has shown to decrease appetite [11]. The production of neuropeptide Y (NPY) and ghrelin—both of which are potent orexigenic hormones—is decreased under the influence of oestrogen [12, 13]. Thus, oestrogen appears to be involved in central regulation of energy balance and has anorexigenic effect on the central nervous system (CNS). Rapid decline in oestrogen levels in menopause can, therefore, be accompanied by an increase in appetite, which can lead to significant weight gain in menopause.

11.3 Risk Factors for Weight Gain

Increased postmenopausal weight gain is caused by a combination of genetic, physiological, psychological, and behavioural factors. According to a number of studies, environmental factors may combine with a genetic vulnerability to cause excessive weight gain in addition to the genetic tendency itself. Various modifiable and non-modifiable characteristics include the following:

1. **Physiologic factors**: Ageing, slow metabolic rate in menopausal women, hypothyroidism, polycystic ovary syndrome, and musculoskeletal disorders
2. **Psychological factors**

   During the menopausal transition, many women assert that they frequently feel unpleasant emotional states (depression, stress, anxiety, tension, and mood disorder), irregular sleep patterns, and sexual issues. Many women experience emotional eating or overeating, which is directly linked to weight gain.
3. **Lifestyle-Related Factors**

   Weight gain results from a favourable energy balance and a diet of inadequate nutritional value. Weight increase during the menopausal transition is positively associated with a diet heavy in high fat, sugar, and salt products and low in dietary fibre. Obesity is also linked to increased consumption of convenience and fried or processed foods because of easy access to these foods. This group of women gains weight as a result of their bad eating habits, physical inactivity, irregular sleeping patterns, and excessive alcohol and tobacco use.
4. **Genetic factors**: Complex interactions between multiple genes and environmental factors that could bring about epigenetic changes leading to obesity (multifactorial obesity) have been poorly understood. Rarely, a clear pattern of inherited obesity may be attributed to a specific variant of a gene (monogenic obesity).

11.4 Implications of Weight Gain

11.4.1 Effect of Obesity on Menopause

A higher body mass index (BMI) has been linked to an earlier onset of menarche, and mounting data indicates that obese women and women with a higher BMI experience menopause later. BMI seems to be directly proportionate to the age of natural menopause: the greater the BMI, the later is the age at which a woman attains menopause. This can be explained by the high levels of circulating oestrogens, secondary to peripheral conversion of androgens in adipose tissues to androgens by the activity of aromatase. Recent evidence suggests that obesity and fat mass have a negative impact on bone health [14].

11.4.2 Effect of Obesity on Menopausal Symptoms

Vasomotor symptoms associated with menopause can be quite bothersome for women, so much so, that she must seek medical help for the same. Not only do these symptoms have adverse impact on sleep; they can have detrimental effects on mood and the overall quality of life.

The incidence of vasomotor symptoms is increased in obesity. A secondary analysis of data from the Study of Women's Health Across the Nation (SWAN) study attempted to identify factors associated with increased menopausal, particularly vasomotor symptoms. Adiposity has shown to be significantly associated with odds of reporting vasomotor symptoms (OR 1.14, 95% CI 1.01–1.28, $p < 0.05$) [15]. It has been hypothesised that an insulating effect of adipose tissues might increase the severity and incidence of hot flashes in obese menopausal women.

11.4.3 Obesity and Cancers

Breast and endometrial cancer development are both independently at risk due to obesity. Obese women with insulin resistance have low SHBG levels, which increased the bioavailable androgens in obese women, which acts a substrate of peripheral aromatization and results in increased oestrogen levels. In contrast to the increased risk of breast cancer in obese postmenopausal women, extended exposure to unopposed oestrogen raised the risk of endometrial cancer at all stages of life. Therefore, obesity is one of the most important modifiable factors in mitigating risk of endometrial and breast cancers in menopausal women.

11.4.4 Menopausal Obesity and Risk of Alzheimer's Disease

Age-related increase in inflammation is worsened by obesity and menopause. As described earlier, oestrogen plays a key role in decreasing proinflammatory cytokines, so lack of oestrogen in menopause contributes to a chronic inflammatory state. Alzheimer's disease is a multifactorial neurodegenerative disorder, and its initiation and onset have been attributed to age-related increase in inflammation and obesity. Recent evidence suggests that onset of menopause elevates the vulnerability of women to cognitive impairment, the pathogenesis of which is probably centred around depletion of oestrogen [16].

11.4.5 Obesity and Risk of Cardiovascular Events in Menopause

Perimenopausal obesity is characterised by adipocyte dysfunction, with a relative increase in proinflammatory adipokines and decreased secretion of anti-inflammatory adipokines, which promote atherosclerotic changes and vascular remodelling. Moreover, an androgenic environment in menopausal women, along with oestrogen deficiency has been associated with left ventricular remodelling [17]. Menopause has been shown to be have an unfavourable cardiovascular disease risk profile that comprises risk factors such as metabolic syndrome, chronic inflammation, insulin resistance, and lipid abnormalities [18].

Most recently, the Atherosclerosis Risk in Communities (ARIC) study has elucidated the influence of obesity on androgenicity and subsequently heart failure development. This study has shown that the absence of excessive adiposity may have a protective effect against heart failure development in menopausal women [19].

11.5 Management

11.5.1 Staging of Obesity in Women

Health check-ups in perimenopausal and menopausal women must include a thorough history taking, with emphasis on her chief complaints and distressing symptoms. A BMI should also be calculated at this time, and women with a BMI more than 23 should be assessed for metabolic syndrome and diabetes. The Women's Preventive Services Initiative advises that BMI measurements be used to check for obesity during routine visits. The Edmonton obesity staging system offers a more comprehensive staging that considers metabolic, physical, and psychological health and has the added advantage of assessing weight-related health and the need and planning for treatment and intervention [20].

11.5.2 Management of Obesity in Perimenopausal Women

Stratification of women according to the grade of obesity and associated comorbidities can help clinicians decide the management strategy that would be best suited for their patient. By considering the BMI and waist circumference, a risk score can be assigned to an obese woman. Scores 3 and above need pharmacological intervention, whereas patients with a score of 4 need surgical intervention [7].

11.5.3 Weight Loss

A structured lifestyle intervention, with proper dietician review and physiotherapist consultation, and motivation go a long way in maintaining compliance to weight loss strategies. It is important to remove the stigma around obesity and avoid weight bias and discrimination that inadvertently leads to psychological stress in our patients, thus demotivating them to approach and seek help for weight loss. As physicians, we must investigate how obesity is viewed in different cultures and use weight-inclusive language and images [20] (Fig. 11.3).

Public health is significantly improved by weight control, and most women, regardless of age, use comparable tactics to accomplish these ends. The benefits of a good diet and regular exercise on both short-term and long-term health are substantial; thus all healthcare providers should take advantage of every chance to promote a healthy lifestyle.

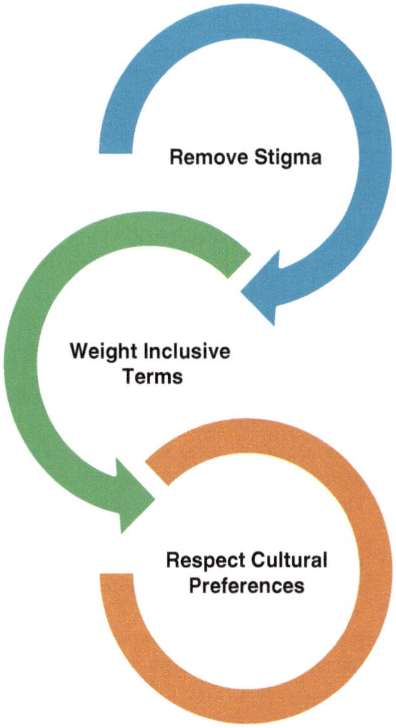

Fig. 11.3 Approaching obese patients with empathy and compassion can go a long way in ensuring compliance and motivation

11.5.4 Role of Menopausal Hormone Replacement Therapy

A decrease in central obesity has been seen with the use of hormone replacement therapy in women. Contrary to popular misconceptions, menopausal hormone replacement therapy (HRT) may even result in a decrease in visceral adiposity and weight gain, both of which are typical misconceptions. HbA1c results demonstrate that oral HRT improves glucose management and delays the onset of diabetes. Planning treatment options for postmenopausal women takes this into account in order to maximise benefits while reducing negative effects. Thus starting HRT in the window of opportunity may prove to have some protective effect in women prone to developing obesity in menopause.

References

1. Prasad JB, Tyagi NK, Verma P. Age at menopause in India: a systematic review. Diabetes Metab Syndr. 2021;15(1):373–7.
2. Banker M, Iglesias C, Mahahan N, Herrero L, Pellicer A, García-Velasco JA. Ethnic differences in ovarian aging between Caucasian and Indian women. Fertil Steril. 2013;100(3):S152–3.
3. Stefanska A, Bergmann K, Sypniewska G. Metabolic syndrome and menopause: pathophysiology, clinical and diagnostic significance. Adv Clin Chem. 2015;72:1–75.
4. Kannel WB, Hjortland MC, McNamara PM, Gordon T. Menopause and risk of cardiovascular disease: the Framingham study. Ann Intern Med. 1976;85(4):447–52.
5. Obesity and overweight [Internet]. [cited 2023 May 15]. https://www.who.int/news-room/fact-sheets/detail/obesity-and-overweight.
6. Pedersen SB, Kristensen K, Hermann PA, Katzenellenbogen JA, Richelsen B. Estrogen controls lipolysis by up-regulating alpha2A-adrenergic receptors directly in human adipose tissue through the estrogen receptor alpha. Implications for the female fat distribution. J Clin Endocrinol Metab. 2004;89(4):1869–78.
7. Lumsden MA, Hor K. Impact of obesity on the health of women in midlife. Obstet Gynaecol. 2015;17(3):201–8.
8. Foryst-Ludwig A, Kintscher U. Metabolic impact of estrogen signalling through ERalpha and ERbeta. J Steroid Biochem Mol Biol. 2010;122(1–3):74–81.
9. Frank A, Brown LM, Clegg DJ. The role of hypothalamic estrogen receptors in metabolic regulation. Front Neuroendocrinol. 2014;35(4):550–7.
10. Tworoger SS, Mantzoros C, Hankinson SE. Relationship of plasma adiponectin with sex hormone and insulin-like growth factor levels. Obesity (Silver Spring). 2007;15(9):2217–24.
11. Nestor CC, Kelly MJ, Rønnekleiv OK. Cross-talk between reproduction and energy homeostasis: central impact of estrogens, leptin and kisspeptin signaling. Horm Mol Biol Clin Investig. 2014;17(3):109–28.
12. Rebouças ECC, Leal S, Sá SI. Regulation of NPY and α-MSH expression by estradiol in the arcuate nucleus of Wistar female rats: a stereological study. Neurol Res. 2016;38(8):740–7.
13. Dafopoulos K, Chalvatzas N, Kosmas G, Kallitsaris A, Pournaras S, Messinis IE. The effect of estrogens on plasma ghrelin concentrations in women. J Endocrinol Invest. 2010;33(2):109–12.
14. Zhao LJ, Liu YJ, Liu PY, Hamilton J, Recker RR, Deng HW. Relationship of obesity with osteoporosis. J Clin Endocrinol Metab. 2007;92(5):1640–6.
15. Thurston RC, Sowers MR, Chang Y, Sternfeld B, Gold EB, Johnston JM, et al. Adiposity and reporting of vasomotor symptoms among midlife women: the study of women's health across the nation. Am J Epidemiol. 2008;167(1):78–85.
16. Christensen A, Pike CJ. Menopause, obesity and inflammation: interactive risk factors for Alzheimer's disease. Front Aging Neurosci. 2015;7:130.

17. Subramanya V, Zhao D, Ouyang P, Lima JA, Vaidya D, Ndumele CE, et al. Sex hormone levels and change in left ventricular structure among men and post-menopausal women: the multi-ethnic study of atherosclerosis (MESA). Maturitas. 2018;108:37–44.
18. Ebong IA, Watson KE, Goff DCJ, Bluemke DA, Srikanthan P, Horwich T, et al. Association of menopause age and N-terminal pro brain natriuretic peptide: the multi-ethnic study of atherosclerosis. Menopause. 2015;22(5):527.
19. Ebong IA, Wilson MD, Appiah D, Michos ED, Racette SB, Villablanca A, et al. Relationship between age at menopause, obesity, and incident heart failure: the atherosclerosis risk in communities study. J Am Heart Assoc. 2022;11(8):e024461.
20. Maxwell CV, Shirley R, O'Higgins AC, Rosser ML, O'Brien P, Hod M, et al. Management of obesity across women's life course: FIGO best practice advice. Int J Gynecol Obstet. 2023;160(S1):35–49.

Lifestyle and Menopause 12

Renu Gupta and Pavika Lal

12.1 Introduction

One of the most notable and significant demographic change that would be observable in the coming decades is the improved life expectancy of women in India due to tremendous advancement in medical care. It is estimated that by the end of 2030, there will be 1.4 billion elderly women [1] in India, necessitating a substantial degree of integrated and holistic approach for preventive care to improve the quality of life [2]. Menopause is a universal natural biological phenomenon that marks the end of reproductive life span due to permanent cessation of menses. There have been various studies and surveys which state that average age of menopause in Indian female is significantly lower (46.2 years) as compared to western population (51 years) [3], thereby majority of the Indian female population spend *30–40%* of their lifespan in menopausal age group.

Menopause brings enormous bodily changes leading to bothersome and troublesome symptoms, namely, *vasomotor, sleep disturbances, fatigue, metabolic syndrome, ischemic heart disease, altered cognitive functions, genitourinary syndrome of menopause (GSM), osteoporosis, and sarcopenia* that can adversely affect the quality of life [4]. The problems arising due to the hypo-estrogenic status can be adequately and appropriately managed by planning a good comprehensive health strategy, involving lifestyle modifications. The perception and social scenario of elderly women in our country is a sad story as they become physically vulnerable, emotionally weak, and dependent on other family members for their day-to-day activities.

Attitude toward the process of biological and chronological aging can be influenced by variables like age and type of menopause (natural, iatrogenic), ethnicity, socioeconomic factors, social and family support, level of education, religion, and

R. Gupta · P. Lal (✉)
Department of Obstetrics and Gynaecology, GSVM Medical College, Kanpur, India

R. Garg (ed.), *Management of Menopause*,
https://doi.org/10.1007/978-981-96-0239-1_12

individual cultural beliefs [5]. They should be made to realize that they can lead their own independent lives by inculcating simple lifestyle modifications which mainly focuses on *nutritional changes* as well as *incorporation of exercises* that can have a positive impact on overall well-being.

12.2 Nutritional Modifications

Dietary changes during the menopausal years are an important adaptation as they contribute significantly to both the longevity and quality of life. A balanced healthy diet comprising of variety of fruits, vegetables, whole grains, lean proteins, and healthy fats should be inculcated during this transition which is worldwide labelled as *Mediterranean diet* (Fig. 12.1).

Current evidence established that the Mediterranean diet pattern (low fat plant-based diet) may have beneficial effect on bone, metabolic, and cardiovascular diseases during this period. Healthy food with anti-inflammatory and antioxidant properties [6] may be associated with significant decrease in blood pressure, blood sugar, and improved cholesterol levels with decrease in body fat.

NHANES study [7] concluded that menopausal transition is associated with loss of lean body mass (LBM) and increase in fat mass (FM) which is associated with major cardiovascular risk. Metabolic flexibility is defined as the capability to switch from fat utilization during fasting to carbohydrate utilization to provide energy [8]. Steroidal hormones like estrogen and progesterone regulate this flexibility [9], and decrease in estrogen in a postmenopausal female affects the metabolic flexibility resulting in accumulation of fat leading to central obesity [10]. Dietary recommendations of FLAMENCO study [11] have emphasized that adherence to Mediterranean diet was associated with decrease in fat mass. Mediterranean diet also seems to have

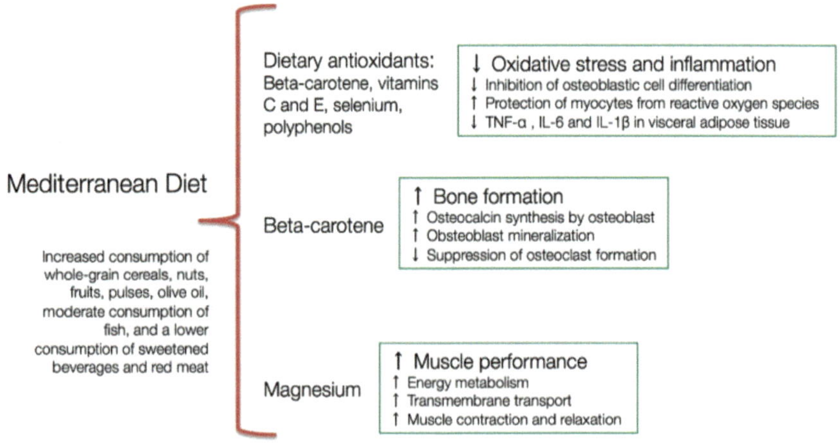

Fig. 12.1 Potential benefits of Mediterranean diet on body composition in postmenopausal women

myoprotective effect linked to increase in vitamin C, vitamin E, and magnesium all of which prevent deleterious effects of oxidative stress, inflammation, insulin resistance, and improved skeletal muscle function [12, 13].

Dietary Proteins: As age advances, protein requirement increases due to inability to synthesize the protein by skeletal mass as a result of increased insulin resistance [14]. Institute of medicine recommends *0.8 g/kg body weight protein for all ages* as increase in protein intake is associated with increase in skeletal mass and decrease in the risk of frailty and sarcopenia [15].

Dietary Carbohydrate: *The most important weightage while planning the carbohydrate amount in the meal should be given to whole grains with high fiber content and with low glycemic index* as it helps in managing a healthier weight and decrease in total fat mass of the body [16]. A meal with increased glycemic index stimulates the pancreas to secrete insulin instantaneously in response to increase blood sugar level causing lowering of blood glucose resulting in hunger and overeating [17].

Avoidance of addiction: Smoking and excessive alcohol consumption can exacerbate menopausal symptoms and increase the risk of stroke and ischemic heart diseases. Quitting smoking and moderating alcohol intake help in improving overall health during menopause [18].

12.3 Bone Health

It is a well-known universal fact that aging has an adverse effect on BMD beyond 32–35 years of age which markedly accelerates especially during the late perimenopause. *NAMS recommends 1000–1500 mg of dietary calcium per day in postmenopausal females for prevention of osteoporosis and fractures along with daily supplement of vitamin D 400–800 IU/kg* [19, 20].

Mediterranean diet also seems to have a protective effect on bone health as beta-carotenoids, vitamin C, and selenium decrease in osteoclast formation and bone resorption. Vitamin K promotes the synthesis of osteocalcin by osteoblasts [21]. In contrast, processed foods such as hamburger, beer, sweets, packed juice, processed meats, and low intake of cruciferous vegetables has been inversely associated with bone mineral content [22].

12.4 Behavioral Modifications [23]

Stress: Practicing relaxation techniques like meditation, yoga, and deep breathing exercises reduces stress and promote mental and emotional well-being.

Dressing in layers helps in managing temperature fluctuations and provides calmness to the body.

Enough quality sleep is crucial during menopause. Creating a bedtime routine, keeping the bedroom cool, and limiting the screen time before bed help to improve the quality of sleep.

Plenty of water intake should be encouraged throughout the day to stay hydrated as it helps in relieving vasomotor symptoms.

Social Support: Surrounding oneself with a supportive network of family and friends and discussing one's experiences and feelings with others can be beneficial during this transitional phase.

12.4.1 Regular Exercise

Postmenopausal females usually gain weight due to the following factors:

- Decreased physical activity owing to weakness of skeletal muscles
- Decrease in basal metabolic rate with aging
- Increase intake of calories as compared to the requirement

It is a well-known established fact that exercise not only promotes physical health but also significantly affects mental and spiritual health. Engaging in regular physical activities helps in maintenance of weight, improves mood, reduces hot flashes, and maintains bone density.

12.4.2 Benefits of Exercise

One of the most desirable and easy to inculcate in one's life is to do exercise. *The aim should be for at least 150 min of moderate-intensity aerobic activity or 75 min of vigorous-intensity aerobic activity per week, along with muscle-strengthening exercises on 2 or more days a week.*

The benefits of exercises are increase in cardiorespiratory function, reduction of metabolic syndrome, reduction in bad cholesterol, i.e., low density lipoprotein (LDL), triglycerides, and fibrinogen with significant improvement in HDL. It is also associated with reduction in risk of hypertension, ischemic heart diseases (IHD), and cerebrovascular accidents. Exercise helps in expenditure of calories creating a calorie deficit thereby minimizing the midlife weight gain. It increases bone mass density as well as preservation of muscle strength [24–26]. It also has a positive impact on mood and helps in relieving stress. It may help to reduce hot flashes, thereby minimizing the "Domino effect" *which states that VMS leads to other problems of menopause such as sexual dysfunction and mood disturbances* [27]. According to the Cochrane review, exercise can be an effective treatment for reducing vasomotor symptoms, although they found weak supportive evidence for exercise when compared to no intervention.

The key while planning an exercise plan is to begin at a slow pace and perform activities which one enjoys such as brisk walking, cycling, swimming, and joining gyms. Even moderate physical activity should be adequate enough to feel one's heart pumping without being tired results in great health benefits [28]. *To determine the maximum heart rate during exercise, one has to subtract the woman's age from 220. For the target heart rate range, multiply maximum heart rate by 50/100 and 80/100.* One should do exercise such that 50% of target zone is achieved and then gradually pace up to 75% of target zone during the 6 months duration. After 6 months of regular physical activities, one can do exercise up to 85 percent of maximum target zone. *A consultation with a physician may be required in patients who have increased blood pressure, ischemic heart disease, or on antihypertensive medications such as beta blockers and target zone may vary in such cases and they may need to exercise at a lower target heart rate.*

Another way to track the intensity of the exercise is the talk test. In moderate-intensity exercise, a woman may be able to talk but unable to sing and should not be panting, whereas in vigorous exercises only a few words can be spoken, and a person is unable to carry out a full clear conversation. Moderate to vigorous intensity exercises help to increase the functional capacity of heart lungs and skeletomuscular system.

12.4.3 Types of Exercises [25]

Various exercises that help in maintaining bone mass density are as follows:

- *Weight-bearing, high-impact exercises:* such as dancing, running/jogging, jumping, and stair climbing, ideal for those females who are strong and non-osteoporotic.
- *Weight-bearing, low-impact exercises:* includes walking (treadmill/outside), stair-step machines. This group of exercises is suitable for women who are unable to perform high-impact exercises.
- *Strength or resistance training exercises:* weight lifting.
- *No weight-bearing, nonimpact activities:* comprises of cycling, swimming, stretching, and flexibility exercises.
- *Nonimpact exercises:* help to maintain balance, gate, posture and attitude.

A postmenopausal female should be motivated for endurance, strength, and balance exercises. Weight-bearing and resistance exercises are very effective in maintaining bone mineral density especially of the vertebral column in postmenopausal female [26].

An effective exercise prescription may be resistance and weight-bearing exercise 3 days a week (on alternate days). Care should be taken to do the exercise for all the muscle groups preferably with a trainer. Brisk walking at the speed of 5–6 kilometers per hour, cycling, treadmill, gardening, or dancing may be done on the remaining days of the week [29]. Warming up beforehand can help to reduce exercise-related injuries and pain following exercise.

12.5 Impact of Exercise on Bone Mineral Density

Active weight-bearing and strength-training exercises also can benefit bone mineral density, reduces the risk of fall, and maintains muscle strength [25, 30]. *To affect areas of the skeleton often involved in osteoporotic fractures, the North American Menopause Society recommends targeting the large extensor muscles of the back, the hip flexors and extensors, and muscles of the thigh, upper arm, and forearm* [31].

12.6 What Not to Do?

Females with osteoporotic changes should not be advised for jumping, jogging, and running as there are possibilities of a fall which may be increase the risk of fragile. Activities which may require repeated movement at the trunk especially flexion and extension (sit ups and toe touches) should always be avoided because of increased workload at the vertebral column which may result in spinal fractures [32].

12.7 When Should Exercise Be Stopped? [33]

This is indeed a warning to all postmenopausal females as one should not ignore the signals of overexhaustion while exercising, which may lead to myocardial injury leading to sudden cardiac arrest. In such cases, one should stop exercising and may switch on to lighter pattern of exercises. It should always be born in mind that one should have adequate calorie and protein intake during excessive workout so as to replenish the requirements by the body.

Conditions when exercise should be avoided include the following:

- Recent electrocardiogram changes or recent myocardial infarction
- Uncontrolled arrhythmia
- Unstable angina
- Third-degree heart block
- Acute progressive heart failure
- Elevated blood pressure
- Cardiomyopathy
- Valvular heart disease
- Complex ventricular ectopy

12.8 Conclusion

Every woman's experience during menopause is unique. If the menopausal symptoms are significantly impacting the quality of life, one must consult the healthcare provider who can provide personalized advice regarding lifestyle modifications. Menopausal Hormone Therapy (MHT) can be considered if the symptoms are unmanageable. Both the gynecologist and the woman herself should be actively involved in planning an integrated and holistic approach. Despite all the physiological changes, menopause should not be considered as a sign of impending decline but a wonderful beginning of new innings. It becomes imperative to plan a comprehensive healthcare strategy including lifestyle modifications of which dietary changes and exercise are an essential and core part of management during this menopausal period. Regular and routine health check-ups with the healthcare provider to monitor the overall health and well-being, to discuss the menopausal symptoms, and to address any concerns are an essential component to stay fit and healthy.

References

1. https://www.who.int/health-topics/ageing#tab=tab_1.
2. Sengupta A. The emergence of the menopause in India. Climacteric. 2003;6(2):92–5. PMID: 12841878.
3. Ahuja M. Age of menopause and determinants of menopause age: a PAN India survey by IMS. J Midlife Health. 2016;7(3):126–31. https://doi.org/10.4103/0976-7800.191012.
4. Nappi RE, Simoncini T. Menopause transition: a golden age to prevent cardiovascular disease. Lancet Diabetes Endocrinol. 2021;9:135–7. https://doi.org/10.1016/S2213-8587(21)00018-8.
5. Schneider HPG, Birkhäuser M. Quality of life in climacteric women. Climacteric. 2017;20:187–94. https://doi.org/10.1080/13697137.2017.1279599.
6. Baumann CW, Kwak D, Liu HM, Thompson LV. Age-induced oxidative stress: how does it influence skeletal muscle quantity and quality? J Appl Physiol (1985). 2016;121:1047–52. https://doi.org/10.1152/japplphysiol.00321.2016.
7. Srikanthan P, Horwich TB, Tseng CH. Relation of muscle mass and fat mass to cardiovascular disease mortality. Am J Cardiol. 2016;117:1355–60. https://doi.org/10.1016/j.amjcard.2016.01.033.
8. Kelley DE, Mandarino LJ. Fuel selection in human skeletal muscle in insulin resistance: a reexamination. Diabetes. 2000;49:677–83. https://doi.org/10.2337/diabetes.49.5.677.
9. Irwin RW, Yao J, Hamilton RT, Cadenas E, Brinton RD, Nilsen J. Progesterone and estrogen regulate oxidative metabolism in brain mitochondria. Endocrinology. 2008;149:3167–75. https://doi.org/10.1210/en.2007-1227.
10. Eaton SA, Sethi JK. Immunometabolic links between estrogen, adipose tissue and female reproductive metabolism. Biology. 2019;8:8. https://doi.org/10.3390/biology8010008.
11. Flor-Alemany M, Marín-Jiménez N, Nestares T, Borges-Cosic M, Aranda P, Aparicio VA. Mediterranean diet, tobacco consumption and body composition during perimenopause. The FLAMENCO project. Maturitas. 2020;137:30–6. https://doi.org/10.1016/j.maturitas.2020.04.002.
12. Silva TRD, Martins CC, Ferreira LL, Spritzer PM. Mediterranean diet is associated with bone mineral density and muscle mass in postmenopausal women. Climacteric. 2019;22:162–8. https://doi.org/10.1080/13697137.2018.1529747.
13. Granic A, Sayer AA, Robinson SM. Dietary patterns, skeletal muscle health, and sarcopenia in older adults. Nutrients. 2019;11:745. https://doi.org/10.3390/nu11040745.
14. Francaux M, Demeulder B, Naslain D, Fortin R, Lutz O, Caty G, Deldicque L. Aging reduces the activation of the mTORC1 pathway after resistance exercise and protein intake in human skeletal muscle: potential role of REDD1 and impaired anabolic sensitivity. Nutrients. 2016;8:47. https://doi.org/10.3390/nu8010047.
15. Trumbo P, Schlicker S, Yates AA, Poos M. Dietary reference intakes for energy, carbohydrate, fiber, fat, fatty acids, cholesterol, protein and amino acids. J Am Diet Assoc. 2002;102:1621–30. https://doi.org/10.1016/S0002-8223(02)90346-9.

16. Augustin LS, Kendall CW, Jenkins DJ, Willett WC, Astrup A, Barclay AW, Björck I, Brand-Miller JC, Brighenti F, Buyken AE, et al. Glycemic index, glycemic load and glycemic response: an international scientific consensus summit from the international carbohydrate quality consortium (ICQC). Nutr Metab Cardiovasc Dis. 2015;25:795–815. https://doi.org/10.1016/j.numecd.2015.05.005.
17. Ludwig DS. Dietary glycemic index and obesity. J Nutr. 2000;130:280s–3s. https://doi.org/10.1093/jn/130.2.280S.
18. Gold EB, Sternfeld B, Kelsey JL, et al. Relation of demographic and lifestyle factors to symptoms in a multi-racial/ethnic population of women 40–55 years of age. Am J Epidemiol. 2000;152:463–73.
19. North American Menopause Society. The role of calcium in peri- and postmenopausal women: 2006 position statement of the North American Menopause Society. Menopause. 2006;13:862–77; quiz 878–880. https://doi.org/10.1097/01.gme.0000243566.25205.0b.
20. Yao P, Bennett D, Mafham M, Lin X, Chen Z, Armitage J, Clarke R. Vitamin D and calcium for the prevention of fracture: a systematic review and meta-analysis. JAMA Netw Open. 2019;2:e1917789. https://doi.org/10.1001/jamanetworkopen.2019.17789.
21. Wang F, Wang N, Gao Y, Zhou Z, Liu W, Pan C, Yin P, Yu X, Tang M. β-Carotene suppresses osteoclastogenesis and bone resorption by suppressing NF-κB signaling pathway. Life Sci. 2017;174:15–20. https://doi.org/10.1016/j.lfs.2017.03.002.
22. Wu F, Wills K, Laslett LL, Oldenburg B, Jones G, Winzenberg T. Associations of dietary patterns with bone mass, muscle strength and balance in a cohort of Australian middle-aged women. Br J Nutr. 2017;118:598–606. https://doi.org/10.1017/S0007114517002483.
23. Caan BJ, Emond JA, Su HI, Patterson RE, Flatt SW, Gold EB, Newman VA, Rock CL, Thomson CA, Pierce JP. Effect of postdiagnosis weight change on hot flash status among early-stage breast cancer survivors. J Clin Oncol. 2012;30:1492–7. https://doi.org/10.1200/JCO.2011.36.8597.
24. Grove KA, Londeree BR. Bone density in postmenopausal women: high impact vs low impact exercise. Med Sei Sports Exerc. 1992;24:1190–4.
25. Shah R. Approches to the prevention of bone health throughout life, target osteoporosis. IMS Insight. 2009;(3):39–46.
26. Bonaiuti D, Cranney A, Iovine R, Kemper HH, Negrini S, Robinson V, et al. Effects of exercise programme on quality of life in osteoporotic and osteopenic postmenopausal women: a systemic review and meta-analysis. Cochrane Database Syst Rev. 2002;2:CD000333.
27. Burleson MH, Todd M, Trevathan WR. Daily vasomotor symptoms, sleep problems, and mood: using daily data to evaluate the domino hypothesis in middle-aged women. Menopause. 2010;17(1):87–95. https://doi.org/10.1097/gme.0b013e3181b20b2d. PMID: 19675506.
28. Bushman BA. Menopause and exercise. ACSM Health Fitness J. 2013;17(3):4–7. https://doi.org/10.1249/FIT.0b013e31828cb232.
29. Ahuja M. Strong bones exercise programme. FOGSIFOCUS-Women and Osteoporosis. pp. 25–27.
30. Lumsden DB, Baccala A, Martire J. T'ai chi for osteoarthritis: an introduction for primary care physicians. Geriatrics. 1998;53:84–8.
31. Unni J. Third consensus meeting of Indian Menopause Society 2008: a summary. J Midlife Health. 2010;1:43–7.
32. Management of osteoporosis in postmenopausal women: 2010 position statement of The North American Menopause Society. Menopause. 2010;17:25–54.
33. Mishra N, Mishra VN, Devanshi. Exercise beyond menopause: dos and don'ts. J Midlife Health. 2011;2(2):51–6. https://doi.org/10.4103/0976-7800.92524. PMID: 22408332; PMCID: PMC3296386.

Menopause and Metabolic Syndrome

13

Sarita Agrawal, Shreya Panda, and Jyotshna Kashibhatla

13.1 Introduction

A woman's life is challenged by a series of events as she enters her fifth decade of life. While menopause is a natural part of aging, a significant effect of natural aging in women is the depletion of sex steroid hormones that may make hormone-responsive tissues such as the brain, bone, and the cardiovascular system more susceptible to diseases. At menopause there is significant increase risk of obesity, type 2 diabetes, cardiovascular diseases, and nonalcoholic fatty liver disease (NAFLD)/metabolic associated fatty liver disease (MFFLD), and metabolic syndrome (MetS).One critical aspect of menopause that has gained attention in recent years is its potential association with metabolic syndrome (MetS) and MetS being identified as good predictor of Type 2 diabetes mellitus (T2DM), coronary artery disease (CAD), and breast cancer in postmenopausal woman. The real challenge is understanding its pathogenesis and identifying effective measures to prevent it either at the level of population or at an individual level in any of the country/region. In this chapter, we will explore the relationship between menopause and metabolic syndrome, understanding the underlying mechanisms, and discuss potential preventive and management strategies to promote women's health during this transitional phase.

S. Agrawal (✉) · S. Panda · J. Kashibhatla
Department of Obstetrics and Gynecology, All India Institute of Medical Sciences, Raipur, Chhattisgarh, India
e-mail: drsaritaagrawal@aiimsraipur.edu.in

R. Garg (ed.), *Management of Menopause*,
https://doi.org/10.1007/978-981-96-0239-1_13

13.2 Metabolic Syndrome

Metabolic syndrome was initially named as "Syndrome X" by Gerald Reaven in 1988, and its features were first described by Vague in 1956. This syndrome has subsequently been termed as insulin resistance syndrome, central obesity syndrome, and deadly quartet. The prevalence of MetS ranges from 32 to 58% in postmenopausal women although it varies with country and race. It is still questionable if obesity and metabolic syndrome progress more rapidly during the transition through menopause or during the postmenopausal period. To clarify this, Gurka et al. [1] did a study on Atherosclerosis Risk in Communities cohort [2]. They concluded that during menopausal transition, women manifested rapid rise in MetS severity across the premenopausal and perimenopausal periods rather than postmenopausal period thus suggesting that higher prevalence of MetS in postmenopausal women may be caused more by changes during the menopausal transition than by postmenopause.

13.3 Diagnostic Criteria of Metabolic Syndrome

The metabolic syndrome is a "constellation of closely related risk factors that together convey substantially increased cardiovascular risk after accounting for traditional cardiovascular disease (CVD) risk factors". MetS is generally defined based on five criteria: increased waist circumference marker of central obesity, hypertension, low high-density lipoprotein-cholesterol (HDL-C), and high triglyceride (TG) concentrations and insulin resistance (IR)/hyperinsulinemi (Fig. 13.1). However, over time, different criteria have been proposed by different organizations (Table 13.1).

In 2009, there was a joint consensus of the International Diabetes Federation Task Force on Epidemiology and Prevention; the National Heart, Lung, and Blood Institute, the American Heart Association, the World Heart Federation, the International Atherosclerosis Society, and the International Association for the Study of Obesity. In this, the IDF criteria were merged with the recommendations of the AHA/NHLBI and 3 out of five criteria were required for the diagnosis of metabolic syndrome [9]. In their joint consensus they have mentioned some additional metabolic criteria in research to define metabolic syndrome (MetS) and named them as "platinum standards." These additional criteria include abnormal body fat distribution, atherogenic dyslipidemia, dysglycemia, insulin resistance, vascular dysregulation, proinflammatory state, prothrombotic state, and hormonal factors. Further research into finding the association with these factors may help in prognosticating the risk of developing cardiovascular diseases, diabetes, breast cancer, and osteoporosis.

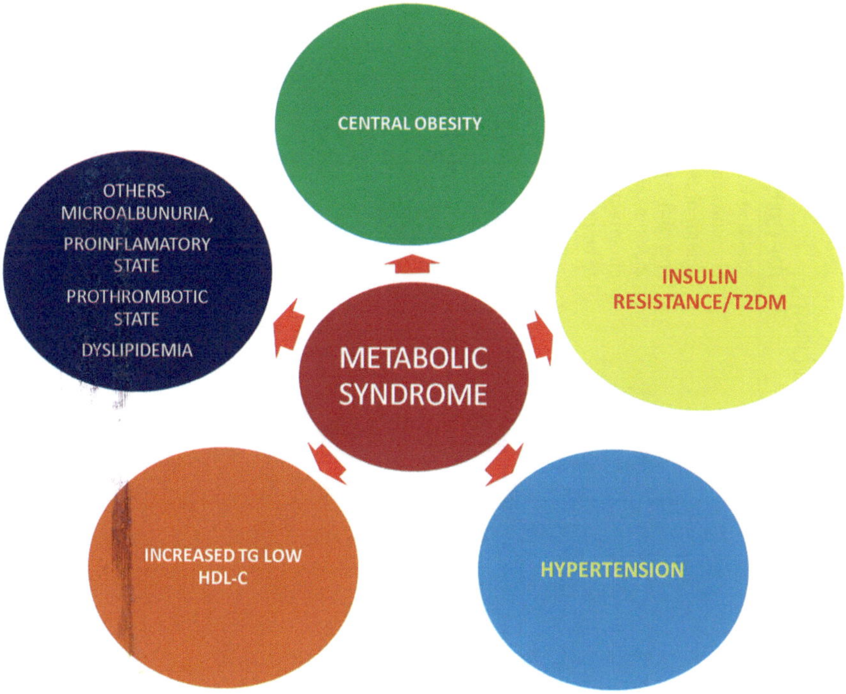

Fig. 13.1 Diagnostic criteria of metabolic syndrome

Table 13.1 Definitions of metabolic syndrome based on different criteria

	WHO (1998) [3]	NCEPT:ATPIII (2005) [4]	AACE (2003) [5]	AHA/NHLBI (2004) [6]	IDF (2005) [7, 8]
Essential criteria	Insulin resistance or its surrogates; impaired glucose tolerance IGT), or diabetes, or impaired fasting glucose (IFG) (>100 mg/dL)				Elevated waste circumference as measure of central obesity (ethnicity-specific)* if body mass index is over 30 kg/m^2, waist circumference does not need to be measured
No. of abnormalities	Plus two of the following:	≥3 of following	Any of the following based on clinical judgment:	≥3 of:	≥2 with central obesity to hormonized any of the 3
Glucose		Fasting glucose ≥100 mg/dL ≥5.6 mmols/L (includes diabetes on drugs)	IGT or IFG (but not diabetes)—Other features of IR (including family history of DM, polycystic ovary syndrome, sedentary lifestyle, advancing age, and ethnic groups susceptible to T2DM)	Fasting glucose ≥100 mg/dL or drug treatment of elevated glucose	Fasting glucose ≥100 mg/dL(5.6 mmols/L) or previously diagnosed T2DM
HDL cholesterol	HDL-C < 50 mg/dL	HDL-C <50 mg/dL in women <40 mg/dL in men, or drug treatment for low HDL-C	HDL-C < 50 mg/dL	HDL-C < 50 mg/dL or specific treatment for lipid abnormality	HDL-C < 50 mg/dL or specific treatment for lipid abnormality

	WHO (1998) [3]	NCEPT:ATPIII (2005) [4]	AACE (2003) [5]	AHA/NHLBI (2004) [6]	IDF (2005) [7, 8]
Triglycerides	≥150 mg/dL	≥1.7 mmols/L (≥150 mg/dL)	≥150 mg/dL	≥150 mg/dL or specific treatment for this lipid abnormality	≥150 mg/dL or specific treatment for this lipid abnormality
Obesity	Abdominal obesity (waist-to-hip ratio >0.9 in men or >0.85 in women, or body mass index (BMI) > 30 kg/m^2	WC > 88 cm in women (35 inch), >102 cm in men	BMI ≥ 25 kg/m^2	WC > 88 cm	Ethnicity-specific in south Asian women >80 cm
Hypertension	≥140/90 mmHg	≥130/85 mmHg or drug treatment for HT	≥130/85 mmHg	≥130/85 mmHg or antihypertensive drug treatment	≥130/85 mmHg or antihypertensive drug treatment
Other	Microalbuminuria: urinary albumin excretion ratio ≥ 20 μg/min or albumin: creatinine ratio ≥ 30 mg/g				

WHO World Health Organization, *NCEPT:ATPIII* the National Cholesterol Education Program Adult Treatment Panel III, *AACE* American Association of Clinical Endocrinologists, *AHA/NHLBI* American Heart Association/National Heart Lung and Blood Institute, *IDF* International Diabetes Federation

13.4 Pathophysiology Underlying Metabolic Syndrome in Menopause

Various studies done till date suggest that the elevated risk of metabolic disorders in women after menopause is contributed by both menopause and temporal aging. Several cross-sectional studies in Europe and Asia have demonstrated an association between metabolic syndrome and menopause. The Study of Women's Health Across Nation (SWAN STUDY) [10] reported the association as independent of aging, ethnicity, BMI, physical activity, and education. The major factors contributing for menopausal metabolic syndrome are transition from predominant estrogen state to predominant androgen state, insulin resistance, central obesity, and altered lipid metabolism. The mechanisms involved in all these are as below:

- Large amounts of androgens are secreted by ovaries for several years after menopause, and also it has been observed that transition from estrogenic state to androgenic state occurs due to increased levels of gonadotropins [11]. Moreover, sex hormone-binding globulin is also decreased with falling levels of estrogen which in turn increases the free androgen levels.
- As estrogen levels decreases, visceral adipocytes express more androgen receptors due to downregulation, thus become more sensitive to androgens and promote visceral fat accumulation. More the bioavailability of testosterone, more is the visceral fat accumulation.
- Furthermore, it is also studied that FSH receptors are expressed in visceral adipocytes. The signaling of these adipocytes could in turn increase lipid synthesis in adipocytes and leptin levels and decrease adiponectin in serum, thus aiding fat accumulation [12].
- It has been shown that insulin activates stem cells of the hypothalamic-pituitary androgen (HPA) axis by enhancing their proliferation and differentiation, leading to augmented hormone production. Also, chronic metabolic stress leads to hyperactivation of the HPA axis.
- The decrease in insulin sensitivity with aging is thought to be largely explained by an increase in adiposity, although aging also results in a decrease in muscle mitochondrial function [6]. Against these views, there are some studies which reflect no effect of age on development of insulin resistance and metabolic syndrome [13]. Thus the increase in insulin resistance can be attributed to the relative hypoestrogenism, developed after menopause.
- Estradiol has been shown in a recent study to enhance glucagon-like peptide-1 secretion through ERb binding, and ovariectomized mice exhibited impaired glucose tolerance during oral glucose tolerance tests (OGTTs), which was associated with decreased GLP-1, highlighting the potential beneficial role of the

estrogenic pathway and, more particularly, of ERβ agonists to prevent type 2 diabetes [14].

- Adipose tissues become more lipolytic in menopause due to absence of estrogen. Visceral adipocytes secrete adipose-specific cytokines which are proatherogenic such as leptin and visfatin and also inflammatory cytokines such as tumor necrosis factor-α, interleukin (IL)-6, prothrombotic factors [plasminogen activator inhibitor 1 (PAI-1)], and vasoconstrictor factors (angiotensin II). Thus, the propensity of visceral adipose tissue for increased inflammation and the subsequent secretion of cytokines that impair insulin signaling may significantly contribute to systemic insulin resistance in central obesity. Visceral adipose tissue also accumulates macrophages that release inflammatory cytokines, which can impair insulin sensitivity [15].
- These hormonal alterations potentially cause hyperinsulinemia, which further increases visceral obesity resulting in lipid dysregulation, hypertension, and Type 2 Diabetes Mellitus. The concentration of serum cortisol has been found to have a stronger correlation with waist circumference, waist-to-hip ratio, triglycerides (TG), total cholesterol (TC), and leptin levels in women with metabolic syndrome (MetS), compared to men. This relationship persists even after adjusting for age and BMI. It is suggested that leptin may have a greater impact on the hypothalamic-pituitary-adrenal (HPA) axis in women than in men [16].
- Studies have indicated that in the general population, lower adiponectin levels are linked to insulin resistance,T2DM and coronary artery disease (CAD) [17]. Most of the adipokines have proinflammatory properties but adiponectin exhibits insulin-sensitizing, anti-inflammatory, anti-atherogenic, cardioprotective, and anti-oxidative stress effects. Here the point to be noted is that adiponectin levels are strongly determined by body composition and are mainly inversely associated with visceral fat, total body fat, body mass index (BMI), and waist circumference.
- In surgical menopause, where both ovaries are removed, there is a rapid decrease in estrogen levels. This results in endothelial dysfunction, an increase in atherogenic lipoproteins, and enhanced lipid oxidation. These changes in lipid metabolism can contribute to the development of metabolic syndrome. The HUNT2 study found that women who underwent bilateral oophorectomy before the age of 50 had a higher prevalence of metabolic syndrome compared to those who did not.

13.5 Effect of Menopausal Changes on Body Metabolism

Key metabolic issues and their impact are shown in Fig. 13.2 and Table 13.2.

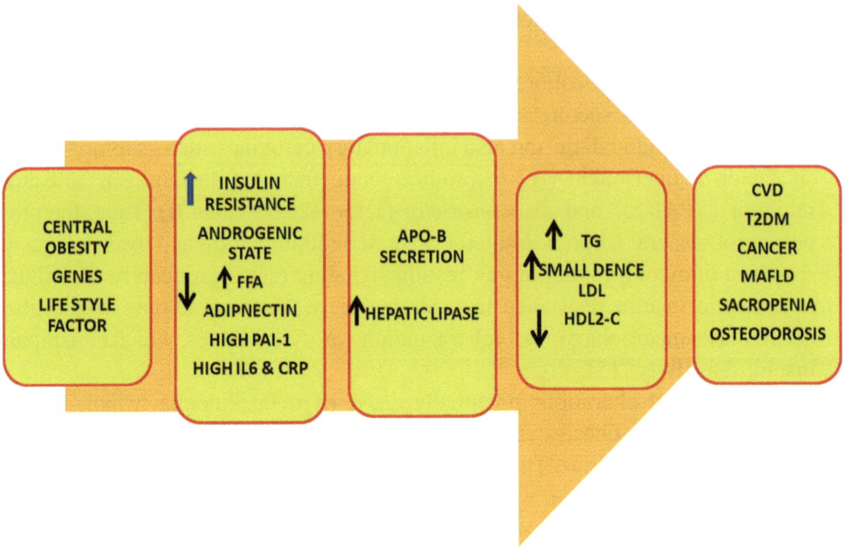

Fig. 13.2 Pathophysiology of metabolic syndrome

Table 13.2 Metabolic abnormalities and associated pathology due to menopausal changes

Metabolic abnormalities	Resulting clinical condition
• Impaired glucose handling/ insulin resistance • Atherogenic dyslipidemia and endothelial dysfunction • Excess ovarian testosterone production • Prothrombotic state • Pro-inflammatory state	• Type 2 diabetes • Essential hypertension • Nonalcoholic fatty liver disease • Central obesity • Cardiovascular disease (myocardial Infraction (MI), peripheral vascular disease (PVD), stroke) • Cancer breast

13.6 Abdominal Obesity

During reproductive years, the fat deposition is concentrated across the periphery in gluteo-femoral region (gynoid or pear shape) is the characteristic of estrogen. After menopause the basic change that occurs is increase in central adiposity as intra-/peri-abdominal fat (android or apple shape) which is characteristic of androgens. Even in the absence of weight gain, body fat distribution changes across the menopause. In perimenopausal period, women with high amounts of visceral fat have an excess of cardiovascular mortality and associated metabolic abnormalities. The reductions in exercise capacity and activity may contribute to reduced muscle mass and increased central adiposity with menopause. Central obesity has emerged as a cardiovascular risk factor independent of overall obesity.

13.7 Lipid Metabolism

High levels of abdominal fat are linked to increased insulin resistance, elevated free fatty acid (FFA) levels, and reduced adiponectin. These factors trigger secretion of Apolipoprotein B containing particles and hepatic lipase. These cause increase in triglyceride levels, increase in small dense low-density lipoprotein (LDL) particles, and decrease in large anti-atherogenic HDL2 particles. The predominance of small, dense LDL particles is associated with a greater risk of myocardial infarction and the progression of cardiovascular disease (CVD). Women with small, dense LDL than in those with large, buoyant LDL [18].

Lindquist et al. reported a prospective increase in TG levels in women who became postmenopausal during a 6-year period, whereas there was no change in TG in the similarly aged women who remained either premenopausal or postmenopausal. TG levels increase with the transition through menopause, and the increase in TG also appears early in the postmenopausal period.

Menopausal changes in HDL metabolism are more complex than the measurement of total HDL reveals, because the more anti-atherogenic cardioprotective HDL2 levels decrease, whereas HDL3 levels increase.

13.8 Insulin Resistance

We have already discussed how insulin resistance develops in menopause. The underlying pathophysiology of insulin resistance is multifaceted and is reinforced by dysregulated lipid metabolism. Insulin resistance, with inadequate compensatory hyperinsulinemia, diminishes the normal suppression of free fatty acids arising from adipose tissue by insulin. The increased levels of FFA may impair peripheral glucose uptake, increase hepatic gluconeogenesis, and reduce hepatic clearance of insulin [18].

13.9 Fibrinolytic and Inflammatory Markers

Fibrinolytic activity is regulated by a balance between plasminogen activators (tPA) and plasminogen activator inhibitors (PAI-1). PAI-1, which is produced by the liver and adipose tissue—especially visceral fat—has been identified as a marker of insulin resistance. With increase in visceral fat in menopause, elevated PAI-1 activity causes prolonged clot lysis times and potentiates thrombosis. High PAI-1 activity is associated with high plasma levels of tPA antigen (which represents t-PA/PAI-1 complexes), which has been found to be independently associated with CVD. Postmenopausal women have higher levels of PAI-1 and tPA antigen than premenopausal women. These data imply that estrogen deficiency and increased visceral adiposity are associated with a decrease in fibrinolytic potential. Given that PAI-1 is positively associated with abdominal fat content and plasma TG, higher PAI-1 levels with menopause may be a marker of women at higher risk of CVD[18].

Similarly inflammatory markers like IL-6 and CRP have positive correlation with abdominal fat and hence are predictors of cardiovascular disease in menopausal women.

13.10 Long-Term Consequences

13.10.1 Cardiovascular Disease

It has been also observed that the CVD risk is significantly increased after menopause, which may be a consequence of menopausal changes in sex hormones, menopausal disturbances in cardiometabolic parameters, as well as chronological aging. Women develop CVD 10 years later than men, with a marked increase after the age of 45–54 years. The mechanism by which MetS increases the risk of CVD is the result of a combination of several different disturbances that intensify atherosclerosis, such as IR, dyslipidemia, peripheral vasoconstriction, and prothrombotic and proinflammatory states. As previously explained, abdominal obesity is more pronounced in postmenopausal women than the changes in the lipid profile that are more atherogenic (increased concentration of small HDL and small dense LDL particles). Additionally, hypertension is a further risk factor for CVD. It remains unclear whether menopause is a universal CVD risk factor for all women or if it primarily affects those genetically predisposed to central obesity.

13.10.2 Type 2 Diabetes Mellitus

MetS is commonly associated with IR and abdominal obesity, which are important pathogenetic factors for prediabetes and T2DM. It has been also observed that IGT was a stronger predictor of diabetes. Additionally, hypertension is a further risk factor for CVD. It remains unclear whether menopause is a universal CVD risk factor for all women or if it primarily affects those genetically predisposed to central obesity.

13.10.3 Breast Cancer

There are several potential mechanisms explaining the positive association between MetS and the risk of breast cancer. Firstly, increased abdominal obesity leads to a greater conversion of androgens to estrogens in adipocytes of postmenopausal women. Moreover, obese insulin-resistant postmenopausal women had lower concentration of SHBG, which is increasing the concentration of free E2, a more biologically active fraction of E2, which is strongly associated with the risk of breast cancer. Secondly, the IR state with a chronic hyperinsulinemia is associated with decreased concentrations of the insulin-like growth factor binding protein1 and IGFBP-2, leading to an increased availability of IGF-I, which may promote cell proliferation in mammary epithelial cells and breast cancer cell lines. Third, abdominal obesity is associated with higher leptin production and lower adiponectin production. Leptin has been found to stimulate tumor cell proliferation, while adiponectin inhibits it. Studies have shown that individual components of MetS are not significantly associated with breast cancer risk, in contrast to the full diagnosis of MetS [19].

13.10.4 Osteoporosis

The association between MetS and osteoporosis is controversial. While some studies have reported lower bone mineral density (BMD) in women with MetS, others have found higher BMD values associated with the condition [20, 21]. Low adiponectin levels and elevated leptin levels have been linked to bone loss. The effect of insulin resistance (IR) on osteoporosis is also mixed. Hyperinsulinemia was recognized as a protective factor, but the IR state was found to be a risk factor for osteoporosis.

13.11 Metabolic Associated Fatty Liver Disease (MAFLD)/ Nonalcoholic Fatty Liver Disease (NAFLD)

In 2020, the term "metabolic-associated fatty liver disease" (MAFLD) was introduced to highlight the role of metabolic abnormalities in fatty liver disease [20]. NAFLD and MAFLD have been used interchangeably, although there is some thought that the definition of MAFLD is more effective than for differentiating FLD patients with high risk of progression. MAFLD could be diagnosed when radiological evidence of hepatic steatosis is accompanied by three metabolic abnormalities: overweight/obesity, DM, or metabolic dysregulation. Visceral fat accumulation is one of the characteristics of FLD. Overweight, obesity, dyslipidemia, insulin resistance, type 2 DM, and sedentary behavior accompanied by lack of physical activity, which are closely related to factors of MetS, are the major causes of the increasing trend of NAFLD/MAFLD worldwide [22].

13.11.1 Sarcopenia

Sarcopenia is characterized by a decline in both the quantity and quality of skeletal muscle and muscle function, and it is particularly common in older adults. Skeletal muscle is relevant to major organs involved in insulin-induced glucose metabolism, and loss of muscle mass is associated with IR and MetS. Skeletal muscle loss and intramuscular fat accumulation cause abnormal muscle contractility and metabolic abnormalities and are thought to be related to various factors, such as oxidative stress, inflammatory cytokines, mitochondrial dysfunction, and insulin resistance [23].

Evaluation for Metabolic Syndrome: Measuring some easily measurable obesity indices, including waist circumference (WC), waist height ratio (WHtR), and waist hip ratio (WHR), in routine practice and monitoring may help to predict the risk early and allow for intervention at an appropriate time to prevent morbidity and mortality associated with these changes in postmenopausal women (Table 13.3).

13.12 Management of Metabolic Disorders in Postmenopausal Women

13.12.1 Prevention of Metabolic Disorders

As we know, the root cause of metabolic syndrome in menopausal women is obesity. So lifestyle modifications, physical activity, and calorie-balanced diet would help in preventing adverse consequences of menopause. A healthy lifestyle with regular moderate physical activity can reverse the changes arising due to metabolic syndrome and improve cardiovascular health.

Physical activity: As abdominal obesity with visceral fat deposition in the prime culprit, it should be targeted with aerobic exercises, walking or endurance exercises. They also help in increasing insulin sensitivity. Regular exercises aiming for at least 150 min of moderate-intensity aerobic activity or 75 min of

Table 13.3 Evaluation of a menopausal woman with metabolic syndrome

General physical examination	Laboratory	Imaging
• Weight gain • Hypertension • Body mass index • Markers for central obesity • Waist circumference (WC) • Hip circumference (HC) • Waste hip ratio (WHR) • Waist height ratio (WHtR) • Lipid accumulation product(LAP): WC (cm) – 58 × TG (mmol/L) • Body shape index: [WC (cm)]/[BMI 2/3 × height (cm) 1/2] • Body roundness index (BRI)	Fasting glucose, lipid profile—HDL-C and TG levels **Additional test** corresponding to the "platinum standards"; markers for risk of CVD; however, they are not essential for diagnosis of MetS: • S. fasting insulin, • apolipoprotein B • non-HDL-C, • low-density lipoprotein • free fatty acid, • HOMA-IR • C-reactive protein, IL6 • fibrinolytic factors clotting factors • **SHBG** • microalbuminuria	**Imaging may be performed but not essential** • DEXA Scan, for the distribution of body fat • Computed tomography or magnetic resonance imaging to determine central fat distribution • Magnetic resonance spectroscopy to check the liver fat content • ECG, 2D-echo

vigorous-intensity aerobic activity per week, along with muscle-strengthening activities on 2 or more days a week, have been shown to be effective. Yoga is a form traditional medicine practiced for more than 4000 years. It is a mind-body discipline that has been successfully used in India for the prevention and management of hypertension, diabetes, and related chronic insulin resistance conditions associated with aging. Apart from yoga, other traditional active mind-body modalities, such as qigong and tai chi chuan (tai chi), may also have promise for the prevention of CVD in postmenopausal women and other at-risk populations. Qigong has many forms; blending meditation and controlled breathing techniques with precise gentle movements and postures have been practiced for hundreds of years by emperors to achieve health and longevity. Tai chi is an ancient Chinese martial art; multiple styles of tai chi (Chen, Yang, Old Wu, Wu, and Sun) all combine deep diaphragmatic breathing with specific postures that are performed in a coordinated, dance-like sequence of slow, graceful movements. Due to the typically slow pace, gentle nature, and low-impact movements characterizing tai chi and qigong, these practices are particularly appropriate for older individuals [24].

Diet: It is a key factor for promoting healthy weight loss and thereby preventing metabolic syndrome. A calorie-restricted diet with low saturated fats and high fiber is found to promote weight loss. Along with this a diet rich in essential nutrients like iron, calcium, and vitamins B6, C, and E was found to be beneficial in preventing metabolic syndrome. The prevalence of MetS in postmenopausal women was significantly lower in women who ate a healthy diet than in those who ate a Western diet [25].The Mediterranean diet is considered particularly healthy in terms of reduced CVD and metabolic risk in contrast with the Western diet. In addition, supplementation, such as foods rich in vitamin D, omega-3 fatty acids, antioxidants, phytochemicals, and probiotics, is recommended for MetS, but further research is needed [26]. Placing an emphasis on whole foods, such as fresh produce, whole grains, lean meats, and healthy fats with reduced consumption of processed foods, sweet drinks, and high-fat snacks in consultation with a registered dietitian for personalized dietary advice, is recommended.

Other preventive strategies include weight reduction, stress reduction techniques, staying hydrated, adequate sleep, quitting smoking, and limiting alcohol intake.

13.13 Treatment of Metabolic Syndrome

In addition to life style modification strategies, the medical management is required for the treatment of various components of metabolic syndrome including hypertension, dyslipidemia, and Type 2 diabetes mellitus. ATP III guidelines—at a glance quick desk reference may be referred while managing metabolic syndrome available at https://www.nhlbi.nih.gov/files/docs/guidelines/atglance.pdf. The target goals for various MetS component as per ATP III guidelines are shown in Table 13.4.

Table 13.4 Target goals for various MetS component as per ATP III guidelines

Targeted area	Goal
CHD and CHD risk equivalent *(10-year risk for CHD >20%)*	<100 mg/dL
Multiple (2+) risk factors and 10-year risk <20%	<130 mg/dL
Institute weight control	−10% from baseline
Institute physical activity	30–60 min/day for 3–7 days/week
Monitor treatment of hypertension	<130/85 mmHg

13.14 Drugs for Hyperglycemia

Diabetes prevention program reported that metformin treatment in patients with prediabetes delayed the development of diabetes mellitus and reduced the cardiovascular mortality in patients with metabolic syndrome. It acts by the activation of AMPK, which plays an important role in the pathogenesis of metabolic syndrome. STOP NIDDM trial has reported that acarbose (α-glucosidase Inhibitor) reduces the progression of impaired glucose tolerance to diabetes mellitus and also reduces the development of cardiovascular disease and hypertension. In the SCALE diabetes trial, liraglutide (glucagon-like peptide-1 analog) apart from treating hyperglycemia showed a mean weight reduction of 6.4 kg when compared to the placebo group which had only 2.2 kg reduction. Thus, the GLP-1 analog is one of the most appropriate treatments for metabolic syndrome [26]. In SELECT trial [27] a randomized, placebo-controlled trial involving patients with preexisting cardiovascular disease and overweight or obesity but without diabetes found that weekly subcutaneous semaglutide at a dose of 2.4 mg was superior to placebo in reducing the incidence of a composite of death from cardiovascular causes with benefit of reducing weight by 9.4%, TG by 18%, and LDL by 5%, and increasing HDL by 4.5% considering this later on reduction weight is added as a new indication for this drug.

13.15 Drugs for Dyslipidemia

The recommended treatment goal is to have low-density lipoprotein (LDL)-c levels less than 130 mg/dL, with an option of target level less than 100 mg/dL in patients with a high risk of cardiovascular morbidity. A study of patients with metabolic syndrome revealed that monotherapy with rosuvastatin had a reduction in the biopsy score for lobar inflammation from 3 to 1, a complete regression of metabolic syndrome, and a large reduction in the plasma glucose. In the same study, a follow-up biopsy taken after 18 months showed no signs of nonalcoholic steatohepatitis (NASH) or metabolic syndrome relapse [28]. Fibrates activate PPAR-α and regulate gene expression that affects fatty acid and lipoprotein metabolism in the skeletal muscle, liver, and kidney and shown to improve microalbuminuria and reduction in cardiovascular risk. Nicotinic acid and fibric acid derivatives are frequently used with statin medications, but caution should be used in combining these drugs. Antagomirs (cholesterol-conjugated antisense oligonucleotides) which target and silence miRNAs, as evidenced by hepatic *miR-122* blockade in vivo [29], have already been successfully tested in a phase I clinical trial. Further studies are needed to explore the full potential of miRNAs as novel biomarkers and therapeutic agents against MetS.

Drugs for Hypertension: All the components of metabolic syndrome activate the renin-angiotensin system, which makes angiotensin receptor blockers and angiotensinogen-converting enzyme inhibitors ideal for treating high blood pressure in these patients [30].

Drugs for Prothrombotic State: Aspirin therapy can be recommended especially when the C-reactive protein levels are above the normal range.

Bariatric Intervention: This can be an option in managing metabolic syndrome patients with body mass index (BMI) of more than 35–40 kg/m^2. It is reported that a reduction in BMI up to 12–14 kg/m^2 decreased the risk of diabetes up to three times and the risk of hypertension and hyperlipidemia up to two times, but only a limited number of trials had good-quality long-term data. The most commonly used bariatric interventions are gastric banding, Roux-en-Y gastric bypass, vertical sleeve gastrectomy, and biliopancreatic diversion with duodenal switch.

Future Perspectives: Two important focuses in this regard are the complement system and the inflammasome [31]. Inflammasome member proteins are involved in the induction of insulin resistance and obesity. The terminal complement pathway involves the proinflammatory anaphylatoxin C5. Monoclonal antibody against C5, eculizumab has shown to effectively inhibit the progression of thrombotic microangiopathy. The final effector molecule in this pathway is IL-β whose action can be blocked with IL-β antagonists like anakinra, rilonacept, and canakinumab.

13.16 Effect of Menopausal Hormone Replacement Therapy (MHT/HRT) on Metabolic Syndrome

It has been observed in various studies that HRT has beneficial effect on various components of metabolic syndrome. The Heart and Estrogen/Progestin Replacement Study (HERS) and the Women's Health Initiative (WHI) studies showed a 35% and 21%, respectively, reduction in incidence of T2DM with HRT. However, it has also been observed that MHT either has no effect in lowering the risk of cardiovascular disease, or in some cases it may even double the risk of developing cardiovascular disease. Having said this, it is also proposed that the age of postmenopausal women and type of HRT (oral or transdermal) can modulate the effect of HRT on CVD risk. One of the remarkable studies is a large meta-analysis by Salpeter et al. [32], summarizing the data from 107 trials with 33,315 subjects, it was seen that HRT increased lean body mass and reduced abdominal fat, HOMA-IR values, and new-onset diabetes in women without diabetes. In the influence of HRT on lipid parameters, blood pressure, inflammation, and thrombotic markers were indifferent to diabetes. HRT increased HDL-C and reduced LDL-C, LDL-C/HDL-C ratio, Lp(a), fibrinogen, and PAI-1. In general, oral therapy had a more favorable effect on these parameters than transdermal therapy. However, oral preparations may increase triglycerides and C-reactive protein which is the major drawback. It was also suggested that the reductions in MetS parameters with HRT could have a more favorable impact on arteriosclerosis, if this therapy is used in healthier and younger postmenopausal women.

Women who are thinking about using MHT should have a thorough conversation with their healthcare practitioner to examine the possible advantages and disadvantages as well as other options for promoting their general health and well-being throughout menopause. Individual reactions to MHT might differ depending on the patient; thus a tailored strategy is necessary with consideration to choice of MHT, duration (long term/short term), and need for HRT. Menopausal women should have regular health checkups to monitor blood pressure, glucose levels, lipid profiles, and other relevant indicators [33].

13.17 Conclusion

Menopause is a significant life transition for women, and understanding its potential association with metabolic syndrome and related adverse health consequences, it is crucial to screen women during perimenopause and menopause for the cardiometabolic risk factors and implementing preventative strategies for improved health and longevity in women. Because MHT improves many of the components of MetS, some consideration should also be given to including MHT as part of this overall prevention strategy. By adopting healthy lifestyle habits and seeking appropriate medical guidance, women can navigate this phase with reduced risks of metabolic syndrome and associated health complications. As research continues to advance, our understanding of menopause and metabolic syndrome, ongoing efforts in education, prevention, and personalized care will continue to empower women to make informed decisions and embrace a healthier and more fulfilling postmenopausal life. Ultimately, through a combination of lifestyle modifications, medical interventions, and holistic support, women can confidently face the challenges of menopause and metabolic syndrome, promoting optimal health and well-being in their later years.

References

1. Gurka MJ, Vishnu A, Santen RJ, et al. Progression of metabolic syndrome severity during the menopausal transition. J Am Heart Assoc. 2016;5:e003609. https://doi.org/10.1161/JAHA.116.003609.
2. The Atherosclerosis Risk in Communities (ARIC) study: design and objectives. The ARIC investigators. Am J Epidemiol. 1989;129(4):687–702. PMID: 2646917.
3. Alberti KG, Zimmet PZ. Definition, diagnosis and classification of diabetes mellitus and its complications. Part 1: diagnosis and classification of diabetes mellitus provisional report of a WHO consultation. Diabet Med. 1998;15:539–53. https://doi.org/10.1002/(SICI)1096-9136(199807)15:7<539::AID-DIA668>3.0.CO;2-S.

4. Saklayen MG. The global epidemic of the metabolic syndrome. Curr Hypertens Rep. 2018;20(2):12. https://doi.org/10.1007/s11906-018-0812-z. PMID: 29480368; PMCID: PMC5866840.
5. Einhorn D, Reaven GM, Cobin RH, Ford E, Ganda OP, Handelsman Y, Hellman R, Jellinger PS, Kendall D, Krauss RM, et al. American College of Endocrinology position statement on the insulin resistance syndrome. Endocr Pract. 2003;9:237–52.
6. Grundy SM, Cleeman JI, Daniels SR, Donato KA, Eckel RH, Franklin BA, Gordon DJ, Krauss RM, Savage PJ, Smith SC Jr, et al. Diagnosis and management of the metabolic syndrome: an American Heart Association/National Heart, Lung, and Blood Institute scientific statement. Circulation. 2005;112:2735–52.
7. Alberti KG, Zimmet P, Shaw J, IDF Epidemiology Task Force Consensus Group. The metabolic syndrome—A new worldwide definition. Lancet. 2005;366:1059–62.
8. Alberti KGMM, Zimmet P, Shaw J. Metabolic syndrome—a new world-wide definition. A consensus statement from the international diabetes federation. Diabet Med. 2006;23(5):469–80.
9. Alberti KG, Eckel RH, Grundy SM, Zimmet PZ, Cleeman JI, Donato KA, Fruchart JC, James WP, Loria CM, Smith SC Jr. Harmonizing the metabolic syndrome: a joint interim statement of the International Diabetes Federation Task Force on Epidemiology and Prevention; National Heart, Lung, and Blood Institute; American Heart Association; World Heart Federation; International Atherosclerosis Society; and International Association for the Study of Obesity. Circulation. 2009;120:1640–5.
10. Scuteri A, Vuga M, Najjar SS, Mehta V, Everson-Rose SA, Sutton-Tyrrell K, Matthews K, Lakatta EG. Education eclipses ethnicity in predicting the development of the metabolic syndrome in different ethnic groups in midlife: the Study of Women's Health Across the Nation (SWAN). Diabet Med. 2008;25(12):1390–9. https://doi.org/10.1111/j.1464-5491.2008.02596.x. PMID: 19046236; PMCID: PMC2607571.
11. Thurston RC, Sowers MR, Chang Y, Sternfeld B, Gold EB, Johnston JM, Matthews KA. Adiposity and reporting of vasomotor symptoms among midlife women: the study of women's health across the nation. Am J Epidemiol. 2008;167:78–85.
12. Liu XM, Chan HC, Ding GL, Cai J, Song Y, Wang TT, Zhang D, Chen H, Yu MK, Wu YT, et al. FSH regulates fat accumulation and redistribution in aging through the Gαi/Ca(2+)/CREB pathway. Aging Cell. 2015;14:409–20.
13. Christakis MK, Hasan H, De Souza LR, Shirreff L. The effect of menopause on metabolic syndrome: cross-sectional results from the Canadian Longitudinal Study on Aging. Menopause. 2020;27:999–1009.
14. Handgraaf S, Dusaulcy R, Visentin F, et al. 17-b estradiol regulates proglucagon-derived peptide secretion in mouse and human a- and L cells. JCI Insight. 2018;3:e98569. https://doi.org/10.1173/jci.insight.98569.
15. Hardy OT, Czech MP, Corvera S. What causes the insulin resistance underlying obesity? Curr Opin Endocrinol Diabetes Obes. 2012;19(2):81–7. https://doi.org/10.1097/MED.0b013e3283514e13.
16. Stefanska A, Bergmann K, Sypniewska G. Metabolic syndrome and menopause: pathophysiology, clinical and diagnostic significance. Adv Clin Chem. 2015;72:1–75.
17. Kuo I-C, Wu P-H, Lin HY-H, Niu S-W, Huang J-C, Hung C-C, et al. The association of adiponectin with metabolic syndrome and clinical outcome in patients with non-diabetic chronic kidney disease. PLoS One. 2019;14(7):e0220158.
18. Carr MC. The emergence of the metabolic syndrome with menopause. J Clin Endocrinol Metabol. 2003;88(6):2404–11.
19. Esposito K, Chiodini P, Capuano A, Bellastella G, Maiorino MI, Rafaniello C, et al. Metabolic syndrome and postmenopausal breast cancer: systematic review and meta-analysis. Menopause. 2013;20(12):1301–9.
20. Hwang DK, Choi HJ. The relationship between low bone mass and metabolic syndrome in Korean women. Osteoporos Int. 2010;21:425–31.
21. Park KK, Kim SJ, Moon ES. Association between bone mineral density and metabolic syndrome in postmenopausal Korean women. Gynecol Obstet Invest. 2010;69:145–52.

22. Molina-Molina E, Furtado GE, Jones JG, Portincasa P, Vieira-Pedrosa A, Teixeira AM, Barros MP, Bachi ALL, Sardao VA. The advantages of physical exercise as a preventive strategy against NAFLD in postmenopausal women. Eur J Clin Invest. 2022;52:e13731.
23. Rubio-Ruiz ME, Guarner-Lans V, Pérez-Torres I, Soto ME. Mechanisms underlying metabolic syndrome-related sarcopenia and possible therapeutic measures. Int J Mol Sci. 2019;20:647.
24. Park CH, Malavasi LM, Wen HJ, et al. Qi gong and tai chi: strategies for developing and implementing community-based programs for older adults: 2300. Med Sci Sports Exerc. 2007;39(5 Suppl):S420.
25. Cho YA, Kim J, Cho ER, Shin A. Dietary patterns and the prevalence of metabolic syndrome in Korean women. Nutr Metab Cardiovasc Dis. 2011;21:893–900.
26. Chatterjee S, Ghosal S, Chatterjee S. Glucagon-like peptide-1 receptor agonists favorably address all components of metabolic syndrome. World J Diabetes. 2016;7(18):441–5. https://doi.org/10.4239/wjd.v7.i18.441.
27. Michael Lincoff A, Brown-Frandsen K, Colhoun HM, Deanfield J, et al. Semaglutide and cardiovascular outcomes in obesity without diabetes. N Engl J Med. 2023;389(24):2221–32. https://doi.org/10.1056/NEJMoa2307563.
28. Kargiotis K. Resolution of non-alcoholic steatohepatitis by rosuvastatin monotherapy in patients with metabolic syndrome. World J Gastroenterol. 2015;21(25):7860. https://doi.org/10.3748/wjg.v21.i25.7860.
29. Krützfeldt J, Rajewsky N, Braich R, Rajeev KG, Tuschl T, Manoharan M, Stoffel M. Silencing of microRNAs in vivo with 'antagomirs'. Nature. 2005;438(7068):685–9. https://doi.org/10.1038/nature04303. Epub 2005 Oct 30. PMID: 16258535.
30. De Kloet AD, Krause EG, Woods SC. The renin angiotensin system and the metabolic syndrome. Physiol Behav. 2010;100(5):525–34. https://doi.org/10.1016/j.physbeh.2010.03.018.
31. Vimala A, Raman PP, Umamaheswari S. Pathogenesis, diagnosis, and management of metabolic syndrome: a comprehensive review. SBV J Basic Clin Appl Health Sci. 2021;4(2):39–45.
32. Salpeter SR, Walsh JM, Ormiston TM, Greyber E, Buckley NS, Salpeter EE. Meta-analysis: effect of hormone-replacement therapy on components of the metabolic syndrome in postmenopausal women, diabetes. Obes Metab. 2006;8:538–54.
33. Jeong HG, Park H. Metabolic disorders in menopause. Metabolites. 2022;12:954.

Cognitive Behavior Therapy in Menopause

14

Cipta Pramana, Soetrisno Soetrisno, and Noor Pramono

14.1 Introduction

Menopause is a physiological change experienced by all women in the process of changing towards old age and a point at the end of the reproductive period. The World Health Organization (WHO) estimates that the number of postmenopausal women worldwide will reach 1.2 billion by 2030, and as many as 47 million women enter the menopause stage each year [1]. The menopausal transition brings with it problems related to the quality of life due to psychological and somatic disorders, and efforts to prevent and control diseases must be carried out [2].

The most frequently recommended treatment for menopausal symptoms is hormonal therapy and is quite effective, especially for vasomotor symptoms and sexual problems. Antidepressants are also effective for treating depression. However, hormonal therapy has unfavorable side effects such as coronary heart disease, venous thromboembolism, and endometrial cancer. Thus, women and healthcare providers will seek effective non-pharmacological treatments [3, 4].

Nonhormonal therapy options can reduce stress with psychological intervention methods such as cognitive behavioral therapy (CBT), behavioral therapy (BT), and mindfulness-based therapies (MBTs) which are possible mechanisms to overcome

C. Pramana (✉)
Department of Obstetrics and Gynecology, KRMT Wongsonegoro Hospital, Semarang, Indonesia

Faculty of Medicine, Universitas Islam Negeri Walisongo, Semarang, Indonesia

S. Soetrisno
Faculty of Medicine, Department of Obstetrics and Gynecology, Universitas Sebelas Maret, Surakarta, Indonesia

N. Pramono
Faculty of Medicine, Department of Obstetrics and Gynecology, Diponegoro University, Semarang, Indonesia

R. Garg (ed.), *Management of Menopause*,
https://doi.org/10.1007/978-981-96-0239-1_14

these problems. Cognitive behavioral therapy (CBT) was originally developed for patients with anxiety and depression disorders. In recent years CBT has also been used to treat insomnia and chronic pain but can now be used for the treatment of women with menopausal symptoms, such as vasomotor symptoms and sleep problems. CBT is a structured psychotherapy program, which is effective in various health problems and mental disorders so that it can be a safe choice for complaints of hot flashes and other vasomotor symptoms such as those complained of by menopausal women [5].

14.2 Signs and Symptoms of Menopause

With increasing life expectancy for women, including in developing countries, one-third to half of women live as postmenopause. So postmenopausal women's health problems need to get very important attention in healthcare centers. Menopausal symptoms result due to a decrease in estrogen levels as women approach menopause. Menopause is associated with changes in body metabolism and causes comorbidities in some middle-aged women or women's general health and psychosocial behavior. Some of the symptoms of estrogen deficiency include disturbances in menstrual patterns, hot flushes, night sweats, genital atrophy, fast and irregular heartbeat, mood swings, sleep disturbances, headaches, muscle aches, joint pain, and problems with concentration and memory. Symptoms and complications of menopause affect a woman's psychological, physical, and emotional well-being, as well as social functioning and family relationships. Quality of life will decrease due to the combination of all these effects [1, 6, 7].

The prevalence and severity of menopausal symptoms differ according to age, marital status, race/ethnicity, geographic location, presence of chronic disease, level and amount and type of physical activity, parity, self-perception of health, and menopausal status [7].

The symptoms that appear in menopausal women are:

14.2.1 Vasomotor Symptoms

Vasomotor symptoms are the main initial symptoms that are common and increasingly disturbing. Symptoms include hot flushes, night sweats, and palpitations. These symptoms are called vasomotor symptoms due to vascular reactivity with prominent initial vasodilation. Hot flushes are temporary periods of intense heat in the upper body that are usually accompanied by sweating. The exact mechanism is unknown, but it is believed to be due to a narrowing of the hypothalamic thermoregulation zone with decreased estrogen levels, with higher norepinephrine, concomitant with lower serotonin levels and upregulation of its receptor (5-HT2A) [8, 9].

14.2.2 Mood Disturbances

Mood swings, anxiety, sleep disturbances, stress, and depression are psychological symptoms during menopausal changes. In this period, women feelings are very sensitive, impatient, and often feel tired and sad. There is a change in serotonin activity after a decrease in estrogen levels which leads to mood changes [10]. The transitional phase of menopause produces psychological, physical, and metabolic changes, which correlate with greater perceived stress [11]. Feelings of stress and anxiety can interfere with work performance and relationships, as well as reduce productivity. Stress is also a risk factor for de novo mood problems and the worsening of preexisting mood disorders during the menopause transition. Furthermore, stress during midlife may be associated with decreased overall satisfaction with life [12].

14.2.3 Genitourinary Symptoms

The urogenital organs, the vagina, the vestibule, and the trigone area of the bladder have a high number of estrogen receptors. After menopause, there is a decrease in estrogen levels, resulting in anatomical and physiological changes in the area resulting in the genitourinary syndrome of menopause (GSM). Genitourinary syndrome of menopause (GSM) is a new term for vulvovaginal atrophy (VVA) with the following complaints: dyspareunia, postcoital bleeding, itching and pain in the vulva/vagina, increased urinary frequency, urgency, nocturia, and recurrent UTI [10].

14.2.4 Osteoporosis

As a result of reduced estrogen, there is increased activity of osteoclasts, reduced activity of osteoblast, and activity of calcitonin. Estrogen is a potent antiresorptive agent on bone, hypoestrogenism in menopause marks a period of increased rate of bone resorption. Loss of estrogen decreases calcium absorption which promotes osteoclast-mediated bone resorption through the upregulation of parathyroid hormone which ultimately causes osteoporosis [8, 10].

14.2.5 Cardiovascular Disease

With the loss of the cardioprotective action of estrogen through its action on fat cells, endothelial function, and anti-inflammatory effects, postmenopausal women are more susceptible to ischemic heart disease. Women with myocardial infarction have atypical symptoms such as fatigue, shortness of breath, and atypical chest pain [8, 10].

14.3 Menopause Management

Treatment options for menopausal symptoms are as follows.

14.3.1 Hormonal Therapy

Hormone therapy with estrogen is the most effective treatment for menopausal VMS and GSM. Women with sleep or mood disorders may benefit significantly during the menopausal transition. HT therapy is considered safe and effective in low-risk women without underlying coronary heart disease or a history of breast cancer, age <60 years, and <10 years since the onset of menopause [8, 13].

14.3.2 Nonhormonal Therapy

In patients who have contraindications to HT, nonhormonal therapy should be selected. The therapies used are selective serotonin reuptake inhibitors (SSRIs), norepinephrine serotonin reuptake inhibitors (SNRIs), gabapentinoids, clonidine, oxybutynin, and neurokinin B antagonists. Paroxetine is an FDA-approved SSRI for treating moderate to severe postmenopausal VMS when given at a dose of 7.5 mg daily, lower than the dose used for psychiatric indications. Side effects include nausea, dizziness, and fatigue, which are dose-dependent [8, 14].

14.3.3 Non-Pharmacological Therapy

The MsFLASH research network conducted several trials, one of which showed that cognitive behavior therapy for insomnia (CBT-I) helped reduce insomnia [15]. Long-term benefits were observed without any effect on VMS. So, it can be concluded that cognitive behavioral therapy for insomnia should be the first-line therapy for women with middle-aged insomnia. In another MsFLASH trial, yoga compared to regular activity was shown to reduce insomnia [8].

14.4 Psychotherapy in Menopause

14.4.1 Cognitive Therapy

Cognitive therapy was first developed in the early 1960s by Aaron T. Beck, a psychiatrist. As a psychoanalyst, Beck conducted a series of experiments in the 1950s that he believed would provide scientific validation of the psychoanalytic concept of depression. He found that depressed patients displayed a characteristic negative bias in their thinking. They persistently have negative spontaneously arising cognitions (verbal or imaginal "automatic thoughts") about themselves, their world, and their future. Beck found that depressed patients rapidly improved when he shifted from free association to a more directive style of treatment in which he and his patients focused on solving current problems and engaging in collaborative empiricism. When patients solve their problems, modify their dysfunctional behaviors, and correct distortions in their thinking, they quickly experience positive change. CT has also been shown to be effective in the treatment of medical conditions such as insomnia, infertility, fibromyalgia, chronic pain, irritable bowel syndrome, erectile dysfunction, obesity, premenstrual syndrome, and migraine headaches [16].

14.4.2 Behavioral Therapy

Behavioral therapy is a newcomer to the psychotherapy scene. It was not until the late 1950s that a systematic approach emerged for the assessment and treatment of psychological disorders. In its early stages, behavioral therapy was defined as the application of modern learning theory to the treatment of clinical problems. The phrase modern learning theory refers to the principles and procedures of classical and operant conditioning. Behavior therapy is seen as a logical extension of behaviorism to complex forms of human activity. Behavioral therapy has undergone significant changes in both nature and scope and has been responsive to advances in experimental psychology and innovations in clinical practice. It has grown more complex and sophisticated. Behavioral therapy can no longer be defined solely as the clinical application of classical and operant conditioning theory. Current behavioral therapy is characterized by a diversity of views. It now comprises a variety of heterogeneous procedures with different theoretical rationales and open debate on conceptual basis, methodological requirements, and evidence of efficacy. As behavioral therapy has evolved, it has increasingly overlapped with other psychotherapeutic approaches. Nevertheless, the basic conceptual characteristics of the behavioral approach are clear and their similarities to and differences from nonbehavioral therapy systems can be easily identified [17].

14.4.3 Cognitive Behavioral Therapy (CBT)

CBT is a new strategy for helping people develop practical ways of managing problems and imparting new, useful skills. Cognitive and behavioral strategies can be used to develop positive views and thoughts about something that is experienced so that you are calmer or accept the situation well. There is one way to get rid of anxiety or stress, write down your thoughts, feelings, and behavioral reactions on the diagram. Then identify the anxiety, is it a threatening event, or our thoughts are too much? However, this is not the case. Then try to write and formulate what solutions might be taken. Is it necessary to consult with close friends and what was discussed [18, 19]?

CBT can be group CBT or guided self-help CBT. Usually it consists of 4–6 sessions, one session per week. More sessions may be required in few women.

Anxiety is one of the symptoms of menopause. There are many psychological theories explaining the occurrence of social anxiety disorder, as well as its treatment. Each of these theoretical perspectives differs from each other in their techniques and goals, but one thing is in common, which is to encourage menopausal women to confront the sources of their anxiety rather than avoid it. Cognitive theoretical perspectives are Biological, Psychoanalytic, Humanistic, Cognitive, and Learning perspectives. One of the theories used to explain social anxiety and often used as the basis for providing therapy to clients is cognitive behavioral theory. This anxiety theory stems from irrational thoughts and beliefs that will form negative thoughts and develop to interpret situations incorrectly. This influences a person's emotional reactions and behavior. The main strategy in administering cognitive behavioral therapy is to change the way of thinking and irrational beliefs with healthier and more positive rational thoughts and beliefs [20].

One of the clinical conditions that can cause anxiety is the state of approaching menopause. The menopausal transition is accompanied by adverse physical changes, including vasomotor symptoms (i.e., hot flashes, night sweats), difficulty sleeping, and sexual problems. Emotional difficulties (e.g., depression, anxiety) also have a significant impact on functioning and quality of life. Women going through menopause are four times more likely to experience a major depressive episode than others [21].

Effective non-pharmacological treatments for women with menopausal symptoms are lacking. One study showed that women on CBT-Meno experienced significantly reduced symptoms of vasomotor disturbances and depression and significantly greater sleep improvements. This advantage was maintained at a 3-month follow-up. A significant reduction in depressive symptoms was observed using the Montgomery-Asberg Depression Rating Scale (MADRS) and measuring anxiety using the Hamilton Anxiety Scale (HAM-A) in both conditions [22].

More comprehensive treatment such as cognitive behavioral group treatment (CBGT) which is a form of psychological and behavioral intervention, focuses not only on vasomotor disorders, but other symptoms that accompany perimenopause or postmenopause, including mental disorders, difficulty sleeping or insomnia, sexual, and urogenital [3].

In patients with breast cancer, CBT is effective in reducing vasomotor symptoms regardless of age, body mass index (BMI), menopausal status, and type of cancer therapy. Therapy is significantly effective in cancer patients without and with chemotherapy [23]. Administration of adjuvant treatment in breast cancer patients causes menopausal symptoms in the form of facial flushing and night sweats. Continued symptoms can interfere with a woman's daily activities and quality. In the medical treatment for menopausal symptoms using gabapentin, clonidine, and selective serotonin reuptake inhibitors, they are quite effective for menopausal symptoms but have quite disturbing side effects. For this reason, women who are induced by breast cancer and other medical treatments are better off doing therapy with nonmedical methods, namely CBT programs to treat anxiety disorders, depression, insomnia, vasomotor symptoms, and sleep problems [24, 25].

A study assessed the benefits of telephone therapy based on cognitive behavioral therapy for insomnia (CBT-I) compared to menopause education controls (MEC) in women with insomnia symptoms of perimenopausal and postmenopausal age. In a randomized clinical trial of 106 women, the Insomnia Severity Index score decreased by 9.9 points in women who received cognitive behavioral therapy and 4.7 points in women who received menopause education controls, showing a significant difference. Telephone-based CBT-I effectively improved sleep quality in perimenopausal and postmenopausal women with insomnia and vasomotor symptoms, both immediately after treatment and at 24 weeks of follow-up [15].

Menopause also causes sexual-related disorders, and this case is quite common. A study developed a CBT protocol specifically designed to address sexual problems during perimenopause as a means of early intervention. CBT is expected to address sexual problems at the start of the menopausal transition to increase sexual satisfaction, thereby improving quality of life. The main objective of this study was to assess the efficacy of weekly, four-session, individual CBT for sexual problems in perimenopause (CBT-SC-Peri). It was hypothesized that the CBT-SC-Peri protocol would significantly improve sexual satisfaction (primary outcome), desire, arousal, relationship satisfaction, body image, vasomotor symptoms, depression, and anxiety (secondary outcome). With increasing client demand for non-pharmacological treatments for perimenopausal symptoms, this form of treatment may be preferred by many people [26].

Psychosocial intervention is an excellent way to treat female sexual dysfunction (FSD) and a combination of biomedical and psychosocial interventions provides optimal results. Psychosocial interventions include basic counseling, physiotherapy, and psychosexual interventions. Basic sexual counseling is an integral part of a health consultation. Cognitive therapy is an important element of psychotherapy. It focuses on individual thoughts, feelings, and behaviors, encouraging patients to become aware of irrational beliefs and also helps in converting wrong thoughts into positive thinking [27].

14.5 Conclusion

Although hormone therapy is the first choice for relieving symptoms of menopause, there are risks to using hormonal therapy that need to be considered. Nonhormonal treatment alternatives have been developed following the publication of Women Health Initiative. Psychological interventions may be a safe and effective alternative option for alleviating symptoms of hot flashes, in women associated with menopause. CBT is one of the psychological interventions that has been developed which is quite effective in reducing menopausal symptoms such as VMS, low mood, insomnia, anxiety, and sexual dysfunction. Research on the effectiveness of CBT still needs to be developed further, to obtain sufficient references to support the benefits of CBT for the treatment of menopausal symptoms.

References

1. Enjezab B, Zarehosseinabadi M, Farzinrad B, Dehghani A. The effect of mindfulness-based cognitive therapy on quality of life in perimenopausal women. Iran J Psychiatry Behav Sci. 2019;13(1):1–9.
2. Stuenkel CA, Santoro NF, Laughlin-Tommaso SK, Black A, Joffe H, Su HI. NAMS 2019 Pre-Meeting Symposium, September 2019, Chicago Illinois: The Perimenopause. Menopause. 2020;27(7):735–45.
3. Ayers B, Smith M, Hellier J, Mann E, Hunter MS. Effectiveness of group and self-help cognitive behavior therapy in reducing problematic menopausal hot flushes and night sweats (MENOS 2): a randomized controlled trial. Menopause. 2012;19(7):749–59.
4. Mehta J, Kling JM, Manson JAE. Risks, benefits, and treatment modalities of menopausal hormone therapy: current concepts. Front Endocrinol. 2021;12(March):1–14.
5. Hunter MS, Chilcot J. Is cognitive behaviour therapy an effective option for women who have troublesome menopausal symptoms? Br J Health Psychol. 2021;26(3):697–708.
6. Thapa R, Yang Y. Menopausal symptoms and related factors among Cambodian women. Women Heal. 2020;60(4):396–411. https://doi.org/10.1080/03630242.2019.1643815.
7. Yim G, Ahn Y, Chang Y, Ryu S, Lim JY, Kang D, et al. Prevalence and severity of menopause symptoms and associated factors across menopause status in Korean women. Menopause. 2015;22(10):1108–16.
8. Santoro N, Roeca C, Peters BA, Neal-Perry G. The menopause transition: signs, symptoms, and management options. J Clin Endocrinol Metab. 2021;106(1):1–15.
9. Thurston RC, Joffe H. Vasomotor symptoms and menopause: findings from the study of women's health across the nation. Obstet Gynecol Clin North Am. 2011;38(3):489–501. https://doi.org/10.1016/j.ogc.2011.05.006.
10. Nasreen SZA. Symptoms of menopause. In: Rangel L, editor. Hormone therapy and replacement in cancer and aging-related diseases. London: IntechOpen; 2019. p. 47–50.
11. Coyoy A, Guerra-Araiza C, Camacho-Arroyo I. Metabolism regulation by estrogens and their receptors in the central nervous system before and after menopause. Horm Metab Res. 2016;48(8):489–96.
12. Sood R, Kuhle CL, Kapoor E, Thielen JM, Frohmader KS, Mara KC, et al. Association of mindfulness and stress with menopausal symptoms in midlife women. Climacteric. 2019;22(4):377–82. https://doi.org/10.1080/13697137.2018.1551344.
13. Shifren JL, Crandall CJ, Manson JE. Menopausal hormone therapy. JAMA. 2019;321(24):2458–9.
14. Madsen TE, Sobel T, Negash S, Allen TS, Marcia L, Manson JE, et al. A review of hormone and non-hormonal therapy options for the treatment of menopause. Int J Womens Health. 2023;15:825–36.
15. McCurry SM, Guthrie KA, Morin CM, Woods NF, Landis CA, Ensrud KE, et al. Telephone-based cognitive behavioral therapy for insomnia in perimenopausal and postmenopausal women with vasomotor symptoms A MsFLASH randomized clinical trial. JAMA Intern Med. 2016;176(7):913–20.
16. Gunderman RB. Cognitive therapy. J Am Coll Radiol. 2006;3(11):835–7.
17. Wilson GT. Behavior therapy. In: Corsini RJ, Wedding D, editors. Current psychotherapies. Washington, DC: Thomson Brooks/Cole Publishing Co.; 2005. p. 202–37.
18. Hunter MS. Cognitive behavioral therapy for menopausal symptoms. Climacteric. 2021;24(1):51–6. https://doi.org/10.1080/13697137.2020.1777965.
19. Hunter M, Smith M. Cognitive behaviour therapy (CBT) for menopausal symptoms. Information for women Myra Hunter and Melanie Smith in collaboration with the British Menopause Society. Post Reprod Heal. 2017;23(2):77–82.
20. Asrori A, Hasanat N, ui. Terapi kognitif perilaku intuk mengatasi gangguan kecemasan sosial. J Ilm Psikol Terap. 2022;3(1):89–107.

21. Bromberger JT, Kravitz HM, Chang YF, Cyranowski JM, Brown C, Matthews KA. Major depression during and after the menopausal transition: study of women's health across the nation (SWAN). Psychol Med. 2011;41(9):1879–88.
22. Green SM, Donegan E, Frey BN, Fedorkow DM, Key BL, Streiner DL, et al. Cognitive behavior therapy for menopausal symptoms (CBT-Meno): a randomized controlled trial. Menopause. 2019;26(9):972–80.
23. Wiley J. Is cognitive behaviour therapy an effective option for women who have troublesome menopausal symptoms? Br J Health Psychol. 2021;26:697–708.
24. Atema V, Van Leeuwen M, Kieffer JM, Oldenburg HSA, Van Beurden M, Gerritsma MA, et al. Efficacy of internet-based cognitive behavioral therapy for treatment-induced menopausal symptoms in breast cancer survivors: results of a randomized controlled trial. J Clin Oncol. 2019;37(10):809–22.
25. Madalinska JB, Van Beurden M, Bleiker EMA, Valdimarsdottir HB, Hollenstein J, Massuger LF, et al. The impact of hormone replacement therapy on menopausal symptoms in younger high-risk women after prophylactic salpingo-oophorectomy. J Clin Oncol. 2006;24(22):3576–82.
26. Green SM, Furtado M. Cognitive behavioral therapy for sexual concerns during perimenopause: a four session study protocol. Front Glob Women's Heal. 2021;2:1–9.
27. Al-Azzawi F, Bitzer J, Brandenburg U, Castelo-Branco C, Graziottin A, Kenemans P, et al. Therapeutic options for postmenopausal female sexual dysfunction. Climacteric. 2010;13(2):103–20.

Menopause and Cardiovascular System 15

Shubhra Agarwal and Ruchika Garg

15.1 Introduction

Menopause is a natural biological process that brings about significant changes in a woman's body and hormone levels, leading to a wide range of physical and emotional symptoms. These symptoms can have a profound impact on a woman's overall well-being and quality of life. Beyond the immediate symptoms, menopause also carries long-term health implications, particularly in relation to the cardiovascular system. Recent years have witnessed growing recognition of the cardiovascular risks associated with menopause. Research has unveiled the intricate relationship between menopause and the cardiovascular system, shedding light on the mechanisms that underlie the increased risk of cardiovascular diseases (CVDs) during this phase. Understanding the significance of menopause in relation to the cardiovascular system is vital for healthcare professionals and women themselves. Cardiovascular diseases are the leading cause of death among women worldwide, and menopause represents a critical period of vulnerability. Recognizing and addressing the cardiovascular risks associated with menopause can lead to targeted interventions and preventive strategies, helping to reduce the burden of CVD and promote healthier aging in women. In this chapter, we will explore the history of menopause, its significance in women's lives, the pathophysiology of menopause and its effects on the cardiovascular system, the importance of understanding this relationship, recent studies and guidelines that provide insights into managing cardiovascular risks during menopause, and the ongoing debates surrounding menopause and the cardiovascular system.

S. Agarwal (✉)
TMMC&RC, Moradabad, India

R. Garg
SN Medical College, Agra, India

R. Garg (ed.), *Management of Menopause*,
https://doi.org/10.1007/978-981-96-0239-1_15

15.2 Pathophysiology

Numerous metabolic alterations that interact with one another lead to cardiovascular disease. Males have twice the risk of developing coronary heart disease (CHD) prior to age 40 than of women. Estrogen in females is a protective agent that causes vasodilatory and antithrombotic activities by endothelial production of nitric oxide and prostacyclin but with menopausal transition this advantage is lost. Cardiovascular disease is made worse by risk factors such as high blood pressure, being overweight, smoking, mellitus type 2 diabetes, abnormal cholesterol, and lipoprotein profiles. Low HDL cholesterol (Avg 55–60 mg/dL) and increased triglyceride level >400 mg/dL increases the risk of CHD. A decrease in HDL even by 10 mg/dL increases CHD risk by 40–50.

15.3 History and Clinical Trials

Long-term use of menopausal hormonal therapy (MHT) for cardiovascular disease went into disrepute following various clinical trials with WHI (Women's Health Initiative) study being at forefront. The results of the clinical trials showed that MHT did not reduce or offer protection against cardiovascular disease; rather, they raised concerns due to an elevated risk of stroke, thrombotic phenomenon, and breast cancer. For a short while, the trials produced a lot of questions and worries about the safety of MHT, which made the study of menopause extremely complex and made it difficult for physicians and patients to make decisions.

15.3.1 WHI

In 40 clinical facilities, 161,809 women aged 50–79 were enrolled in the WHI between 1993 and 1998. There were two groups: one received treatment with progestin and estrogen together, and the other received treatment with estrogen alone. A total of 16,608 women were randomized to receive therapy or a placebo in the combined estrogen-progestin arm, which involved daily doses of 2.5 mg of medroxyprogesterone acetate and 0.625 mg of conjugated estrogens. The other hormone experiment randomized 10,739 hysterectomized women to therapy or a placebo. The estrogen-only arm of the trial had daily doses of 0.625 mg conjugated estrogens. The Data and Safety Monitoring Board (DSMB) released recommendations on July 9, 2002, after its to end the daily combination hormone trial arm because of a statistically increase in cardiovascular events and aggressive breast cancer and to keep the hysterectomized women in the trial arm by giving them daily unopposed estrogen [1]. Due to a higher chance of a stroke similar to the one reported by the canceled estrogen progestin arm of the WHI, the National Heart, Lung, and Blood Institute of the United States canceled the estrogen-only arm of the study on March 2, 2004. The outcomes in the estrogen-only arm of the trial were comparable with those in the estrogen-progestin arm, with the possible exception of breast cancer and CHD.

Direct comparisons are inappropriate because, as Table 15.1 makes clear, these were two distinct trials via two distinct populations and treatments.

A reanalysis of the CHD data, which was released 7 years after the original report, verified that women who were 10 years or older away from menopause were the only ones who experienced a rise in coronary heart events. WHI does not support the conclusion that hormone therapy raises the chance of coronary cardiac events among all postmenopausal women; rather, results from the estrogen-only arm indicated that younger women benefitted from estrogen treatment in terms of CHD.

15.3.2 Nurses' Health Study

It provided an update on treatments for hormones and stroke, with particular attention to when to start treatment and how much estrogen to take at first. It was reported that as estrogen dosage increased, so did the risk of stroke [2]. It is advisable to use small amounts of estrogen in women who have stroke risk factors. As a result, it makes sense to advise older women to use HT transdermally rather than otherwise.

15.3.3 The Heart and Estrogen-Progestin Replacement Study (HERS)

It studied the effect of daily treatment of 0.625 mg conjugated estrogens and 2.5 mg medroxyprogesterone acetate as secondary prevention in women with preexisting coronary disease [3–5]. No noticeable distinctions existed between the treatment and placebo groups. Among the treatment and placebo groups receiving aspirin and statins, there was no statistically significant rise in thrombosis of deep veins or pulmonary embolism during the follow-up period. HERS clinical trial results are compromised because of decreased compliance and drop-out problems.

Table 15.1 Comparison of the two arms of WHI trial

	Estrogen and progestin arm	Only estrogen arm
Average age	63.3	63.6
Drop-out rate	42%	53.8%
<5 years of menopause	<16.5%	
Demographic profile	1. More sedentary 2. More obese 3. Higher rates of preexisting cardiovascular disease	1. Premature births 2. Bilateral oophorectomy 3. Longer and more extensive prior hormone treatment

15.3.4 Estrogen Replacement and Atherosclerosis (ERA) Trial

It looked at how postmenopausal hormone therapy affected angiography-measured coronary atherosclerosis progression [6, 7]. A total of 309 women were randomized to receive a placebo, unopposed estrogen, or a daily dose of progestin plus estrogen. Similar to the HERS study, there were no documented rises in cardiac incidents in each of the three therapy groups.

15.4 Timing Hypothesis

The age at which clinical events begin is determined by the slope of the atherosclerosis development trajectory that each woman has. In monkeys, estrogen therapy started right after menopause reduced the rate of coronary artery atherosclerotic by almost 70%; however, no impact was seen if the treatment was postponed for 2 years, or roughly 6 years in women. According to WHI's measurements of coronary artery calcium, women who had bilateral oophorectomies but did not get estrogen therapy had a higher incidence of subclinical coronary heart disease [8]. The relative hazards for cardiovascular events were, in fact, 30–38% lower in the WHI observational arm than in the clinical trials once confounding variables such dietary, behavioral, activity levels, and cardiovascular risk factors were taken into account. When hormonal therapy was started in the Nurses' Health Study, the risk of coronary heart disease was significantly lower for women under 60 years old, whereas there was no discernible difference in the risk for women over 60. The timing theory was examined in the Kronos Early Estrogen Prevention Study (KEEPS), a double-blind, randomized, placebo-controlled experiment. Comparing early and late intervention the trial involving estradiol (ELITE) evaluated the impact of early HT treatment on the onset and progression of atherosclerosis. After 5 years, it was shown that the early postmenopausal group's carotid artery intima-media thickness (CIMT) increased far more slowly in response to oral E2, with or without vaginal progesterone, than in response to placebo [9]. The ELITE trial's findings, which showed that earlier HT initiation—that is, closer to menopause—was linked to better cardiovascular outcomes, lend support to the timing hypothesis. Cardioprotection by itself shouldn't be used as a reason to prescribe hormone therapy until further information is obtained.

15.5 Menopausal Hormone Therapy

The menopause, which signifies the end of a woman's reproductive years, is a normal stage of life. While it is a significant and inevitable transition, it often comes with a host of physical and emotional challenges that can impact a woman's quality of life. Menopausal hormone therapy (MHT), also known as hormone replacement therapy (HRT), has emerged as a valuable medical intervention designed to alleviate the symptoms and discomfort associated with menopause. This therapy involves the use of hormones, such as estrogen and progestin, to manage the hormonal imbalances that occur during this life stage.

The Role of MHT: Menopausal hormone therapy has been a cornerstone of menopausal symptom management for decades. By replenishing declining hormone levels, MHT can effectively alleviate many of the discomforts associated with menopause. Beyond symptom relief, it has also shown potential benefits in preventing bone loss, reducing the risk of fractures, and maintaining cardiovascular health.

Personalized Approach: It's important to recognize that menopause is a highly individualized experience. What works for one woman may not be suitable for another. The decision to undergo MHT requires careful consideration, taking into account a woman's medical history, risk factors, and personal preferences. Factors such as the type of hormones used, the method of administration, and the duration of therapy are all key components that should be tailored to meet the specific needs and goals of each woman.

Controversies and Risks: While menopausal hormone therapy offers numerous benefits, it has not been without controversy. Past studies have raised concerns about potential risks, including an increased risk of breast cancer and blood clots in some women. These concerns have led to a shift towards a more conservative and individualized approach to MHT, emphasizing the importance of weighing the potential benefits against the associated risks.

A series of clinical trials raised doubts about the long-term use of MHT as a treatment for cardiovascular disease. The results of the clinical trials not only showed that MHT did not prevent cardiovascular disease, but they also gave rise to worries about possible negative effects, such as an increased risk of stroke, thrombotic phenomena, and breast cancer. The decades that followed WHI brought up issues with hormone therapy prescriptions. The various hormones and routes that can be used in MHT are described below:

1. **Oral and transdermal route:**

   No matter how ethinyl estradiol is administered, the 17α-ethinyl group has an impact on liver function [10]. For CEEs, the same holds true. Therefore, it appears that the mode of delivery primarily affects the metabolic reactions when it comes to certain estrogens, most notably estradiol. The levels of estrone and estradiol in commercial preparations including estriol, estradiol, and estrone are sufficient to cause normal clinical effects [11].

   One can apply transdermal estradiol via a patch, gel, emulsion, or spray. There are two different dosages of the patches available: Vivelle and Climatera. The gel can be administered once daily to the arm, wrist, shoulder, or thigh. It is also marketed under different brand names (Divigel, EstroGel, Estreva Gel) and in different doses. Estrasorb is an emulsion that comes in foil bags; two packets are typically applied to each thigh each day and thoroughly massaged in. Evamist is a transdermal spray; a single daily dose is applied to the forearm (many sprays are applied to different sites if several daily doses are needed). There is a metered dispenser for elestrin.

When transdermal estradiol is administered, the circulation estrone to estradiol ratio is one, while when oral estradiol is administered, it is roughly five. Nonetheless, the first-pass impact has a significant lipoprotein effect, showing a reduction in cholesterol and LDL and a rise in HDL. There is insufficient information on how low-dose estrogen regimens can reduce the risk of fracture, despite the fact that they can effectively suppress vasomotor symptoms and improve bone mineral density [12]. Although it is challenging to quantify, the first-pass hepatic effect may contribute to variations in clinical effectiveness, making it impossible to compare the clinical efficacy of oral and transdermal estrogen delivery with any degree of accuracy.

Transdermal estrogen reduces factor VII, oral estrogen increases prothrombin 1 and 2 fragment, MMP 2, MMP 9, and APC resistance [13]. Given this distinction, it stands to reason that transdermal rather than oral estrogen administration would be less likely to cause VTE.

Oral estrogen causes noticeably higher rises in HDL cholesterol and triglycerides as compared to transdermal estrogen, while transdermal estrogen lowers triglyceride levels. In fact, when medication is switched to transdermal administration, triglyceride levels that were noticeably raised in response to oral therapy return to normal [14]. Furthermore, progestin supplementation somewhat reduces the risk of gallstones, which is linked to oral estrogen therapy.

C-Reactive protein (CRP) levels are higher in women using oral estrogen than in those taking transdermal estrogen [15]. Oral hormone therapy actually lowers the levels of other inflammatory markers (electin, intercellular binding molecule-1, vascular cell adhesion molecule-1, monocyte chemoattractant protein-1, and necrosis factor-α) in the bloodstream while raising CRP, although its effects on IL-6 are not always constant. The association between baseline CRP levels and an increased risk of CHD was validated by a WHI trial; however, the risk was not increased further by the rise in CRP brought on by oral hormone therapy [16].

There is insufficient data to conclude that postmenopausal smokers respond better to transdermal estrogen than to oral estrogen. This includes higher vascular responsivity, greater reductions in norepinephrine levels, vascular sympathetic tone, and total peripheral resistance. Smokers might be among the women for whom transdermal estrogen might be beneficial, notwithstanding the paucity of data [17].

2. **Implants:**

   Two times a year, subcutaneous injection in doses of 25, 50, and 75 mg of estradiol pellets is provided. Considering that using transdermal distribution reduces the incidence of thrombotic events associated with the use of exogenous estrogen. Furthermore, transdermal distribution of estradiol may be preferred in women with poor sexual function due to its lack of influence on blood sex hormone binding globulin (SHBG) levels and thus little impact on free androgen levels.

3. **Vaginal Administration:**

   Vaginal creams containing estrogen are easily absorbed from immature and atrophic vaginas, but when the epithelium grows after 3–4 months, the absorption of estrogen diminishes. Progesterone addition is generally not recommended with low-dose therapy; nevertheless, endometrial observation is necessary if vaginal cream treatment is continued for more than 12 months. Low-level estrogen found in vaginal rings is adequate to relieve urogenital problems. Estring is a silicone ring with a diameter of 55 mm that releases 2 mg of estradiol at a rate of 7.5 μg each day for a period of 90 days. Now available in the USA, the Vagifem tablet [18] (10 μg estradiol) relieves atrophic symptoms in 2 weeks and can be used twice a week after that. The issue is that none of the studies have been lengthy enough to establish endometrial safety over the long run. For the purpose of relieving vasomotor symptoms, we feel that long-term treatment necessitates ultrasonographic evaluation of the thickness of the endometrium with biopsy when necessary, despite the fact that the alteration in blood levels is incredibly minor and hence ineffective.

15.6 Estrogen Dose

For a long time, the suggested dosage of estrogen was

1. 0.625 mg of conjugated estrogens
2. 1–2 mg of micronized estradiol
3. 1–2 mg of valerate estradiol.

or comparable amounts of other estrogens, like 5 μg of ethinyl estradiol.

Bone density increases when 1.5 mg of medroxyprogesterone acetate is administered with 0.3 or 0.45 mg of conjugated estrogens; 0.5 mg of micronized estradiol produces results comparable to these [19]. Both the 0.45/1.5 mg and 0.3/1.5 mg conjugated estrogens/medroxyprogesterone acetate combinations improve vaginal atrophy, reduce hot flushes, and improve indices of sexual function in a way that is statistically and subjectively comparable to high dose [20]. These lower-dose combos are associated with less breakthrough bleeding while preserving the advantageous lipid profile changes. When assessing response, care should be used because women's higher rates of metabolism and clearance may cause them to react adversely to lower dosages.

15.7 Menopausal Hormone Therapy: Progestational Component

A gestational agent may be administered either continuously or sequentially. Depression, bloating, and breast tenderness are among the negative effects of progestational hormones. For women who have trouble falling asleep, progestational drugs in the form of micronized progesterone can be used at night. Because progesterone has a first-pass effect on the uterus, it can also be given as a vaginal gel (90 mg), which can successfully preserve the endometrium. Most patients experience amenorrhea after applying the 4% commercial solution (Crinone) twice a week to preserve the endometrium. The 4% formulation is administered every day for at least 14 days a month in a sequential regimen.

15.7.1 Infrequent Progestational Exposure: Long Sequential Regimens

Such regimens reduce the length of progestin exposure and serve to lessen the number of withdrawal bleeding episodes. Though there is a dearth of data regarding prolonged cycle regimens. One study found that taking medroxyprogesterone acetate every 3 months was linked to longer, heavier menses, unplanned bleeding, and a 1.5% risk of hyperplasia at 1 year. In contrast, another study found that there was less total bleeding but a 4% incidence of hyperplasia [21]. After 3 years, the 5-year Scandinavian Long Cycle Study was stopped due to a 12.5% incidence of endometrial pathology and one case of endometrial cancer [22]. Endometrial monitoring is recommended in patients at risk for endometrial hyperplasia, including as obese, insulin-resistant, and diabetic women, due to the paucity of data regarding the safety of prolonged regimens.

15.7.2 The Progestin Intrauterine Device

Progesterone administered intrauterine is known to efficiently protect the endometrium while limiting systemic negative effects. For instance, the beneficial lipid benefits of estrogen are not diminished when progesterone is administered intrauterine. Within the first 6 months, there may be irregular breakthrough bleeding, and 60–70% of the women experience amenorrhea after a year.

15.8 Sequential and Continuous Regimens

The successive regimens mirror the menstrual cycle's cyclical patterns of progesterone and estrogen. In the consecutive regimen, progestogens are given at similar levels for 2 weeks each month while estrogen is given daily. When progestin was added to estrogen once a day, the progestin dose may be lowered and still effectively prevent endometrial hyperplasia. Eighty to ninety percent of patients experienced amenorrhea within a year of starting treatment [23].

Progestins and estrogen are mixed in the daily continuous regimen at the following equivalent doses:

0.35 mg norethindrone
1.5 or 2.5 mg medroxyprogesterone acetate
0.5 or 1.0 mg of acetate norethindrone
Progesterone micronized in 100 mg

Drosperinone 2 mg
Dienogest 2 mg

Indication of combination of estrogen and progestational agent:

- Hysterectomy after endometriosis as patients with pelvic endometriosis who received unopposed estrogen treatment have been documented to have adenocarcinomas.
- Treatments that might leave endometrial behind, such as supracervical hysterectomy.
- Patients who have undergone endometrial ablation.
- Hysterectomy for early stage endometrial adenocarcinoma.
- Individuals receiving treatment for ovarian endometrioid cancers.

15.9 Impact of MHT on Cardiovascular System

1. **Effect on Lipoproteins and Lipids:**
   MHT raises HDL cholesterol while lowering LDL cholesterol. The suppression of hepatic lipase activity, which converts HDL2 to HDL3, is mostly responsible for the rise in HDL cholesterol levels, especially because of the HDL2 subfraction.
2. **Apolipoprotein:**
   A decrease in the amounts of lipoprotein in circulation is also brought about by postmenopausal estrogen therapy, whether or not additional progestin is administered [24]. While the levels of apolipoprotein A-I, the main apolipoprotein of HDL, rise in response to estrogen, those of apolipoprotein B, the primary surface protein of LDL, decrease. Concomitant dosing of estrogen with an HMG-CoA reductase inhibitor has a stronger positive effect on the lipid profile. Therapy with estrogen alone or in conjunction with progesterone decreased atherosclerosis as compared to no hormone therapy [25].
3. **Endothelium-Dependent Vasodilation and Antiplatelet Aggregation:**
   Endothelium-derived relaxing and contracting factors are responsible for maintaining dilation. Nitric oxide the relaxing factor in hypertension is increased by hormonal therapy which inhibits adhesion and aggregation of platelets [26].
4. **Actions on the Heart and Large Blood Vessels:**
   Estrogen treatment by its direct inotropic action increases left ventricular diastolic filling and stroke volume. In a three-month study, medroxyprogesterone acetate (5 mg daily for 10 days each month) did not attenuate the increase in left ventricular output (systolic flow velocity) observed with estrogen treatment. On the other hand, others have detected attenuation of estrogen's beneficial effects on compliance (stiffness) associated with combined estrogen-progestin treatment [27]. And others have not been able to demonstrate an effect of short-term oral estrogen or long-term transdermal estrogen treatment on cardiac structure and function [28].

5. **Actions on Glucose Metabolism:**
   Menopause is associated with increase in body fat, especially central (android) body fat. Insulin resistance and circulating insulin levels increase in women after menopause, and impaired glucose tolerance predicts an increased risk of CHD. The WHI randomized clinical trial documented improvements in fasting glucose and insulin levels in the estrogen-progestin treated group [29]. Hyperinsulinemia also has a direct atherogenic effect on blood vessels, perhaps secondary to insulin propeptides. Insulin directly stimulates the secretion of endothelin-1 in endothelial cells, and the circulating levels of endothelin-1 are correlated with insulin levels [29].
6. **Inhibition of Lipoprotein Oxidation:**
   Estrogen is an antioxidant. Estradiol directly inhibits LDL cholesterol oxidation in response to copper and decreases the overall formation of lipid oxides. In addition, estrogen may regenerate circulating antioxidants (tocopherols and beta-carotene) and preserve these antioxidants within LDL cholesterol particles. Estrogen thereby preserves endothelial-dependent vasodilator function by preventing the deleterious effect that oxidized LDL cholesterol has on endothelial production of vasoactive agents [30].
7. **A Favorable Impact on Fibrinolysis:**
   Menopause is associated with increase in factor VII, fibrinogen, and plasminogen activator inhibitor-1 (PAI-1) thereby producing a relatively hypercoagulable state. Oral estrogen alone or combined with a progestin prevents increase in clotting factors associated with menopause thereby creating a favorable impact on fibrinolysis [31].

15.10 Conclusion

In conclusion, menopause represents a significant and complex phase in a woman's life, characterized by a myriad of physical and emotional symptoms that can impact her well-being and quality of life. Beyond the immediate symptoms, research has increasingly highlighted the intricate relationship between menopause and the cardiovascular system. The transition into menopause brings about hormonal changes that can increase the risk of cardiovascular diseases, which are the leading cause of death among women globally.

Understanding the pathophysiology of this relationship is crucial. Estrogen, which plays a protective role in the cardiovascular system by promoting vasodilation and reducing thrombotic activity, decreases during menopause. The field of menopause and its relationship with the cardiovascular system requires further research to elucidate the intricate mechanisms at play. It's important to distinguish between endogenous and exogenous estrogens, and studies with the right design are required to learn more about the components that contribute to postmenopausal women's cardiovascular disease.

In conclusion, recognizing the significance of menopause in relation to the cardiovascular system is essential for healthcare professionals and women themselves.

By addressing the cardiovascular risks associated with menopause through targeted interventions and preventive strategies, we can reduce the burden of cardiovascular disease and promote healthier aging in women.

References

1. The Women's Health Initiative Steering Committee. Effects of conjugated equine estrogen in postmenopausal women with hysterectomy. The women's health initiative randomized controlled trial. JAMA. 2004;291:1707.
2. Grodstein F, Manson JE, Stampfer MJ, Rexrode K. Postmenopausal hormone therapy and stroke. Role of time since menopause and age at initiation of hormone therapy. Arch Intern Med. 2008;168:861.
3. Hulley S, Grady D, Bush T, Furberg C, Herrington D, Riggs B, Vittinghoff E, for the Heart and Estrogen/progestin Replacement Study (HERS) Research Group. Randomized trial of estrogen plus progestin for secondary prevention of coronary heart disease in postmenopausal women. JAMA. 1998;280:605.
4. Grady D, Herrington D, Bittner V, Blumenthal R, Davidson M, Hlatky M, Hsia J, Hulley SB, Herd A, Khan S, Newby LK, Waters D, Vittinghoff E, Wenger N, Heart and Estrogen/progestin Replacement Study Follow-up (HERS II): 1. Cardiovascular outcomes during 6.8 years of hormone therapy. JAMA. 2002;288:49.
5. Hulley S, Furberg C, Barrett-Connor E, Cauley J, Grady D, Haskell W, Knopp R, Lowery M, Satterfield S, Schrott H, Vittinghoff E, Hunninghake D, Heart and Estrogen/progestin Replacement Study Follow-up (HERS II): 2. Non-cardiovascular disease outcomes during 6.8 years of hormone therapy. JAMA. 2002;288:58.
6. Herrington DM, Reboussin DM, Brosnihan KB, Sharp PC, Shumaker SA, Snyder TE, Furberg CD, Kowalchuk GJ, Stuckey TD, Rogers WJ, Givens DH, Waters D. Effects of estrogen replacement on the progression of coronary-artery atherosclerosis. N Engl J Med. 2000;343:522.
7. Clarkson TB. Estrogen effects on arteries vary with stage of reproductive life and extent of subclinical atherosclerosis progression. Menopause. 2007;14:373.
8. Allison MA, Manson JE, Langer RD, Carr JJ, Rossouw JE, Pettinger MB, Phillips L, Cochrane BB, Eaton CB, Greenland P, Hendrix S, Hsia J, Hunt JR, Jackson RD, Johnson KC, Kuller LH, Robinson J, Women's Health Initiative and Women's Health Initiative Coronary Artery Calcium Study Investigators. Oophorectomy, hormone therapy, and subclinical coronary artery disease in women with hysterectomy: the women's health initiative coronary artery calcium study. Menopause. 2008;15:639.
9. Hodis HN, Mack WJ, Henderson VW, Shoupe D, Budoff MJ, Hwang-Levine J, Li Y, Feng M, Dustin L, Kono N, Stanczyk FZ, Selzer RH, Azen SP, ELITE Research Group. Vascular effects of early versus late postmenopausal treatment with estradiol. N EnglJ Med. 2016;374(13):1221.
10. Hodis HN, Mack WJ, Henderson VW, Shoupe D, Budoff MJ, Hwang-Levine J, Li Y, Feng M, Dustin L, Kono N, Stanczyk FZ, Selzer RH, Azen SP, ELITE Research Group. Vascular effects of early versus late postmenopausal treatment with estradiol. N Engl J Med. 2016;374(13):1221.
11. Fugh-Berman A, Bythrow J. Bioidentical hormones for menopausal hormone therapy: variation on a theme. J Gen Intern Med. 2007;22(7):1030.
12. Utian WH, Burry KA, Archer DF, Gallagher JC, Boyett RL, Guy MP, Tachon GJ, Chadha-Boreham HK, Bouvet AA. Efficacy and safety of low, standard, and high dosages of an estradiol transdermal system (Esclim) compared with placebo on vasomotor symptoms in highly symptomatic menopausal patients. The Esclim study group. Am J Obstet Gynecol. 1999;181:71.
13. Vehkavaara S, Silveira A, Hakala-Ala-Pietilä T, Virkamäki A, Hovatta O, Hamsten A, Taskinen M-R, Yki-Järvinen H. Effects of oral and transdermal estrogen replacement therapy on markers of coagulation, fibrinolysis, inflammation and serum lipids and lipoproteins in postmenopausal women. Thromb Haemost. 2001;85:619.

14. Canonico M, Oger E, Plu-Bureau G, Conard J, Meyer G, Lévesque H, Trillot N, Barrellier MT, Wahl D, Emmerich J, Scarabin PY, for the Estrogen and Thromboembolism Risk (ESTHER) Study Group. Hormone therapy and venous thromboembolism among postmenopausal women. Impact of the route of estrogen administration and progestogens: the ESTHER study. Circulation. 2007;115:840.
15. Silvestri A, Gebara O, Vitale C, Wajngarten M, Leonardo F, Ramieres JA, Fini M, Mercucro G, Rosano GM. Increased levels of C-reactive protein after oral hormone replacement therapy may not be related to an increased inflammatory response. Circulation. 2003;107:3165.
16. Pradhan AD, Manson JE, Rossouw JE, Siscovick DS, Mouton CP, Rifai N, Wallace RB, Jackson RD, Pettinger MB, Ridker PM. Inflammatory biomarkers, hormone replacement therapy, and incident coronary heart disease. Prospective analysis from the women's health initiative observational study. JAMA. 2002;288:980.
17. Girdler SS, Hinderliter AL, Wells EC, Sherwood A, Grewen KM, Light KC. Transdermal versus oral estrogen therapy in postmenopausal smokers: hemodynamic and endothelial effects. Obstet Gynecol. 2004;103:169.
18. Rigg LA, Hermann H, Yen SSC. Absorption of estrogens from vaginal creams. N Engl J Med. 1978;298:195.
19. Lindsay R, Gallagher JC, Kleerekoper M, Pickar JH. Effect of lower doses of conjugated equine estrogens with and without medroxyprogesterone acetate on bone in early postmenopausal women. JAMA. 2002;287:2668.
20. Utian WH, Shoupe D, Bachmann G, Pinkerton JV, Pickar JH. Relief of vasomotor symptoms and vaginal atrophy with lower doses of conjugated equine estrogens and medroxyprogesterone acetate. Fertil Steril. 2001;75:1065.
21. Ettinger B, Selby J, Citron JT, Vangessel A, Ettinger V, Hendrickson MR. Cyclic hormone replacement therapy using quarterly progestin. Obstet Gynecol. 1994;83:693.
22. Bjarnason K, Cerin Å, Lindgren R, Weber T, for the Scandinavian Long Cycle Study Group. Adverse endometrial effects during long cycle hormone replacement therapy. Maturitas. 1999;32:151.
23. Speroff L, Rowan J, Symons J, Genant H, Wilborn W, for the CHART Study Group. The comparative effect on bone density, endometrium, and lipids of continuous hormones as replacement therapy (CHART study). JAMA. 1996;276:1397.
24. Munk-Jensen N, Ulrich L, Obel E, Nielsen S, Edwards D, Meinertz H. Continuous combined and sequential estradiol and norethindrone acetate treatment of postmenopausal women: effect on plasma lipoproteins in a two-year placebo-controlled trial. Am J Obstet Gynecol. 1994;171:132.
25. Davidson MH, Testolin LM, Maki KC, von Duvillard S, Drennan KB. A comparison of estrogen replacement, pravastatin, and combined treatment for the management of hypercholesterolemia in postmenopausal women. Arch Intern Med. 1997;157:1186.
26. Bar J, Tepper R, Fuchs J, Pardo Y, Goldberger S, Ovadia J. The effect of estrogen replacement therapy on platelet aggregation and adenosine triphosphate release in postmenopausal women. Obstet Gynecol. 1993;81:261.
27. Liang Y-L, Teede H, Shiel L, Thomas A, Craven R, Sachithanandan N, McNeil JJ, Cameron JD, Dart A, McGrath B. Effects of oestrogen and progesterone on age-related changes in arteries of postmenopausal women. Clin Exp Pharmacol Physiol. 1997;24:457.
28. Snabes MC, Payne JP, Kopelen HA, Dunn JK, Young RL, Zoghbi WA. Physiologic estradiol replacement therapy and cardiac structure and function in normal postmenopausal women: a randomized, double-blind, placebo-controlled, crossover trial. Obstet Gynecol. 1997;89:332.
29. Chlebowski RT, Wactawski-Wende J, Ritenbaugh C, Hubbell FA, Ascensao J, Rodabough RJ, Rosenberg CA, Taylor VM, Harris R, Chen C, Adams-Campbell LL, White E, for the women's Health Initiative Investigators. Estrogen plus progestin and colorectal cancer in postmenopausal women. N EnglJ Med. 2004;350:991.

30. Keaney J Jr, Shwaery G, Xu A, Nicholosi R, Loscalzo J, Foxall T, Vita J. 17 beta-estradiol preserves endothelial vasodilator function and limits low-density lipoprotein oxidation in hypercholesterolemic swine. Circulation. 1994;89:225.
31. Gebara OCE, Mittleman MA, Sutherland P, Lipinska I, Matheney T, Xu P, Welty FK, Wilson PW, Levy D, Muller JE, Tofler GH. Association between increased estrogen status and increased fibrinolytic potential in the Framingham offspring study. Circulation. 1995;91:1952.

Memory and Menopause

16

P. Pallavee and R. Ashwini

16.1 Introduction

Menopause is a well-known natural process in a woman's life with important connotations for its quality. Menopause is cessation of menstruation for at least a year, as the functioning of the ovaries and consequently ovulation gets progressively impaired [1]. This pathway of attenuation of ovarian function, can be a process that is either natural or surgical (following removal of the ovaries). In addition to the key role of supporting the reproductive function, estrogen and progestogen play a major role in brain-mediated actions, like cognition [2]. These steroid hormones are present in the brain and can be even synthesized, in the presence of the respective receptors [3]. Menopause is associated with many undesirable symptoms that affects the day-to-day activities of a woman. Many women experience cognitive complaints during their midlife [4] and these become well pronounced as the women goes through the menopause transition. While exogenous hormonal therapy can be used to alleviate these symptoms (e.g., sleep disturbances, vasomotor symptoms, vaginal atrophy, osteoporosis etc.), menopausal hormonal therapy is currently not approved for aiding cognitive functions as there aren't enough clinical data to support its benefits [5]. There are also important deficiencies in our understanding of whether this impaired cognition can predict the risk of dementia and whether menopausal hormonal transition increases the risk or protects against late-onset dementia.

P. Pallavee (✉) · R. Ashwini
Department of Obstetrics and Gynaecology, Mahatma Gandhi Medical College and Research Institute, Sri Balaji Vidyapeeth Deemed-to-be-University, Puducherry, India

R. Garg (ed.), *Management of Menopause*,
https://doi.org/10.1007/978-981-96-0239-1_16

16.2 What Is Cognition?

Cognition is described as "all forms of knowing and awareness, like perceiving, conceiving, remembering, reasoning, judging, imagining, and problem solving" [6]. Changes in cognition happening during the menopausal transition are reliably validated and well documented. They are of concern as whether the alterations in cognition may signify an underlying serious and a long-term cognitive disorder as some research suggest that these problems are a part of alterations in cerebral function which are insidiously progressive and finally leading to dementia [7–9].

16.3 Menopause Brain Fog

The cluster of alterations in cognition happening around menopause is referred to as "brain fog." This includes trouble in daily life (like misplacing things such as keys), difficulty in concentrating (easily distracted, being absent-minded, losing the train of thoughts), difficulty in recalling words, increased forgetfulness and manifestations representative of attention deficit hyperactivity disorder [10, 11]. Hence the condition is defined as "the constellation of cognitive symptoms experienced by women around the menopause, which most frequently manifest in memory and attention difficulties and involve symptoms such as difficulty encoding and recalling words, names, stories or numbers, difficulty maintaining a train of thought, distractibility, forgetting intentions (reason for coming into a particular room), and difficulty switching between tasks" [12]. However, these changes are not to be taken for dementia, as true dementia occurring prior to 64 years is extremely uncommon.

Neuropsychological analysis in substantial samples of women from a premenopausal state to postmenopause have reported that verbal learning and memory, and less apparent and less definitive impact on psychomotor performance, working memory and attention as the major cognitive domains affected through menopausal transition [13–19]. Higher-order cognitive functions like strategic thinking, planning and other executive functions remain unaltered across the menopausal transition [19]. The aspects differentiating postmenopausal females likely to be affected by cognitive diminution in the menopausal transition from others, are still not well-appreciated. Women with lower educational status/occupation and reduced leisure activities are reported to be more prone for decline in cognitive function and dementia [20].

16.4 Biology of Sexual Steroids in the Central Nervous System (CNS)

All women experience perceptible alterations in the proportions of different sexual steroids namely, estradiol, progesterone, and androgens, during their lifetime from menarche to menopause. A progressive fluctuation in the ovarian activity is seen in middle-aged women, that starts 4–6 years before menopause, also known as the menopause transition period. These changes have important influences on all organ systems including the central nervous system (CNS). The neurosteroids, which are the steroid hormones of the CNS, act at the level of cortical and subcortical structures via non-genomic and genomic pathways [21]. They are responsible for several neurological functions like cognition, memory, behavior, mood, sleep, pain, etc. apart from other functions like regulating formation of myelin with a significant role in demyelinating diseases. Different hormones play a role on regulation of brain function in a particular way, such as, estrogen with neuroprotective effect that is more pronounced in females than males, androgen being more active in males that is evident during recovery from demyelinating diseases and progestogens which are effective in limiting apoptosis or atypical proliferation following a CNS insult like traumatic brain injury or cerebrovascular accident [22].

The function of estrogens involves neurotransmitters like acetylcholine, serotonin, glutamate, and noradrenaline. The estrogen receptors are distributed in various sites of the brain involving memory and executive functions. Estrogen-mediated cholinergic action includes neurotrophic and neuroprotective actions, protecting against apoptosis and other neural injury, in addition to DNA repair and antioxidant effect [23, 24]. Like estrogen, progestogens also play a role in neurogenesis, bioenergetic systems, and cell survival. However, they are not known to have synergistic effects and concomitant administration can result in reduced effects, as compared to when it is used as a single agent. Progesterone, particularly allopregnanolone, acts by promoting GABAergic inhibiting synaptic transmission and hence lower proportions of allopregnanolone are associated with depression. This GABAergic action of progesterone on the hippocampus explains the negative impact on cognitive performance with exogenous intake of progestins. The androgen dihydrotestosterone is also locally produced in brain. In animal model, they are capable of effecting neurogenesis and spine synapses at the level of the hippocampus. Similar to estrogens, androgens also exert a neuroprotective action and studies have shown that testosterone (through its conversion to estradiol) produce increase serotonergic tone. Dehydroepiandrosterone (DHEA) exerts neuroprotective, anti-glucocorticoid, and antioxidant effects, thereby playing a role in improved cognitive deficits, reduce anxiety and depressive symptoms.

16.5 Role of Menopausal Hormonal Therapy

Many women experience changes in cognition such as forgetfulness, difficulty with words etc., during the menopausal transition period suggesting the role of hormonal changes happening around the perimenopausal period. Though women in early midlife are known to have better performance in memory tasks, elderly women are more vulnerable for age-related dementia when compared to age-matching men. A recent study has demonstrated that higher plasma estradiol levels was associated with better cognitive performance and lower impairment even in women who were already reporting cognitive decline [25]. Though the longitudinal data regarding the memory and cognitive changes with menopausal transition are less, there are two studies reporting the minute reductions in cognition. The Kinmen Women-Health Investigation (KIWI) found no striking deterioration in cognition except in verbal fluency over 18 months in a follow-up study of women from their premenopausal state [26]. The Study of Women's Health Across the Nation (SWAN) delineated cognitive decline as learning disabilities during the menopausal transition which improved to the premenopausal state in the postmenopausal period, once menopause was fully established [14]. The Women's Health Initiative (WHI) provided 5-year data to prove that combination of conjugated equine estrogen (CEE) and medroxyprogesterone acetate (MPA) resulted in a twofold increased risk of all-cause dementia [27], while CEE alone did not show any effect on risk of all-cause dementia [28].

In addition to the changes happening around menopausal transition, the long-term hormonal fluctuations also contribute to the cognitive changes in later life. In a meta-analysis of observational studies, menopausal hormonal transition was associated with 29% reduction in Alzheimer's disease though the results of clinical trials like Women's Health Initiative (WHI) and Women's Health Initiative Memory Study (WHIMS) were not reflective of the same [23]. The limitations of these studies were that women included were above 65 years, and the supposed "timing hypothesis" was not taken into consideration. Long-term users (5–10 years duration) of estrogen or estrogen-progestin combination have demonstrated an elevated risk of cognitive impairment. On the contrary, further studies have suggested that estrogen is neuroprotective exclusively when started a little while following the initiation of menopause [29, 30]. Nevertheless, hormone treatment is presently not advocated, as a means of alleviating cognitive impairment related to menopause, as the available medical evidence till date does not favor the usefulness of menopausal hormonal transition in allaying cognitive impairment or improving clinical outcomes from dementia.

16.6 Role of Mind-Body Medicine in Enhancing Cognition

The period of menopausal transition is associated with a wide variety of disturbing symptoms like stress, anxiety, sexual dysfunction, vasomotor symptoms, depression, and sleep alterations all of which result in cognitive dysfunction. Though MHT can alter the levels of estrogen and provide symptomatic relief, it is always associated with increased risk of cardiovascular diseases and malignancies like breast cancer. Hence an alternative approach, in the form of mind-body interventions are proven to alleviate the symptoms of menopausal transition in peri- and postmenopausal women. Mind-body medicine addresses the woman as a whole with the aim of improving the mental health without the intake any exogenous hormones. It is not associated with troubling side effects or serious drug interactions and are frequently effective at treating more than one symptom simultaneously. The different types of mind-body therapies are mindfulness, meditation, yoga, and hypnosis. These modalities are effective by directly targeting the memory/cognitive concerns and increase the self-reliance of the women.

In a pilot study involving menopausal women, two, 90-min weekly meditation session, for a period of 8 weeks, in the form of self-affirmation, guided imagery and silent reflection were offered and the results showed that there was significant reduction in hot flashes (67%) and depression (70%), though sleep quality and quantity were not assessed [31].

In a recent study by Carmody et al., women in late stages of perimenopause or early stages of postmenopause were randomized to either an 8-week mindfulness-based stress reduction (MBSR) or a wait-list control group. This MBSR included interventions like supine body scans, mindful stretching, seated meditation, education, and an all-day retreat during the sixth week of intervention. The results indicated a greater degree of improvement of hot flashes in the MSBR group during the course of study and at follow-up (32.25 and 44.56% vs. 20.69 and 26.97%), sleep thereby improving the overall quality of life, as measure by Menopause-Related Quality of Life Scale and sleep quality, as measured by Women's Health Initiative Insomnia Rating Scale [32].

Hypnosis therapy has also shown promising results for managing menopausal symptoms linked to cognitive dysfunction. In a randomized control trial, postmenopausal women were randomized to either a hypnosis intervention like coolness and relaxation or a structured attention group. The intervention included weekly 45-min therapy. Results proved a greater reduction of hot flashes among women who received hypnosis intervention (69%) than the control group (18%) and this was measured by Hot Flash Related Daily Interference Scale (HFRDIS), along with improvement in sleep (53.63 vs. 10.34%) as measured by PSQI [33].

The most commonly used method of mind-body therapy is yoga. A recent meta-analysis has shown that yoga can result in small, but significant decrease in psychological and vasomotor symptoms including hot flashes, depression, sleep disturbances, thereby improving the cognitive function [34].

Therefore, the available research works indicate that mind-body interventions may be beneficial in treating menopausal concerns and reducing the cognitive problems. However larger studies will need to be conducted for utilization of a holistic approach to help peri- and postmenopausal women cope with the complaints of cognitive impairment during menopause.

16.7 Optimizing Brain Health

The major concern for women with cognitive complaints at menopause is the risk of dementia in later life. Women must be made aware that the cognitive issues or dementia can be delayed by addressing the modifiable risk factors like smoking, cognitive activity, social interaction, obesity, hypertension, diabetes, and depression. To optimize brain health, the ideal time for intervention is during the midlife focusing on the above modifiable factors. The following methods can be advised:

- Counselling women about the significance of weight reduction, physical activity, and dietary management by maintaining a systematic plan for workout for a minimum of 150 min a day of adequate aerobic exercises and healthy BMI of 18.5–25.

- To evaluate and manage hypertension, dyslipidemia, diabetes, etc.
- Advise on avoiding excessive alcohol intake, quit smoking.
- To maintain social engagements, particularly if there is history of depression.
- Encourage to challenge the brain-reading, learning new language, learning new skill to increase cognitive reserve.
- A brain-friendly diet that is rich in polyunsaturated fatty acids like Omega 3 and Omega 6, antioxidants like vitamins A, C, and E to get rid of free radicals and reduce the negative impact on brain cells.
- Good sleep habits like limiting screen time before bed, use of pillow sprays/aromatherapy, comfortable sleep room have shown dramatic effects by boosting energy levels, mood and concentration thereby lifting the cloud of brain fog.

Hence a multi-pronged approach is recommended for dementia prevention and to achieve an optimal brain health.

16.8 Conclusion

Most women report cognitive changes or memory disturbances associated with menopause transition which are collectively referred to as "brain fade" or "brain fog" due to perceptible variations in the sexual hormones namely estradiol, progestins as well as androgens. The timing of these changes implies an underlying hormonal etiology secondary to declining ovarian function. The most frequently affected cognitive abilities include learning and recall of words, working memory, and attention. However, these cognitive performances also depend on several other factors like age at menopause, severity of vasomotor symptoms, psychological symptoms etc. Unfortunately, menopausal hormonal transition is not advocated as therapy, or for prevention of cognitive dysfunction in any age group, during menopause, though estrogen therapy might be valuable in sustaining cognitive performance and lessening the threat of dementia if started at the onset of menopause. This lack of proper pharmacological options to deal with cognitive issues at menopause necessitates a focused life style modification approach, in the form of mind-body interventions, to maintain optimal brain health. A multidisciplinary approach that includes gynecologists, psychiatrists, and specialist nurses should be adopted to provide individualized support, taking into consideration the aftermath of the manifestations on the woman's aptitude to operate normally in her day-to-day life.

References

1. Shifren JL, Gass MLS, NAMS Recommendations for Clinical Care of Midlife Women Working Group. The North American Menopause Society recommendations for clinical care of midlife women. Menopause. 2014;21(10):1038–62.

2. Koebele SV, Bimonte-Nelson HA. The endocrine-brain-aging triad where many paths meet: female reproductive hormone changes at midlife and their influence on circuits important for learning and memory. Exp Gerontol. 2017;94:14–23.
3. Micevych P, Sinchak K. Estradiol regulation of progesterone synthesis in the brain. Mol Cell Endocrinol. 2008;290(1–2):44–50.
4. Greendale GA, Karlamangla AS, Maki PM. The menopause transition and cognition. JAMA. 2020;323(15):1495–6.
5. The NAMS 2017 Hormone Therapy Position Statement Advisory Panel. The 2017 hormone therapy position statement of the North American Menopause Society. Menopause. 2017;24(7):728–53.
6. APA Dictionary of Psychology [Internet]. American Psychological Association; [cited 2023 Aug 9]. https://dictionary.apa.org/.
7. Rettberg JR, Yao J, Brinton RD. Estrogen: a master regulator of bioenergetic systems in the brain and body. Front Neuroendocrinol. 2014;35(1):8–30.
8. Jett S, Malviya N, Schelbaum E, Jang G, Jahan E, Clancy K, et al. Endogenous and exogenous estrogen exposures: how women's reproductive health can drive brain aging and inform Alzheimer's prevention. Front Aging Neurosci. 2022;14:831807.
9. Scheyer O, Rahman A, Hristov H, Berkowitz C, Isaacson RS, Diaz Brinton R, et al. Female sex and Alzheimer's risk: the menopause connection. J Prev Alzheimers Dis. 2018;5(4):225–30.
10. Sullivan Mitchell E, Fugate Woods N. Midlife women's attributions about perceived memory changes: observations from the Seattle midlife Women's health study. J Womens Health Gend Based Med. 2001;10(4):351–62.
11. Epperson CN, Shanmugan S, Kim DR, Mathews S, Czarkowski KA, Bradley J, et al. New onset executive function difficulties at menopause: a possible role for lisdexamfetamine. Psychopharmacology. 2015;232(16):3091–100.
12. Maki PM, Jaff NG. Brain fog in menopause: a health-care professional's guide for decision-making and counseling on cognition. Climacteric. 2022;25(6):570–8.
13. Cao Q, Tan CC, Xu W, Hu H, Cao XP, Dong Q, et al. The prevalence of dementia: a systematic review and meta-analysis. J Alzheimers Dis. 2020;73(3):1157–66.
14. Greendale GA, Huang MH, Wight RG, Seeman T, Luetters C, Avis NE, et al. Effects of the menopause transition and hormone use on cognitive performance in midlife women. Neurology. 2009;72(21):1850–7.
15. Epperson CN, Sammel MD, Freeman EW. Menopause effects on verbal memory: findings from a longitudinal community cohort. J Clin Endocrinol Metab. 2013;98(9):3829–38.
16. Kilpi F, Soares ALG, Fraser A, Nelson SM, Sattar N, Fallon SJ, et al. Changes in six domains of cognitive function with reproductive and chronological ageing and sex hormones: a longitudinal study in 2411 UK mid-life women. BMC Womens Health. 2020;20(1):177.
17. Maki PM, Springer G, Anastos K, Gustafson DR, Weber K, et al. Cognitive changes during the menopausal transition: a longitudinal study in women with and without HIV. Menopause. 2021;28(4):360–8.
18. Weber MT, Rubin LH, Schroeder R, Steffenella T, Maki PM. Cognitive profiles in perimenopause: hormonal and menopausal symptom correlates. Climacteric. 2021;24(4):401–7.
19. Maki PM, Weber MT. A research primer for studies of cognitive changes across the menopause transition. Climacteric. 2021;24(4):382–8.
20. Stern Y. Cognitive reserve. Neuropsychologia. 2009;47(10):2015–28.
21. Denley MCS, Gatford NJF, Sellers KJ, Srivastava DP. Estradiol and the development of the cerebral cortex: an unexpected role? Front Neurosci. 2018;12:245.
22. Zárate S, Stevnsner T, Gredilla R. Role of estrogen and other sex hormones in brain aging. Neuroprotection and DNA repair. Front Aging Neurosci. 2017;9:430.
23. Morgan KN, Derby CA, Gleason CE. Cognitive changes with reproductive aging, perimenopause, and menopause. Obstet Gynecol Clin N Am. 2018;45(4):751–63.
24. Bethea CL, Kohama SG, Reddy AP, Urbanski HF. Ovarian steroids regulate gene expression in the dorsal raphe of old female macaques. Neurobiol Aging. 2016;37:179–91.

25. Lui LY, Stone K, Cauley JA, Hillier T, Yaffe K. Bone loss predicts subsequent cognitive decline in older women: the study of osteoporotic fractures. J Am Geriatr Soc. 2003;51(1):38–43.
26. Fuh JL, Wang SJ, Lee SJ, Lu SR, Juang KD. A longitudinal study of cognition change during early menopausal transition in a rural community. Maturitas. 2006;53(4):447–53.
27. Shumaker SA, Legault C, Rapp SR, Thal L, Wallace RB, Ockene JK, WHIMS Investigators, et al. Estrogen plus progestin and the incidence of dementia and mild cognitive impairment in postmenopausal women: the women's health initiative memory study: a randomized controlled trial. JAMA. 2003;289(20):2651–62.
28. Shumaker SA, Legault C, Kuller L, Rapp SR, Thal L, Lane DS, Women's health initiative Memory Study, et al. Conjugated equine estrogens and incidence of probable dementia and mild cognitive impairment in postmenopausal women: women's health initiative memory study. JAMA. 2004;291(24):2947–58.
29. Coker LH, Espeland MA, Rapp SR, Legault C, Resnick SM, Hogan P, et al. Postmenopausal hormone therapy and cognitive outcomes: the women's health initiative memory study (WHIMS). J Steroid Biochem Mol Biol. 2010;118(4–5):304–10.
30. Marder K, Sano M. Estrogen to treat Alzheimer's disease: too little, too late? So what's a woman to do? Neurology. 2000;54(11):2035–7.
31. Manocha R, Semmar B, Black D. A pilot study of a mental silence form of meditation for women in perimenopause. J Clin Psychol Med Settings. 2007;14(3):266–73.
32. Carmody JF, Crawford S, Salmoirago-Blotcher E, Leung K, Churchill L, Olendzki N. Mindfulness training for coping with hot flashes: results of a randomized trial. Menopause. 2011;18(6):611–20.
33. Elkins GR, Fisher WI, Johnson AK, Carpenter JS, Keith TZ. Clinical hypnosis in the treatment of postmenopausal hot flashes: a randomized controlled trial. Menopause. 2013;20(3):291–8.
34. Cramer H, Lauche R, Langhorst J, Dobos G. Effectiveness of yoga for menopausal symptoms: a systematic review and meta-analysis of randomized controlled trials. Evid Based Complement Alternat Med. 2012;2012:863905.

Skin and Menopause

17

K. Geetha

17.1 Introduction

The skin is one of the most important organs in the body, and the physiological effects of ageing and menopause have a big impact on it. In most cases, menopause happens between the ages of 45 and 55. Menopause is an oestrogen-deficient hormonal condition distinguished by physical degradation of the skin due to the absence of oestrogen's beneficial qualities. Skin structure and function are influenced by postmenopausal low oestrogen levels, with up to 64% of women seeking menopause clinics suffering dermatological disorders [1].

17.2 Definition

Menopause and perimenopause are separate stages in the life of a woman. Menopause is defined in medicine as the appearance of the last menstrual bleeding, after which it ceases for approximately 1 year [2].

17.3 Role of Hormones on Skin and Hair

17.3.1 Oestrogens

From systemic steroid hormones produced by the adrenals, skin cells generate sex hormones and other steroids such as oestrogens, androgens, and glucocorticoids. During menopause, sex hormones fluctuate. Menopause pathogenesis has been

K. Geetha (✉)
Dermatology Department, ESIC Medical College and Hospital, Chennai, India

R. Garg (ed.), *Management of Menopause*,
https://doi.org/10.1007/978-981-96-0239-1_17

linked to the androstenedione/sex-hormone-binding globulin ratio, cortisol, melatonin, insulin-like growth factor-1 (IGF-1), as well as norepinephrine [3].

Oestrogen receptors (ERs) often are found in the dermis and epidermis, with a significant density in the genitalia, face, and lower abdomen. There are two isoforms of ER (ER α and ER β). ER β can be detected in dermal papilla cells, dermal fibroblasts, sebocytes, adipocytes, melanocytes, and keratinocytes of the outer root sheath. The effect of oestrogen decline during menopause on skin ageing has been widely studied. The adrenals produce systemic steroid hormones, and skin cells produce sex hormones and other steroids such as oestrogens, androgens, and glucocorticoids.

During menopause, oestrogen deficiency induces skin barrier dysfunction, lack of moisture, reduced sebum production on the face and scalp, diminished antioxidant function and wound healing, and decreased collagen and elastin synthesis, which causes wrinkles and dermal thinning on both skin and genital mucosa. Furthermore, it impairs the extracellular matrix's ability to bind glycosaminoglycans such as hyaluronic acid, reducing skin turgescence and moisture. It also impairs the body's capacity to regulate temperature, resulting in pallor, decreased vascularity, and hot flushes caused by vasodilation that occurs within the blood capillaries of the papillary dermis [4–6].

17.3.2 Androgens

The production of sebum and the development of hair in the pilosebaceous unit are both regulated by androgens. A considerable rise in androgens after menopause causes clinical hyperandrogenism, which presents as sebaceous gland enlargement and androgenetic alopecia of the female pattern due to local deficits in hair regeneration and growth [7].

17.4 Normal Structural and Functional Changes in the Skin After Menopause

The reproductive hormones impede cell proliferation at the epidermis and skin levels, resulting in atrophy in both the epidermis and vascular bed. Reduced collagen and elastin fibre activity lowers glucose-amine-glucans concentration, resulting in collagen and elastin fibre destruction as well as elastosis. Collagen loses physical and chemical characteristics as it ages, but it gains hydroxyproline content and calcium binding capacity. Collagen density decreases by 2% every year on average during the postmenopausal period. The number of melanocytes and Langerhans cells in the epidermis reduces due to diminished blood circulation. Skin loses its ability to resist external or internal forces and becomes more permeable [8].

The hypodermic tissue also gets impacted by alterations in sexual hormones. When peroxisomes and the so-called peroxisome proliferator-activated receptor (PPAR) receptors are damaged, adipocyte activity is diminished. This mechanism results in the breakdown or atrophy of fatty tissue. The superciliary arch, orbits, temples, and cheek bones all experience unique changes. The jaw, nasolabial folds, and chin are also transformed into fatty tissue reservoirs [9].

Table 17.1 Normal structural and physiological changes in the components of skin after menopause

S. no	Structure	Structural and physiological changes
1.	Epidermis	• Atrophy of epidermis • Decrease in the number of Langerhans cells and melanocyte activity
2.	Dermis	• Decreased collagen and elastic fibres along with reduced blood flow and fibroblast function • Increased activity of matrix metalloproteinase (MMPs)
3.	Subcutaneous fat	• Reduction in the volume and distribution
4.	Other changes	• Defective barrier function and reduced defence against oxidative stress

Table 17.2 Classification of dermatoses associated with menopause

S. no	Dermatoses	
1.	Dermatoses due to physiological structural and functional changes	Increased dryness of the skin, pruritis, flushing, hyperhidrosis, thinning and atrophy of skin, increase in the wrinkles, impaired wound healing, increase in the ageing changes, decrease in skin tone and turgor, decreased barrier function, and immunological function
2.	Dermatoses aggravated with aging	Senile xerosis and eczema, leg ulcers, decubitus ulcers, post-herpetic neuralgias, skin tumours like seborrheic keratosis, skin tags, actinic keratosis, basal cell carcinoma, squamous cell carcinoma, and lentigo maligna
3.	Dermatoses associated with oestrogen deficiency	Atrophic vulvovaginitis, vulvar lichen sclerosus, dysaesthetic vulvodynia, burning mouth syndrome (orodynia), hirsutism, alopecia (female pattern hair loss), keratoderma climactericum (thickening of the soles), vulvovaginal candidiasis
4.	Dermatoses not specific to menopause	Generalised or localised pruritis, pemphigus vulgaris, psoriasis, lichen planus, dermatophyte fungal infections etc.
5.	Dermatoses associated with hormone replacement therapy	Melasma, darkening of nevi, acanthosis nigricans, urticarial, increased skin sensitivity, erythema multiforme, pompholyx (hand eczema)

The normal structural and functional changes in the skin that occur after menopause is given in Table 17.1 [5].

17.5 Classification of Dermatoses Associated with Menopause

The cutaneous dermatoses seen with menopause can be classified as in Table 17.2 [10, 11].

The most common dermatoses in postmenopausal females observed in an Indian study by Pragya et al. included genital dermatoses such as atrophic vaginitis, lichen sclerosus et atrophicus, and lichen simplex chronicus, followed by extragenital dermatoses such as dermatophytosis, lichen planus, psoriasis, and eczema [10].

17.6 Common Dermatoses After Menopause

17.6.1 Xerosis and Eczema

The reduction in oestrogen levels after menopause causes dry, fragile, and sensitive skin, rendering it more susceptible to eczema. The loss of barrier function and an increase in transepidermal water loss (TEWL) may also worsen it [12]. Postmenopausal women tend to suffer from pruritus, which is frequently accompanied by xerosis. Oestrogen hormone replacement treatment (HRT) and preventative measures, including staying away from triggers, taking fewer baths, utilising humidifiers, and applying low pH emollients once a day, may be beneficial [13].

17.6.2 Flushing

According to theory, the "hot flush" of menopause is triggered on by changes in oestrogen levels causing hypothalamus thermoregulatory failure. The thermoneutral zone, which has been restricted in women who have hot flushes, is said to be recovered by oestrogen when taken daily in doses of 0.31–1.25 mg. Women who have moderate to severe hot flushes might consider therapy with any of the following medications if oestrogen is contraindicated or poorly tolerated: Along with behavioural therapy, patients should take paroxetine 7.5 mg, venlafaxine 36.5–75 mg, desvenlafaxine 50–100 mg, citalopram 10 mg, escitalopram 10–20 mg, gabapentin 300–900 mg, and pregabalin 10–50 mg daily [14, 15].

17.6.3 Acne and Rosacea

Acne, which is most common in teenagers, is now more common in adults. There are often papules, pustules, inflammatory nodules, open and closed comedones, and other abnormalities. Rosacea is a significant differential diagnosis; but unlike rosacea, the presence of comedones in acne can help differentiate the two illnesses. The exact cause of menopausal acne is uncertain; however, it is thought to be caused by an imbalance of the hormones oestrogen and androgen, which results in a relative hyperandrogenic state. As therapeutic options, standard topical medicine and anti-androgenic therapy, such as spironolactone and isotretinoin, are available [7]. A few studies have looked into the association between menopause and rosacea, but menopausal flushes can aggravate or even induce rosacea.

17.6.4 Hirsutism

Hirsutism, or excessive hair growth in women, corresponds to a male hair pattern, such as a moustache and chin, or hair that grows thicker on the limbs than normal. It is an inheritable disorder caused by an excess of testosterone [16]. Androgen therapy, including testosterone therapy and androgen-oestrogen hormone therapy, has also been associated to postmenopausal hirsutism. The main objective is to correct any hormonal imbalances, reduce the appearance of excess hair, and improve overall quality of life.

Anti-androgens such as cyproterone acetate (CPA) 2 mg/day in combination with ethinyl oestradiol (35 gm/day), spironolactone (50–200 mg/day), drospirenone (3 mg/day), flutamide and bicalutamide (250–750 mg/day), oral contraceptive pill (OCP), enzyme inhibitors such as finasteride (2.5 mg/day), metformin (insulin-sensitising agent), gonadotropic-releasing hormone (GnRH) analogues like leuprolide acetate and nafarelin, eflornithine (13.9% topical cream), physical and chemical epilation (shaving, waxing, sugaring, threading), electrolysis, laser, intense pulse light (IPL), and thermolysis are among the therapeutic options available [17].

17.6.5 Alopecia (Female Pattern Hair Loss)

The condition is an inheritable disorder that results from a genetic susceptibility to the effects of dihydrotestosterone (DHT). Female pattern hair loss (FPHL) is the most prevalent type of alopecia in elderly women. It is progressive and often increases during or after menopause, especially if it is pre-existing. It damages hair follicles in the parietal or fronto-vertical areas, resulting in bitemporal hair loss but with unaffected frontal hairline [18]. Women with hormonal dysfunction are treated with systemic spironolactone, finasteride, and flutamide [19]. Through an androgen-independent mechanism, minoxidil (2–5%) can be used to treat postmenopausal women with or without hyperandrogenism. For FPHL cases that have not responded to medical treatment, hair transplantation may be considered [20].

17.6.6 Keratoderma Climactericum

The disorder, also known as acquired plantar keratoderma, occurs during menopause and is characterised by palmar and plantar hyperkeratosis. Frequently obese and hypertensive menopausal women experience it. Therapy alternatives include topical oestradiol 0.05% cream, urea 40% cream, and systemic retinoids [21].

17.6.7 Dermatoses Associated with Oestrogen Deficiency

17.6.7.1 Atrophic Vulvovaginitis

This is distinguished by the thinning (atrophy) of the vaginal skin. The vulva is comparatively unaltered because it contains lesser oestrogen receptors than the vagina. Vaginal skin atrophy results in itching, soreness, burning sensation, painful intercourse (dyspareunia), and painful urination [22].

17.6.7.2 Vulval Lichen Sclerosis (LS)

Vulval LS is a postmenopausal inflammatory scarring dermatosis. Although the precise aetiology is uncertain, autoimmune factors and genetic predispositions are thought to be associated. It manifests with white, atrophic, polygonal papules with flat surfaces that coalesce into plaques and extend in a figure-eight pattern into the vulva and perianal skin. It is possible to notice skin thickening in the vulva, perineum, labia majora, labia minora, fourchette, and clitoris. Architectural abnormalities brought about by severe disease consist of fusion of the labia, clitoral tethering, along with introitus narrowing. A greater risk of squamous cell carcinoma has been associated with LS [23]. Treatment with topical medications like potent steroids, emollients, oestrogens, retinoids, tacrolimus (0.03–0.1%) and lignocaine (5%) along with intralesional steroids, oral retinoids or surgery are found to be useful in various studies [24].

17.6.7.3 Dysaesthetic Vulvodynia

The condition is characterised by distinguishing features like widespread spontaneous discomfort in the vulvar region, labia, clitoris, vestibule, perineum, mons pubis, and inner thighs. Touch or pressure on the vulva does not trigger pain, and activities such as bicycling and riding a horse may aggravate the symptoms [25]. To reduce muscle spasms, it is usually treated with one or more of the following therapies: avoiding irritating substances, regular local anaesthetic use, physiotherapy, strengthening exercises for the pelvic floor, oral amitriptyline, pregabalin, carbamazepine, or gabapentin.

17.6.7.4 Vulvovaginal Candidiasis

It is a vaginal fungal infection caused by candida albicans overgrowth. The use of oral contraceptive pills (OCP), hormonal therapy, type 2 diabetes, steroid therapy, and an oral antibiotic worsens the condition. It is distinguished by profuse white curd-like vaginal discharge, along with a burning sensation in the vagina and vulva, and pruritus. Treatment comprises primarily of oral antifungal medicines and vaginal suppositories [26].

17.6.7.5 Burning Mouth Syndrome

Burning mouth syndrome (BMS) is a heterogeneous condition which occurs in 10–40% of perimenopausal women. Symptoms include burning sensations at the front of the tongue, hard palate, or lower lip mucosa [27]. Treatment alternatives consist of alpha lipoic acid 200 mg thrice daily, topical clonazepam, gabapentin 300–1200 mg, or a combination of these medicines [28].

17.6.8 Dermatoses Associated with Hormone Replacement Therapy (HRT)

According to studies, only 25% of women who experience symptoms consult a physician, emphasising the importance of for increased understanding about ways to take care of menopausal symptoms. Considering the Women's Health Initiative (WHI) trial results in 2002 among elderly women led to a substantial reduction in the number of women using hormone replacement treatment (HRT), it has become evident that the potential hazards of HRT are negligible for healthy women [29]. HRT comprises oestrogen (17b-oestradiol or conjugated equine oestrogen [CEE]), and progestogen is additionally needed to protect the endometrium in women with an intact uterus. SERMs are nonsteroidal synthetic medications that possess varying oestrogen agonist and antagonist activities in different target tissues as an alternative to progestogens [30].

HRT improves dermal collagen material, elasticity, as well as skin surface texture [31]. Systemic hazards of HRT use include venous thromboembolism as well as breast and endometrial cancer. However, the advantages frequently outweigh the risks, which are generally regarded as insignificant. Cutaneous adverse events of HRT include acne, androgenic hair loss, hirsutism and regional hypersensitivity. Oestrogen therapy can also exacerbate some dermatoses, including chloasma, naevi darkening, acanthosis nigricans, skin sensitivity, and hand eczema [32]. After menopause, systemic lupus erythematosus flares less often and more mildly; but there's a potential possibility that HRT may trigger flares [25].

17.7 General Management of Skin, Hair, and Mucosal Symptoms

HRT can be used alone or in conjunction with skin cosmetics and individualised dermatological care for the skin over the face and other sites. Preventing photoaging and melanoma and non-melanoma skin cancers can possibly be accomplished through photoprotection with sunscreen. Dermatological cosmetics may consist of collagen stimulators, antioxidants, or oestrogen to hydrate and treat dryness of the skin. For hair care, customised shampoos can be applied either prior to or after using prescription drugs. In order to preserve hair density, active components in dermocosmetics like aminoxil and the antioxidant stemoxydine can reduce the ratio of hair in the inactive telogen phase.

Topical oestrogen preparation is an essential component of treatment for genitourinary syndrome of menopause (GSM). Oestriol and oestradiol are the two main formulations. Symptoms and the patient's preference are used to define the formulations, which can be pessaries, creams, or gels. Topical oestrogen should be used in conjunction with lubricants and moisturisers. It has been repeatedly proved to be the most effective strategy to treat GSM symptoms, notably vulvovaginal atrophy [33]. Smoking cessation, stress reduction, photoprotection, proper nutrition, weight reduction, and regular exercise may possibly help to alleviate symptoms and reduce the likelihood of further decline before menopause is medically acknowledged [34].

17.8 Cosmetic Procedural Management

Cosmetic therapies attempt to slow down the ageing process by promoting the skin's natural renewal and repair processes. The enhancement of skin microcirculation and stimulation of collagen or elastin fibres make the skin more resistant to the effects of endo- or exogenic agents [35]. Traditional cosmetic massage comprises of five progressive techniques such as stroking, rubbing, pressing, patting, and vibrating. The procedure concludes with a gentle final stroke. Chemical peels containing fruit acids such as glycolic acid can be used. Microdermabrasion, or controlled mechanical peeling of the epidermis, is another procedure that may be advised to women during or after menopause. Regular microdermabrasion therapies eliminate scars, make wrinkles shallower, promote tissue regeneration, combat collagen, fibre, and elasticity loss, and get the skin prepared to accommodate the introduction of active ingredients [35].

Thermage systems are contemporary radio wave generators. This monopolar technique is used to carry out the treatment at a frequency of around 6 MHz. Skin elasticity is increased, wrinkles are filled, and cheeks and facial features are moulded through a series of radiofrequency procedures. Devices that output DC current are used primarily to regenerate mature skin. These methods are advised in the treatment of atrophic skin in order to tighten muscles, enhance skin microcirculation, and encourage adequate cell oxygenation. Iontophoresis, another method utilising DC current, allows active compounds to enter tissues [5, 35].

In order to combat the signs of ageing, ultrasounds can be used. Ultrasound waves have a frequency that is higher than the human auditory range (16 kHz). On the skin's surface, ultrasound waves have a variety of general therapeutic effects, including the stimulation of blood and lymph circulation, restoration of sebaceous gland activity, elimination of wrinkles, pigmentation marks, enhancement of rigidity and elasticity, stimulation of enzymes, improvement of cell membrane permeability along with antibacterial action [5]. Needle mesotherapy is an innovative therapy that includes intradermal injections while concurrently delivering numerous lyophilic therapeutic substances to areas of aesthetic deficit. These injections contain "conditioning substances," which include organic silica, hyaluronic acid (HA), micronutrients complex, rutin and artichoke extracts, phosphatidylcholine, L-carnitine, and caffeine. Based on the epidermal electroporation phenomenon, no needle mesotherapy is a replacement alternative to needle intradermotherapy [5, 35]. Acupuncture, cryotherapy, cryolift, injectables such as botulinum toxin and hyaluronic acid fillers, and other cosmetic procedures can also be provided. Modern cosmetology constantly searches for the most efficient treatments for dealing with skin ageing.

17.9 Conclusion

Hormone changes in menopausal women often lead to unpleasant physical, psychological, and sexual changes, which may affect their quality of life. Women at this point of their lives will feel less burdened and have a higher quality of life if they have better knowledge of the skin, hair, and mucosal changes that occur with menopause and how to control or prevent them. Evidence suggests that HRT can lessen or undo some of these alterations. Other possibilities for treatment depend on the specific issue but are typically within the purview of dermatologists.

References

1. Duarte GV, Trigo AC, Paim de Oliveira Mde F. Skin disorders during menopause. Cutis. 2016;97:E16–23.
2. Herman J, Rost-Roszkowska M, Skotnicka-Graca U. Skin care during the menopause period: non-invasive procedures of beauty studies. Postepy Dermatol Alergol. 2013;30(6):388–95. https://doi.org/10.5114/pdia.2013.39430. Epub 2013 Dec 18. PMID: 24494002; PMCID: PMC3907896
3. Slominski A, Zbytek B, Nikolakis G, et al. Steroidogenesis in the skin: implications for local immune functions. J Steroid Biochem Mol Biol. 2013;137:107–23.
4. Hall G, Phillips T. Estrogen and skin: the effects of estrogen, menopause, and hormone replacement therapy on the skin. J Am Acad Dermatol. 2005;53:555–68.
5. Lephart ED, Naftolin F. Menopause and the skin: old favorites and new innovations in cosmeceuticals for estrogen-deficient skin. Dermatol Ther (Heidelb). 2021;11(1):53–69. https://doi.org/10.1007/s13555-020-00468-7. Epub 2020 Nov 26. PMID: 33242128; PMCID: PMC7859014
6. El Mohtadi M, Whitehead K, Dempsey-Hibbert N, et al. Estrogen deficiency—a central paradigm in age-related impaired healing? EXCLI J. 2021;20:99–116.
7. Khunger N, Mehrotra K. Menopausal acne—challenges and solutions. Int J Women's Health. 2019;11:555–67.
8. Wojnowska D, Juszkiewicz-Borowiec M, Chodorowska G. Menopause impact to skin ageing [polish]. Postep Derm Alergol. 2006;3:149–56.
9. Donorfio LM. Fat distribution: a morphologic study of the ageing face. Dermatologic Surg. 2000;26:1107–12.
10. Nair P, Pariath K. A cross-sectional study on the dermatoses in postmenopausal patients at a rural-based tertiary health care center. Indian J Dermatol. 2019;64:360–5.
11. Nair PA. Dermatosis associated with menopause. J Midlife Health. 2014;5(4):168–75. https://doi.org/10.4103/0976-7800.145152. PMID: 25540566; PMCID: PMC4264279.
12. Brincat M, Muscat Baron Y, Galea R. Estrogens and the skin. Climacteric. 2005;8:110–23.
13. Kamp E, Ashraf M, Musbahi E, DeGiovanni C. Menopause, skin and common dermatoses. Part 2: skin disorders. Clin Exp Dermatol. 2022;47(12):2117–22.
14. Santoro N, Epperson C, Mathews S. Menopausal symptoms and their management. Endocrinol Metab Clin N Am. 2015;44:497–515.
15. Borda L, Wong L, Tosti A. Bioidentical hormone therapy in menopause: relevance in dermatology. Dermatol Online J. 2019;25:13030/qt4c20m28z.
16. Mofid A, Seyyed Alinaghi SA, Zandieh S, Yazdani T. Hirsutism. Int J Clin Pract. 2008;62:433–43.
17. Blume-Peytavi U, Atkin S, Gieler U, Grimalt R. Skin academy: hair, skin, hormones and menopause—current status/knowledge on the management of hair disorders in menopausal women. Eur J Dermatol. 2012;22:310–8.
18. Dinh QQ, Sinclair R. Female pattern hair loss: current treatment concepts. Clin Interv Aging. 2007;2:189–99.
19. Trüeb RM, Swiss Trichology Study Group. Finasteride treatment of patterned hair loss in normoandrogenic postmenopausal women. Dermatology. 2004;209:202–7.
20. Blumeyer A, Tosti A, Messenger A, Reygagne P, Del Marmol V, Spuls PI, European Dermatology Forum (EDF), et al. Evidence-based (S3) guideline for the treatment of androgenetic alopecia in women and in men. J Dtsch Dermatol Ges. 2011;9:S1–57.
21. Scheinfeld NS. Obesity and dermatology. Clin Dermatol. 2004;22:303–9.
22. Versi E, Cardozo L, Brincat M, Cooper D, Montgomery J, Studd J. Correlation of urethral physiology and skin collagen in postmenopausal women. Br J Obstet Gynaecol. 1988;95:147–52.
23. Spring A, Griffiths D, Nirmal D, et al. Identification and management of vulval problems of the postmenopausal woman—tips and tricks. Post Reprod Health. 2020;26:155–61.
24. Tasker GL, Wojnarowska F. Lichen sclerosus. Clin Exp Dermatol. 2003;28:128–33.

25. Wines N. Willsteed Menupause and the skin. Austral J Dermatol. 2001;42:149–60.
26. Musbahi E, Kamp E, Ashraf M, DeGiovanni C. Menopause, skin and common dermatosis. Part 3: genital disorders. Clin Exp Dermatol. 2022;47(12):2123–9.
27. Friedlander AH. The physiology, medical management and oral implications of menopause. J Am Dent Assoc. 2002;133:73–81.
28. Liu Y, Kim Y, Yoo T, et al. Burning mouth syndrome: a systematic review of treatments. Oral Dis. 2018;24:325–34.
29. Langer RD, Hodis HN, Lobo RA, et al. Hormone replacement therapy—where are we now? Climacteric. 2021;24(1):3–10.
30. Pinkerton JV, Conner EA. Beyond estrogen: advances in tissue selective estrogen complexes and selective estrogen receptor modulators. Climacteric. 2019;22(2):140–7.
31. Reus TL, Brohem CA, Schuck DC, et al. Revisiting the effects of menopause on the skin: functional changes, clinical studies, in vitro models and therapeutic alternatives. Mech Ageing Dev. 2020;185:111193.
32. Graham-Brown R. Dermatologic problems of the menopause. Clin Dermatol. 1997;15:143–5.
33. Lethaby A, Ayeleke RO, Roberts H. Local oestrogen for vaginal atrophy in postmenopausal women. Cochrane Database Syst Rev. 2016;2016:CD001500.
34. Zouboulis CC, Blume-Peytavi U, Kosmadaki M, Roó E, Vexiau-Robert D, Kerob D, Goldstein SR. Skin, hair and beyond: the impact of menopause. Climacteric. 2022;25(5):434–42.
35. Kasprzak W, Mańkowska A. Physiotherapy in cosmetology and esthetic medicine [polish]. Warsaw: Wydawnictwo Naukowe PZWL; 2010.

Cognition at Menopause

18

Archana Kumari and Akansha Gupta

Menopause represents the final phase in a woman's reproductive life. With the life expectancy of Indian women reaching up to 70 years as of 2020, it is crucial to ensure that the postmenopausal years are as comfortable as possible.

Neurological symptoms experienced during perimenopause indicate disruptions in multiple estrogen-regulated systems, including thermoregulation, sleep, circadian rhythms, sensory processing, and cognitive functions. Estrogen plays a pivotal role as a master regulator in brain function, operating through a network of estrogen receptors to maintain effective brain function. It regulates brain energy metabolism through coordinated signalling and transcriptional pathways.

Estrogen provides the following neurological benefits:

- Protection against neuronal cytotoxicity induced by oxidative stress.
- Reduction in serum concentrations of amyloid P components, associated with Alzheimer's disease.
- Enhancement of synaptic formation and neuronal growth, particularly dendritic spasticity.
- Protection against cerebrovascular toxicity caused by amyloid peptides, and promotion of neuronal survival and growth [1].

During the perimenopausal transition, the estrogen receptor network may become uncoupled and weakened, potentially leading to a hypometabolic state that increases the risk of developing neurodegenerative diseases later in life. However, this transition could also present an opportunity to prevent age-related neurological diseases [2].

Recent evidence suggests that women who undergo surgical menopause at a younger age (≤45 years) may experience a faster decline in global cognition,

A. Kumari (✉) · A. Gupta
Department of Obstetrics and Gynaecology, AIIMS, New Delhi, India

R. Garg (ed.), *Management of Menopause*,
https://doi.org/10.1007/978-981-96-0239-1_18

semantic and episodic memory, worse performance in verbal fluency and executive function, and an accumulation of Alzheimer's neuropathology. Further large-scale cohort studies are necessary to validate these findings [3].

Several studies have shown inconsistent declines in verbal memory during the menopausal transition, with some suggesting a possible rebound during the post-menopausal stage. Clinical studies that investigate memory changes following hormonal withdrawal and hormone therapy (HT) have demonstrated that estradiol is crucial for memory retention. Despite the common belief that memory issues are linked to menopausal symptoms, research shows that memory problems occur during the transition even when menopausal symptoms are controlled. While self-reported vasomotor symptoms (VMS) do not correlate with objective memory performance, emerging evidence indicates that VMS significantly affect memory performance, brain activity during rest, and white matter hyperintensities. In clinical practice, it is helpful to reassure women experiencing significant VMS that their memory may improve with treatment [4].

A systematic review and meta-analysis of literature over the past century indicate that hormone replacement therapy (HRT) may have specific cognitive effects, though many studies suffer from significant methodological limitations. The meta-analysis found a decreased risk of dementia in HRT users [5].

The WHIMS (Women Health Initiative Memory Study), a landmark randomized double-blind placebo-controlled clinical trial, compared estrogen plus progestin therapy with a placebo in postmenopausal women aged 65 and older. The study concluded that estrogen plus progestin therapy increased the risk of probable dementia and did not prevent mild cognitive impairment, suggesting that the risks outweigh the benefits [6].

Given the adverse effects associated with HT, the Cognitive and Affective Study (KEEPS-Cog) of the Kronos Early Estrogen Prevention Study (KEEPS) explored the impact of up to 4 years of menopausal hormone therapy (MHT) on cognition and mood in recently postmenopausal women. Although the study did not find a significant impact on cognition, it noted mood benefits in women who received oral conjugated equine estrogens (o-CEEs). However, these findings are limited to recently postmenopausal women with low cardiovascular risk profiles [7].

The ELITE (Early versus Late Intervention Trial) study supported the notion that starting MHT during early in perimenopause might offer cognitive and cardiovascular benefits [8]. Conversely, a study by Henderson et al. in 2016 reinforced the neutral effect of combined estrogen and progesterone therapy on cognitive function, indicating that estradiol neither benefits nor harms cognitive abilities, regardless of the time since menopause [9].

Contrasting evidence from a Finnish nationwide case-control study showed that long-term use of systemic hormone therapy was associated with a 9–17% increased risk of Alzheimer's disease in postmenopausal women, which is not related to the type of progestogen or the age at initiation of systemic hormone therapy. However, the use of vaginal estradiol did not show the same risk. Researchers concluded that while the absolute risk increase is small, this information should be shared with current and prospective hormone therapy users [10]. The FINGER trial demonstrated that a multidomain lifestyle intervention could benefit cognition in elderly individuals at elevated risk of dementia. While other trials did not show a statistically significant benefit from preventive interventions, secondary analyses among participants at risk of dementia revealed positive effects of intervention [11].

18.1 Conclusion

There is no definitive evidence supporting or refuting the use of MHT in early postmenopausal women, but it appears to be safe, with no harmful cognitive effects later in life. MHT may be particularly beneficial for younger women who have undergone surgical menopause, as opposed to those who experience spontaneous menopause. Therefore, it should be considered for these women.

Postmenopausal cognitive decline is influenced by various factors beyond age, including comorbidities like diabetes, hypertension, Coronary artery disease (CAD), psychological factors such as depression and anxiety, and vasomotor symptoms. To prevent cognitive decline in postmenopausal women, a multipronged approach should be adopted at least 10 years before menopause. This approach includes a healthy diet, regular physical activity, social engagement, and cognitive training through learning new skills.

References

1. Diaz Brinton R. The women's health initiative estrogen replacement therapy is neurotrophic and neuroprotective. Neurobiol Aging. 2000;21(3):475–96.
2. Brinton RD, Yao J, Yin F, Mack WJ, Cadenas E. Perimenopause as a neurological transition state. Nat Rev Endocrinol. 2015;11(7):393–405.
3. Georgakis MK, Beskou-Kontou T, Theodoridis I, Skalkidou A, Petridou ET. Surgical menopause in association with cognitive function and risk of dementia: a systematic review and meta-analysis. Psychoneuroendocrinology. 2019;106:9–19.
4. Maki PM. Verbal memory and menopause. Maturitas. 2015;82(3):288–90.
5. LeBlanc ES, Janowsky J, Chan BKS, Nelson HD. Hormone replacement therapy and cognition: systematic review and meta-analysis. JAMA. 2001;285(11):1489.
6. Shumaker SA, Legault C, Rapp SR, Thal L, Wallace RB, Ockene JK, et al. Estrogen plus progestin and the incidence of dementia and mild cognitive impairment in postmenopausal women: the women's health initiative memory study: a randomized controlled trial. JAMA. 2003;289(20):2651.
7. Gleason CE, Dowling NM, Wharton W, Manson JE, Miller VM, Atwood CS, et al. Effects of hormone therapy on cognition and mood in recently postmenopausal women: findings from the randomized, controlled KEEPS–cognitive and affective study. Brayne C, editor. PLOS Med. 2015;12(6):e1001833.
8. Hodis HN, Mack WJ, Shoupe D, Azen SP, Stanczyk FZ, Hwang-Levine J, et al. Methods and baseline cardiovascular data from the early versus late intervention trial with estradiol testing the menopausal hormone timing hypothesis. Menopause. 2015;22(4):391–401.
9. Henderson VW, St. John JA, Hodis HN, McCleary CA, Stanczyk FZ, Shoupe D, et al. Cognitive effects of estradiol after menopause: a randomized trial of the timing hypothesis. Neurology. 2016;87(7):699–708.

10. Savolainen-Peltonen H, Rahkola-Soisalo P, Hoti F, Vattulainen P, Gissler M, Ylikorkala O, et al. Use of postmenopausal hormone therapy and risk of Alzheimer's disease in Finland: nationwide case-control study. BMJ. 2019;364:l665.
11. Ngandu T, Lehtisalo J, Solomon A, Levälahti E, Ahtiluoto S, Antikainen R, et al. A 2 year multidomain intervention of diet, exercise, cognitive training, and vascular risk monitoring versus control to prevent cognitive decline in at-risk elderly people (FINGER): a randomised controlled trial. Lancet. 2015;385(9984):2255–63.

Menopause and Antiaging: A Novel Strategy for Life Extension

19

Igor Victorovich Lakhno and Ruchika Garg

Humankind is getting older gradually. The human search for universal interventions to achieve longevity lies in the field of translational medicine. Aging is known as a sum of diseases [1]. Antiaging is based on disease prevention. Cardiovascular disease (CVD) has its origin in the antenatal period of life. The hypothesis of "fetal programming" explains the nature of the diseases of an adult period of life [2]. However, active atherogenic vasculopathy is known to be started during perimenopausal years. Therefore, hypoestrogenicity is a trigger for CVD in women.

Menopause is a current issue of great medical and social significance. Most women in their transitional period of life are very concerned due to increased body weight, type II diabetes mellitus (DM), CVD, and its complications. The majority of studies support the importance of monitoring risk factors for type 2 DM and CVD in mid-life to older women to reduce morbidity and mortality associated with estrogen deficiency [3]. The level of DM increased four times over the last three decades [4]. Undoubtedly, a decreased level of estradiol changes the emphasis on the action of testosterone. Hyperandrenogenicity provokes obesity and insulin resistance. These changes contribute to the progression of carbohydrate metabolism disturbances and dyslipidemia [5]. The decrease in the level of estradiol stimulates the appetite [6].

Adipose tissue is a "field" for the synthesis of mediators of chronic inflammation and oxidative stress. Since lipid metabolism disorders are involved in the development of endothelial malfunction, the pathogenesis of CVD in perimenopausal women has becomes completely understood [7]. Hypertrophied adipocytes have a significant number of genes involved in inflammation and cytokines production.

I. V. Lakhno (✉)
Department of Obstetrics and Gynecology No 3 at Kharkiv National Medical University, Kharkiv, Ukraine
e-mail: iv.lakhno@knmu.edu.ua

R. Garg
Department Obstetrics and Gynaecology, SN Medical College, Agra, India

R. Garg (ed.), *Management of Menopause*,
https://doi.org/10.1007/978-981-96-0239-1_19

The attack of tissue hypoxia may contribute to the accumulation of macrophages and other immune cells in adipose tissue. The inflammatory events in adipose tissue cause a disturbed hepatic carbohydrate metabolism and reduces the sensitivity of skeletal muscles to insulin. All obese patients demonstrate elevated levels of pro-inflammatory substances: IL-6 and C-reactive protein (C-RP) [8]. Pro-inflammatory cytokines: TNF-α, IL-6, and IL-1β have a paracrine effect that contributes to insulin resistance. The increased blood level of pro-inflammatory cytokines is involved in the development of atherosclerosis and chronic inflammation. IL-18, TNF-α, IL-6, and C-RP are the main markers of inflammation found in women with hyperandrogenicity. However, the fact of increased levels of pro-inflammatory substances both in obese and slim women is of interest. Thus, chronic inflammation plays an active role in the scenario of insulin resistance, atherosclerosis, and arterial hypertension. The elevated level of C-RP was found in women with hyperandrogenicity. This relationship gets more strong in older and obese women [9]. Il-6 is known as an indicator of the risk of atherosclerosis, coronary heart disease, and arterial hypertension [10]. IL-6 is a potential inducer of C-reactive protein hepatic synthesis. Increased C-RP is a marker for severe atherosclerosis, the risk of myocardial infarction and stroke [11].

The level of IL-6 and C-RP is also elevated in women with hyperandrogenicity and insulin resistance [12]. Since leukocytes are located in visceral adipose tissue, and white blood cells are a source of pro-inflammatory cytokines, it can be assumed that insulin resistance stimulates the activity of leukocytes. The correlation between C-RP, IL-6, and body mass index was found [13]. The detection of C-RP blood serum levels could be an important addition to the traditional screening for the prediction of metabolic syndrome X in women. Pro-inflammatory cytokines could be thought an early marker of insulin resistance and atherosclerosis [14]. There are also other known markers of inflammation in women with hyperandrogenicity. Chemerin affects metabolic risk factors and blood pressure. The level of this novel adipokine is increased in women with hyperandrogenicity. The elevated levels of visfatin were found to be associated with beta-cell damage in type 2 DM. The visfatin level is elevated and correlates with body mass index, insulin resistance, and hyperinsulinemia in patients with hyperandrogenicity [15]. The increased concentrations of vaspin, leptin, and resistin were also found. However, the level of irisin ("hormone of physical activity") is reduced in this category of patients. This myokine improves cognitive impairment [16]. Therefore, menopause contributes to the development of metabolic syndrome X. The following issue remains relevant: "Is it sufficient to prescribe only hormone replacement therapy (HRT) drugs for the correction of metabolic disorders in menopause, and which pathogenic pathways should be additionally taken into account for the development of novel approaches to the management of menopausal women?"

Aging is a significant risk factor for type 2 DM. Obesity, decreased physical inactivity, an unbalanced diet, smoking, excessive alcohol consumption, and some medications contribute to the development of this disease. Vitamin D3 and calcium deficiency increase the risk of both types of DM [17]. Women with polycystic ovary syndrome (PCOS) are a major risk group for metabolic disorders. The history of PCOS is about 40,000 years old. During the Paleolithic period, the harsh human living conditions led to the suppression of fertility and the accumulation of fat reserves [18]. The wave of migration of primitive people from Africa to Europe led to the necessity to survive in conditions of cold winters and food shortages. The storage of additional energy reserves was facilitated by insulin resistance and excessive development of fat. Declining fertility also increased the survival of women at the time. Therefore, PCOS contributed to the preservation of humankind and can be considered an endocrinopathy of the surviving descendants of insulin-resistant ancestors [9]. The hyperandrogenicity persists even after menopause in women with PCOS. Increased levels of C-RP and other markers of inflammation were also found in this population [10]. Early or late menarche can also lead to metabolic disorders in menopause [11]. The osteopenic syndrome and osteoporosis are separate problems. Disturbed gut microbiota was found in women with osteopenia recently [19].

Unfortunately, HRT is not recognized as an efficient method for metabolic syndrome X prevention [15]. Since metabolic disorders reduce the active working capacity and life period in general, it is necessary to develop a therapeutic strategy focused on their negative impact on a woman's health prevention or reduction. Women with a normal weight before the onset of menopause should be recommended to increase physical activity, and obese patients additionally should be asked for a diet [20]. Diet was found to be associated with a reduction in incident cardiovascular and coronary adverse events, as well as heart failure [21]. The daily consumption of 400 g of vegetables for 3 weeks was found in one study to improve lipid metabolism and glycemic control in obese menopausal women [22]. The Mediterranean diet may help in the primary prevention of bone, metabolic, and cardiovascular diseases in the postmenopausal period [17]. Interestingly, CVD risk in postmenopausal women appears to be sensitive to a change to a low-fat dietary pattern and, among healthy women, includes both coronary heart disease benefit and stroke risk [6]. The existing experience of wellness anti-aging programs indicates the use of medical nutrition and physical education. However, the issue of emotional and physical comfort in the process of weight loss remains open.

The state of moderate ketosis is known to reduce the patient's appetite in the process of medical diet therapy [4]. However, ketosis leads to the predominance of anaerobic glycolysis, the accumulation of lactate, and lipid peroxidation tissue products. This supports oxidative stress and adversely affects hepatic lipid metabolism. Increased ketogenesis is dangerous for people with DM and requires adjustment of insulin dose or a sulfonylurea drug. How can these deviations be prevented? The obvious prospect is the use of xylitol preparations, which is not an insulin-dependent source of energy and could prevent the transition from the Krebs cycle to other metabolic pathways [23].

Xylitol is known as a source of energy to achieve balance with an excellent anti-catabolic effect. Xylitol can reduce constipation, DM, obesity, and other diseases. This polyol has a stimulating effect on digestion and the immune system. The level of xylitol was found to be used as a predictor of the prospect of weight loss without surgical interventions in patients with morbid obesity [3]. After the use of xylitol, the glycemia level stays constant, and the processes of gluconeogenesis prevail over glycolysis. The long-term experience of using xylitol in the food industry supports its anti-inflammatory and antibacterial effects. It is capable of counteracting the etiological microbial factors of gingivitis, pneumonia, and media otitis. The dose-dependent antimicrobial effect of xylitol is known. Xylitol can compensate for NADH deficiency in patients with hemolytic anemia. There is also evidence that xylitol can reduce the proliferation of cancer cells [23]. Xylitol enhances the processes of lipolysis, contributing to the reduction of adipose tissue, and has a therapeutic effect on dyslipidemia. It protects the heart, liver, kidneys, and pancreas from the negative effects of oxidative stress. Xylitol promotes a better metabolism of calcium and phosphorus and prevents the occurrence of osteoporosis after bilateral oophorectomy in experimental animals. Xylitol was found to have a beneficial effect on gut microbiota and increased the absorption of phytoestrogens in another experimental study. These findings could support its possible use for the prevention and treatment of osteoporosis [5].

Prevention of endothelial malfunction is one of the main tasks in management of menopause. Formerly, HRT was found to have a protective effect on the endothelium [16]. However, this effect is critically dependent on the NO-system. Estrogen-mediated effects, including increasing nitric oxide bioavailability and attenuating oxidative stress and inflammation, contribute to preserving cardiovascular health. The level of nitric oxide was found to be decreased in women of transitional age. The lack of this vasodilating agent induces vasculopathy. HRT is known to contribute to the restoration of the lipid profile, increase the activity of nitric oxide synthase, and release this powerful vasodilator from the endothelium. The level of nitric oxide synthase is the key to the vasorelaxant effect of estradiol [7]. Since L-arginine is a substrate for the synthesis of nitric oxide, its use could be a promising option for women obtaining HRT. The application of L-arginine could provide anti-inflammatory, metabolic, and vasoactive effects [24]. L-arginine deficiency possibly plays a key role in the progress of endothelial malfunction after menopause. A combination of aerobic exercise and regular L-arginine intake contributed to decreased blood pressure (BP) and inflammatory markers in older women [25].

The development of a therapeutic and preventive strategy including HRT, physical activity, diet therapy, and the use of xylitol and L-arginine preparations could make a favor in improving the quality of life of women over 45 years old. Xylitol solution with micronutrients should be administered in the form of infusions from the first days of the reduction diet once for 5 days. Administration of L-arginine should be started intravenously at 200 mL once a day for a week, and then be continued in oral form for another 3 weeks. The results of 1-month and 3-month programs including physical training, diet, xylitol, and L-arginine were already reported [26, 27]. The findings showed a real prospect of such a strategy for life extension. But the emphasis should be done.

Seventy-one perimenopausal women were enrolled in the study. Thirty-six patients with or without periods from Group II received sequential or continuous combined HRT. Thirty-five women of transitional age (Group III) additionally to HRT received a diet, of L-arginine infusions 200.0 mL once daily for a week, and 20 mL of oral L-arginine solution for 3 weeks, and also xylitol solution 200.0 mL once daily during the 5 days of treatment were included in Group III. A low-carbohydrate and mild-fat diet (less than 26% carbohydrates or less than 130 g/day) was used in the study [12]. The distribution of the nutrients was 20% carbohydrates, 40% fat, and 40% protein. This diet featured a low glycemic index, slow ketogenesis, and anti-atherogenic effects [20]. Thirty-five healthy reproductive-aged women were included in Group I (control).

The obtained results showed that obesity plays an important role in the pathogenesis of climacteric syndrome. The findings of the study demonstrated a moderate positive correlation between BMI and diastolic BP, BMI, and Cooperman's score, BMI and glucose level, and BMI and C-RP (Fig. 19.1). The results of the multivariate regression model with C-RP showed a statistically significant relationship with BMI and insulin (Table 19.1). The model itself was meaningful. The role of chronic inflammation and insulin-resistance in metabolic disorders among perimenopausal women was shown.

The reduction of BMI was found in patients from Group III (Fig. 19.2). The declining Cooperman's score in these patients supported the opinion of the use of diet in the treatment of early menopausal disorders. The reduction of BP was possibly associated with the improved metabolic profile of patients in Group III (Fig. 19.3). However, the effect could be also associated with autonomic tone restoration by reducing sympathetic regulation [26]. The decrease of atherogenicity, improved carbohydrate metabolism, and complete history of chronic inflammation was found in perimenopausal women (Fig. 19.3). These findings support available data on the relationship between insulin resistance, atherogenicity, and systemic inflammation [28].

Since the effect of HRT on BP is multifactorial, the use of estrogens is not definitely postulated. Some studies showed the increased risk of complications of CVD in elderly women who obtained HRT [16]. The proposed 3 months program demonstrated its

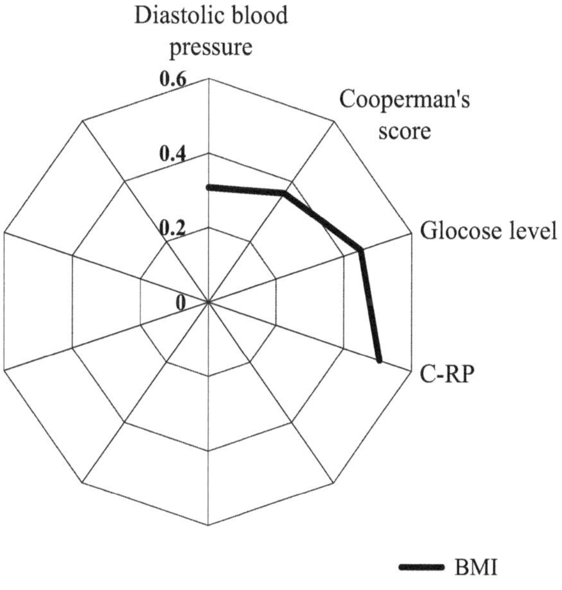

Fig. 19.1 The correlation between BMI and diastolic BP, BMI and Cooperman's score, BMI and glucose level, BMI and C-RP

Table 19.1 Multivariate logistic regression model with C-RP coefficient

	Unstandardized coefficients	Standardized coefficients				95% Confidence interval for *B*	
Model	*B*	Beta	Standard error	*t*	*p*	Lower bound	Upper bound
(Constant)	−414.44		165.63	−2.5	0.017	−749.52	−79.35
BMI	13.49	0.27	4.83	2.79	0.008	3.72	23.27
Cooperman's score	0.31	0.01	2.58	0.12	0.905	−4.9	5.52
HOMA index	−0.23	−0.17	0.17	−1.37	0.178	−0.57	0.11
Insulin	0.25	0.69	0.04	5.97	<0.001	0.16	0.33
Glucose	0.18	0.21	0.12	1.5	0.143	−0.06	0.43
Triglycerides	0.13	0.04	0.46	0.28	0.782	−0.81	1.07
Atherogenic index	0.09	0.06	0.17	0.52	0.608	−0.25	0.42

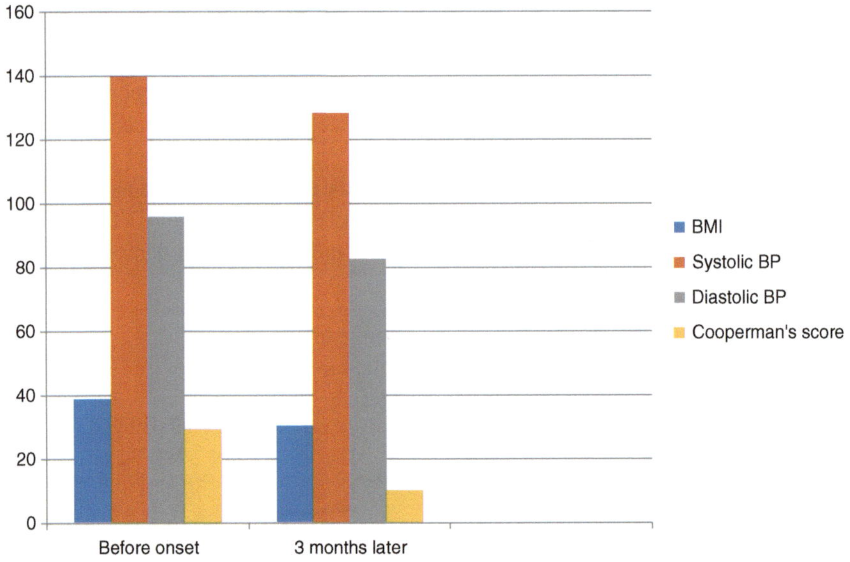

Fig. 19.2 The changes of BMI, systolic BP, diastolic BP, and Cooperman's score in Group III

positive vasoactive effect. This method of management for perimenopausal women has a positive synergistic with estradiol effect on endothelium. Thus, L-arginine donation could be thought as an efficient intervention for improved cardiovascular health in perimenopausal women. Thus, the use of diet, L-arginine, and xylitol could be an important supplement to HRT. The findings emphasize the possible options for the prevention of atherogenicity. Weight gain and increased BMI was the main factor for insulin resistance, atherogenicity, and menopausal disorders. The use of diet, xylitol, and L-arginine improved metabolic processes and reduced menopausal disorders [26, 27].

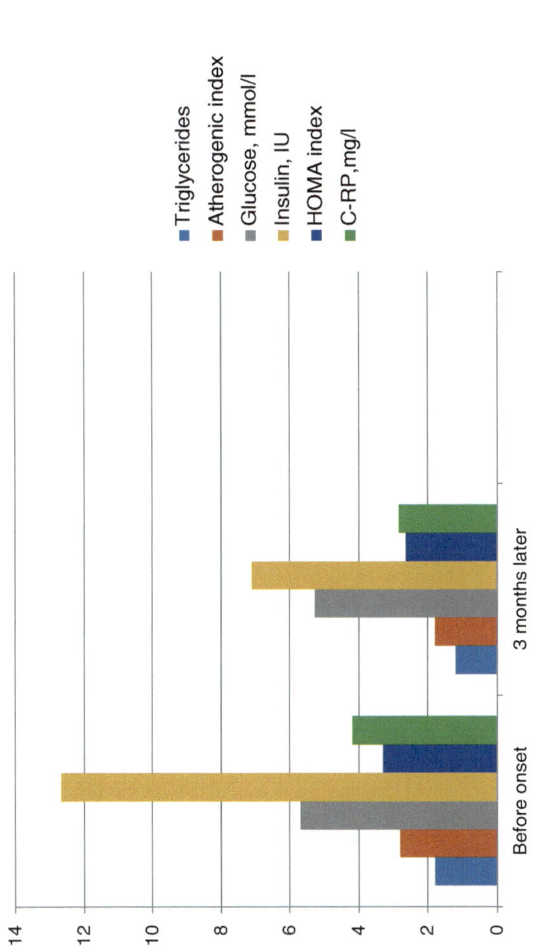

Fig. 19.3 The level of triglycerides, atherogenic index, glucose, insulin, HOMA index, and C-RP before and after 3 months program

Weight gain was the main factor for insulin-resistance, atherogenicity, and menopausal disorders. The use of diet, xylitol, and L-arginine improved metabolic processes and reduced menopausal disorders.

BMI in perimenopausal women was responsible for BP, menopausal Cooperman's score, carbohydrate metabolism, and inflammatory response. The use of a 3-month program including diet, xylitol, and L-arginine solutions contributed to the reduction of Cooperman's score, chronic inflammation, and restoration of lipid and carbohydrate metabolism. This program could help us to make another step in the march towards improving women's health during their perimenopausal years.

References

1. Blagosklonny MV. As predicted by hyperfunction theory, rapamycin treatment during development extends lifespan. Aging (Albany NY). 2022;14(5):2020–4. https://doi.org/10.18632/aging.203937.
2. Hoyer D, Żebrowski J, Cysarz D, Gonçalves H, Pytlik A, Amorim-Costa C, Bernardes J, Ayres-de-Campos D, Witte OW, Schleußner E, Stroux L, Redman C, Georgieva A, Payne S, Clifford G, Signorini MG, Magenes G, Andreotti F, Malberg H, Zaunseder S, Lakhno I, Schneider U. Monitoring fetal maturation-objectives, techniques and indices of autonomic function. Physiol Meas. 2017;38(5):R61–88. https://doi.org/10.1088/1361-6579/aa5fca.
3. Berikhanova RR, Minenko IA, Bondarev SA. Carbohydrate metabolism in women with metabolic syndrome with multimodal non-drug correction of menopausal disorders. Arch Gerontol Geriatr. 2020;28(91):104205. https://doi.org/10.1016/j.archger.2020.104205.
4. Proietto J. Obesity and weight management at menopause. Aust Fam Physician. 2017;46(6):368–70.
5. Bermingham KM, Linenberg I, Hall WL, Kadé K, Franks PW, Davies R, Wolf J, Hadjigeorgiou G, Asnicar F, Segata N, Manson JE, Newson LR, Delahanty LM, Ordovas JM, Chan AT, Spector TD, Valdes AM, Berry SE. Menopause is associated with postprandial metabolism, metabolic health and lifestyle: the ZOE PREDICT study. EBioMedicine. 2022;85:104303. https://doi.org/10.1016/j.ebiom.2022.104303.
6. Silva TR, Oppermann K, Reis FM, Spritzer PM. Nutrition in menopausal women: a narrative review. Nutrients. 2021;13(7):2149. https://doi.org/10.3390/nu13072149.
7. Nair AR, Pillai AJ, Nair N. Cardiovascular changes in menopause. Curr Cardiol Rev. 2021;17(4):e230421187681. https://doi.org/10.2174/1573403X16666201106141811.
8. Geidenstam N, Al-Majdoub M, Ekman M, et al. Metabolite profiling of obese individuals before and after a one year weight loss program. Int J Obes (Lond). 2017;41(9):1369–78. https://doi.org/10.1038/ijo.2017.124.
9. Marciniak A, Nawrocka Rutkowska J, Brodowska A, et al. Cardiovascular system diseases in patients with polycystic ovary syndrome—the role of inflammation process in this pathology and possibility of early diagnosis and prevention. Ann Agric Environ Med. 2016;23(4):537–41.
10. Patel SS, Truong U, King M, et al. Obese adolescents with polycystic ovarian syndrome have elevated cardiovascular disease risk markers. Vasc Med. 2017;22(2):85–95.
11. Glintborg D, Rubin KH, Nybo M, et al. Cardiovascular disease in a nationwide population of Danish women with polycystic ovary syndrome. Cardiovasc Diabetol. 2018;17:37. https://doi.org/10.1186/s12933-018-0680-5.
12. Stamatelopoulos K, Papavagelis C, Augoulea A, Armeni E, Karagkouni I, Avgeraki E, Georgiopoulos G, Yannakoulia M, Lambrinoudaki I. Dietary patterns and cardiovascular risk in postmenopausal women: Protocol of a cross-sectional and prospective study. Maturitas. 2018;116:59–65. https://doi.org/10.1016/j.maturitas.2018.07.006.

13. Rangel-Huerta OD, Pastor-Villaescusa B, Gil A. Are we close to defining a metabolomic signature of human obesity? A systematic review of metabolomics studies. Metabolomics. 2019;15:93. https://doi.org/10.1007/s11306-019-1553-y.
14. Paschou SA, Anagnostis P, Pavlou DI, Vryonidou A, Goulis DG, Lambrinoudaki I. Diabetes in menopause: risks and management. Curr Vasc Pharmacol. 2019;17(6):556–63. https://doi.org/10.2174/1570161116666180625124405.
15. Stuenkel CA. Menopause, hormone therapy and diabetes. Climacteric. 2017;20(1):11–21. https://doi.org/10.1080/13697137.2016.1267723.
16. Somani YB, Pawelczyk JA, De Souza MJ, et al. Aging women and their endothelium: probing the relative role of estrogen on vasodilator function Review. Am J Physiol Heart Circ Physiol. 2019;317(2):H395–404. https://doi.org/10.1152/ajpheart.00430.2018.
17. Hirahatake KM, Jiang L, Wong ND, Shikany JM, Eaton CB, Allison MA, Martin L, Garcia L, Zaslavsky O, Odegaard AO. Diet quality and cardiovascular disease risk in postmenopausal women with type 2 diabetes mellitus: the women's health initiative. J Am Heart Assoc. 2019;8(19):e013249. https://doi.org/10.1161/JAHA.119.013249.
18. Azziz R. Introduction: determinants of polycystic ovary syndrome. Fertil Steril. 2016;106(1):4–5. https://doi.org/10.1016/j.fertnstert.2016.05.009.
19. Rettedal EA, Ilesanmi-OyelereB L, Roy NC, et al. The gut microbiome is altered in postmenopausal women with osteoporosis and osteopenia. JBMR Plus. 2021;5(3):e10452. https://doi.org/10.1002/jbm4.10452.
20. Prentice RL, Aragaki AK, Van Horn L, Thomson CA, Beresford SA, Robinson J, Snetselaar L, Anderson GL, Manson JE, Allison MA, Rossouw JE, Howard BV. Low-fat dietary pattern and cardiovascular disease: results from the women's health initiative randomized controlled trial. Am J Clin Nutr. 2017;106(1):35–43. https://doi.org/10.3945/ajcn.117.153270.
21. Glenn AJ, Lo K, Jenkins DJA, Boucher BA, Hanley AJ, Kendall CWC, Manson JE, Vitolins MZ, Snetselaar LG, Liu S, Sievenpiper JL. Relationship between a plant-based dietary portfolio and risk of cardiovascular disease: findings from the women's health initiative prospective cohort study. J Am Heart Assoc. 2021;10(16):e021515. https://doi.org/10.1161/JAHA.121.021515.
22. Sari IK, Utari DM, Kamoshita S, et al. Increasing vegetable intake 400 g/day to control body weight and lipid profile in overweight hyperlipidemia menopausal women. J Public Health Res. 2020;9(3):1733. https://doi.org/10.4081/jphr.2020.1733.
23. Benahmed AG, Gasmi A, Arshad M, et al. Health benefits of xylitol review. Appl Microbiol Biotechnol. 2020;104(17):7225–37. https://doi.org/10.1007/s00253-020-10708-7.
24. Klawitter J, Hildreth KL, Christians U, et al. A relative L-arginine deficiency contributes to endothelial dysfunction across the stages of the menopausal transition. Physiol Rep. 2017;5(17):e13409.
25. Puga GM, Novais IP, Katsanos CS, et al. Combined effects of aerobic exercise and l-arginine ingestion on blood pressure in normotensive postmenopausal women: a crossover study. Life Sci. 2016;151:323–9. https://doi.org/10.1016/j.lfs.2016.02.091.
26. Lakhno I. State of metabolic processes and ways to improve them in premenopausal women due to the life extension strategy. Rep Endocrinol. 2021;61:51–4. https://doi.org/10.18370/2309-4117.2021.61.
27. Lakhno I, Korovai S, Struk T, Pak S. The pathogenic pathways of cardiovascular disease in perimenopausal women. Prz Menopauzalny. 2023;22(2):59–63. https://doi.org/10.5114/pm.2023.127902.
28. Welten SJGC, Onland-Moret NC, Boer JMA, Verschuren WMM, van der Schouw YT. Age at menopause and risk of ischemic and hemorrhagic stroke. Stroke. 2021;52(8):2583–91. https://doi.org/10.1161/STROKEAHA.120.030558.

Contraception for Middle-Aged Women 20

Priyanka Rai, Sweta Singh, and Ruchika Garg

20.1 Introduction

In the United States, the era of modern contraception began in 1960 with the reintroduction of intrauterine contraceptive devices (IUDs) and oral contraception was first approved by the Food and Drug Administration. It took 12 years following this approval for the social and legal landscape in the USA to evolve sufficiently to make widespread access to contraception possible [1]. For all age groups, the unwanted pregnancy rate in developed countries is 44 per 1000 females [2]. In America, middle-aged women had 46% of unplanned pregnancies aborted between 2008 and 2011, which was the highest percentage of any age group [3]. The unplanned pregnancy rate in this population is 16 per 1000 women [3]. The increased usage of long-acting reversible contraception (LARC) is the most significant modification to contraception in the United States before 2010 and now. A total of 62% of women in the USA who are of reproductive age presently use contraception. Ninety percent of all women at risk of unwanted pregnancies use contraceptives [4].

Despite their decreasing fertility, middle-aged women need an effective form of contraception if they want to prevent pregnancy. Women in the middle-aged group who have relationships or are married, the majority having vaginal intercourse.

P. Rai (✉)
Department of Obstetrics and Gynaecology, All India Institute of Medical Sciences, Deoghar, India
e-mail: priyanka.obgy@aiimsdeoghar.edu.in

S. Singh
Department of Obstetrics and Gynaecology, All India Institite of Medical Sciences, Bhubaneswar, India
e-mail: obgyn_sweta@aiimsbhubaneswar.edu.in

R. Garg
Department Obstetrics and Gynaecology, SN Medical College, Agra, India

R. Garg (ed.), *Management of Menopause*,
https://doi.org/10.1007/978-981-96-0239-1_20

However, these populations have unique characteristics that affect contraceptive choice [5]. These women may be experiencing perimenopausal symptoms that could be managed with contraceptives. Additionally, in this age group, many women may have suffered from any of the medical illness that make some contraceptive methods inappropriate. Finally, due to their reduced fecundity (chance of having a live birth per menstrual cycle), decreased frequency of sexual activity, and higher compliance with contraceptive regimens, women of late reproductive age experience lower rates of contraceptive failure than younger women [5, 6].

20.2 Efficacy of Contraception

It is generally assessed by the Pearl Index and Life-Table Analysis methods.

Pearl Index: The Pearl Index, originated by Raymond Pearl in 1933, and is defined as the number of contraception failures per 100 women years of exposure [7]. The Pearl Index is often based on a long exposure (about 1 year) and it cannot accurately compare methods with different durations of exposure. The life-table analysis method is used to overcome this limitation.

Life-Table Analysis: For each month of contraceptive use, the failure rate is calculated by the life-table analysis. Then for any specific exposure length, a cumulative failure rate can be compared [1].

20.3 Contraception Failure

Contraception failure can occur, for many of the reasons. The efficacy of incorrect and correct use of contraception methods is designated with "method effectiveness" and "use effectiveness". Women more than 30 years of age and married women will experience less failure rate than younger women. The most important factors of oral contraceptive pills (OCP) and condom failure were age, parity, marital status, and intention towards future birth [8].

20.4 Contraception for Middle-Aged Women

The methods of contraception used by middle-aged women vary by country [9–11]. According to data female sterilization is more common in the United States as compared to other developed nations (2006–2008). The use of condom and OCP was more common in middle-aged women in Canada (2006). An intrauterine device is more common in the United Kingdom (2008–2009) [8–10]. Female sterilization is the most common method of contraception globally (23 per 100 women) followed by male condoms (22%). It is extensively used in India, as it accounts for 48% of the global number of women [12]. It may be a good choice for middle-aged women or couples who do not require children (Fig. 20.1). IUDs (intrauterine devices) are also more common among women over 40 years, especially hormone-releasing IUDs, the LNG-IUS 20 (levonorgestrel-releasing intrauterine system, Mirena). Oral

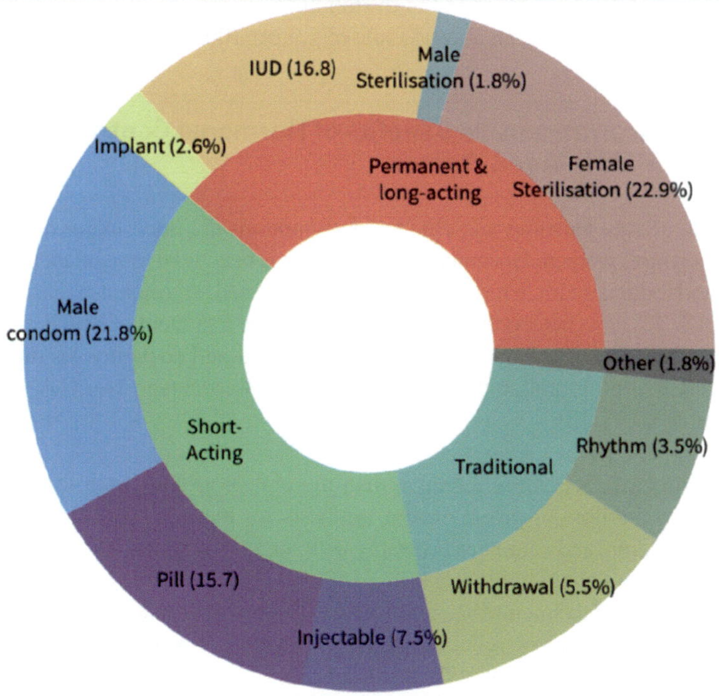

Fig. 20.1 Distribution of contraception practices. Calculation is based on the United Nations, Department of Economics and Social Affairs, Population Division (2022)

contraception is also popular among middle-aged women in developed countries [13]. Progesterone only pills (POPs) are safer than COCs (combined oral contraceptive pills) in women over 40 years even by smokers and with other vascular diseases but using POPs may cause some intermenstrual bleeding [14].

20.5 WHO Consideration for Middle-Aged Women

According to WHO 2022 update 96% of women have reached menopause by the age of 55 years. A middle-aged woman can use any kind of contraception to avoid unwanted pregnancies until menopause if she has no medical conditions that would prevent it from being used [15].

20.6 Risk of Fertility in Middle-Aged Women

Fertility decreases in middle-aged women, but they still have a chance to conceive, and most of the time that pregnancy is unplanned and unwanted [14]. The chances of spontaneous abortion and chromosomal abnormalities were high in this group of patients. However, the age-related decline in fertility is not a solid basis for effective contraception [13]. Compared to the overall abortion rate of 13 per 1000 women, middle-aged women have an abortion rate of 2.9 per 1000 [13].

20.7 Noncontraceptive Benefits of Hormonal Contraception in Middle-Aged Women

Abnormal uterine bleeding and climacteric symptoms are often major concerns in perimenopausal women. Hormonal contraception is beneficial to regulate menstrual cycles and reducing climacteric symptoms in this period. Hormonal-releasing IUDs (LNG-IUS 20) have been proven most effective in the treatment of heavy menstrual bleeding including when it is associated with fibroid and adenomyosis due to the local release of progestin on the endometrium and its advantage over CuT is as follows (Table 20.1) [13].

- The Mirena IUS is more effective than the oral progestins, steroid contraceptives, or inhibitors of prostaglandin synthesis for the treatment of heavy menstrual bleeding, and compares favorably with surgical treatment like hysterectomy or endometrial ablation [16].
- It decreases the dysmenorrhea and menstrual blood loss (about 40–50%). Up to 90% of bleeding can be reduced and about 30–40% of women become amenorrheic 1 year after insertion [17].

Table 20.1 Risk factors and noncontraceptive benefits of various contraceptive methods

Methods of contraception	Risk factors (>40 years)	Noncontraceptive benefits	When to stop in perimenopausal age group (age in years)
COCs	Smokers, migraine, severe hypertension, cardiovascular diseases	Effective in heavy menstrual bleeding, reduces risk of ovarian and endometrial and colorectal Ca, bone loss and vasomotor symptoms	50 years
POPs	Risk of developing osteoporosis and fracture bone in later life	Effective in heavy menstrual bleeding, reduces risk of ovarian and endometrial Ca and vasomotor symptoms	55 years
Cu IUD	Sometimes risk of infrequent bleeding, infection during insertion	Decreases risk of endometrial cancer	Safe up to menopause
Hormonal IUD	Benefits outweigh risks	Beneficial in heavy menstrual bleeding	Safe up to menopause
Female sterilization	Benefits outweigh risks	Decreases ovarian cancer risk	Surgical procedure done after completion of family
Condom	Failure rate is high	Prevents sexually transmitted infections	Safe up to menopause

- It has been used successfully to treat endometriosis, especially dysmenorrhea associated with endometriosis [18].
- It protects the endometrium against polyps and hyperplasia in women using tamoxifen or postmenopausal estrogen therapy.
- The Mirena can be used to treat endometrial hyperplasia [19].

20.8 Major Concern at Perimenopause

The majority of women are anxious about when they can safely stop taking contraception. It has been suggested that COC should be stopped at 50 and POP at 55 years [14]. International guidelines state that up to menopause Cu IUD is safe unless bleeding abnormalities begin [13]. According to European guidelines, amenorrheic women could assume natural sterility after the age of 55. Menopause can also be assumed in women who are not taking hormonal contraception after 1 year of amenorrhea in those over 50 or after 2 years of amenorrhea in those under 50 [20].

20.9 Risk of Contraceptive Use in Middle-Aged Women (Table 20.1)

Cardiovascular Symptoms: The risk of thromboembolism with COCs increases with age and is rare in the reproductive age group. The risk of thromboembolism is lower with POPs. Estrogen-containing method may be avoided in middle-aged women. A total of 5–10 per 10,000 woman-year, incidence of venous thromboembolism among reproductive-age women has been reported and it increases with age [21]. Use of estrogen-containing pills will double the risk of thromboembolism [22].

Risk of Fracture: With increasing age bone mineral density decreases due to inadequate production of endogenous estrogen. The use of POPs (DMPA) may cause relative hypoestrogenic status and a further decline in bone mineral density, raising the possibility of fracture risk in users [23].

Cancer: The risk of cancer increases with age. It has been found that the risk of endometrial cancer and ovarian cancer decreases with the use of oral contraception [13]. There is no association between past or current use of breast cancer and oral contraceptives as found by the Royal College of General Practitioners study [24]. According to a systematic review long-term use of oral contraceptives may cause an increased risk of cervical cancer (relative risk [RR] 1.6, 95% CI 1.4–1.7) and DMPA (RR 1.2, 95% CI 1.0–1.6) [25].

20.10 Conclusion

This article contributed to an existing understanding of which contraception is better for women approaching menopause and also demonstrated that the use of contraception settles over time and that they frequently switch to more effective methods. Sometimes sociodemographic factors and medical conditions also affect a woman's choice of contraception. A contraceptive review may be beneficial for women in the perimenopausal stage so that they are given the contraceptive options most suitable to their unique circumstances, even though fertility declines with age and some women continue to use short-acting contraception.

References

1. Taylor HS, Pal L, Seli E. Speroff's clinical gynaecologic endocrinology and infertility. 9th ed; 2020. p. 2028–490.
2. Sedgh G, Singh S, Hussain R. Intended and unintended pregnancies worldwide in 2012 and recent trends. Stud Fam Plan. 2014;45:301.
3. Finer LB, Zolna MR. Declines in unintended pregnancy in the United States, 2008–2011. N Engl J Med. 2016;374:9.
4. Guttmacher Institute. Fact sheet: contraceptive use in the United States. 2016. https://www.guttmacher.org/fact-sheet/contraceptive-use-united-states.
5. Herbenick D, Reece M, Schick V, et al. Sexual behaviors, relationships, and perceived health status among adult women in the United States: results from a national probability sample. J Sex Med. 2010;7(Suppl 5):277–90.
6. Trussell J, Guthrie K. Choosing a contraceptive: efficacy, safety, and personal considerations. In: Hatcher RA, Trussell J, Nelson AL, et al., editors. Contraceptive technology. 20th ed. Valley Stream, NY: Ardent Media Inc; 2011. p. 45–74.
7. Pearl R. Factors in human fertility and their statistical evaluation. Lancet. 1933;222:607.
8. Mosher WD, Martinez GM, Chandra A, Abma JC, Willson SJ. Use of contraception and use of family planning services in the United States: 1982–2002. Adv Data. 350, 2004:1–36.
9. Mosher WD, Jones J. Use of contraception in the United States: 1982–2008. Vital Health Stat 23. 2010:1–44.
10. Lader D. Contraception and sexual health, 2008–9. London: Office for National Statistics; 2009. www.ons.gov.uk/ons/rel/lifestyles/contraception-and-sexual-health/2008-09/index.html. Accessed 26 June 2012.
11. Black A, Yang Q, Wu Wen S, et al. Contraceptive use among Canadian women of reproductive age: results of a national survey. J Obstet Gynaecol Can. 2009;31:627–40.
12. Expanding choices and ensuring rights in a diverse and changing world: UNFPA Strategy for Family Planning, 2022–2030. p. 17–18.
13. Allen RH, Cwiak CA, Kaunitz AM. Contraception in women over 40 years of age. CMAJ. 2013;185(7) https://doi.org/10.1503/cmaj.121280.
14. Ruan X, Mueck AO. Oral contraception for women of middle age. Maturitas. 2015;82:266–70. https://doi.org/10.1016/j.maturitas.2015.06.030.
15. World Health Organization Department of Sexual and Reproductive Health and Research (WHO/SRH) and Johns Hopkins Bloomberg School of Public Health/Center for Communication Programs (CCP) Knowledge Success. Family Planning: a global handbook for Providers (2022 updates). Baltimore/Geneva: CCP and WHO; 2022.
16. Kaunitz AM, Meredith S, Inki P, Kubba A, Sanchez-Ramos L. Levonorgestrel-releasing intrauterine system and endometrial ablation in heavy menstrual bleeding. A systematic review and meta-analysis. Obstet Gynecol. 2009;113:1104.
17. Baldszti E, Wimmer-Puchinger B, Loschke K. Acceptability of the long-term contraceptive levonorgestrel-releasing intrauterine system (Mirena): a 3-yearfollow-up study. Contraception. 2003;67:87.
18. Bahamondes L, Petta CA, Fernandes A, Monteiro I. Use of the levonorgestrel-releasing intrauterine system in women with endometriosis, chronic pelvic pain and dysmenorrhea. Contraception. 2007;75:S134.

19. Bahamondes L, Ribeiro-Huguet P, de Andrade KC, Leon-Martins O, Petta CA. Levonorgestrel-releasing intrauterine system (Mirena) as a therapy for endometrial hyperplasia and carcinoma. Acta Obstet Gynecol Scand. 2003;82:580.
20. European Society of Human Reproduction and Embryology. Female contraception over 40. Hum Reprod Update. 2009;15:599–612.
21. Heinemann LA, Dinger JC. Range of published estimates of venous thromboembolism incidence in young women. Contraception. 2007;75:328–36.
22. Reid RL, Westhoff C, Mansour D, et al. Oral contraceptives and venous thromboembolism: consensus opinion from an international workshop held in Berlin, Germany in December 2009. J Fam Plann Reprod Health Care. 2010;36:117–22.
23. Isley MM, Kaunitz AM. Update on hormonal contraception and bone density. Rev Endocr Metab Disord. 2011;12:93–106.
24. Hannaford PC, Selvaraj S, Elliott AM, et al. Cancer risk among users of oral contraceptives: cohort data from the Royal College of General Practitioner's oral contraception study. BMJ. 2007;335:651.
25. Smith JS, Green J, Berrington de Gonzalez A, et al. Cervical cancer and use of hormonal contraceptives: a systematic review. Lancet. 2003;361:1159–67.

Postmenopausal Bleeding

21

Pradnya Changede and Dinesh Wade

21.1 Introduction

A woman is said to have menopause when she has not had periods for 12 months in a row. Menopause is said to have occurred when menstruation stops permanently due to loss of ovarian follicular activity. A clinical diagnosis of menopause is made after 12 months of amenorrhea. The ovaries of postmenopausal women stop secreting estrogen resulting in increased Follice stimulating hormone (FSH). Fifty-one years is the average age when menopause occurs in females.

Post menopausal bleeding accounts for 5% of office gynecology presentations [1].

Postmenopausal bleeding is defined as any bleeding from the genital tract that occurs more than a year after a woman's last menstrual period [2]. Vaginal bleeding is noted in about 10% of women of postmenopausal age. Postmenopausal bleeding is a common reason for early referral to gynecological services for further evaluation.

Till date many updates have come up for evaluation of women with PMB with advent transvaginal ultrasound (TVUS) and outpatient hysteroscopy.

Completely asymptomatic patients have coincidental findings such as fibroids, polyps or thick endometrium and are referred for further management. It is a must to have knowledge of normal physiological changes and ultrasound appearance of the endometrium during menopause (Fig. 21.1).

P. Changede (✉)
Department of Obstetrics and Gynecology, Lokmanya Tilak Municipal Medical College and General Hospital, Sion, Mumbai, India

D. Wade
Progenesis IVF, Pune, India

R. Garg (ed.), *Management of Menopause*,
https://doi.org/10.1007/978-981-96-0239-1_21

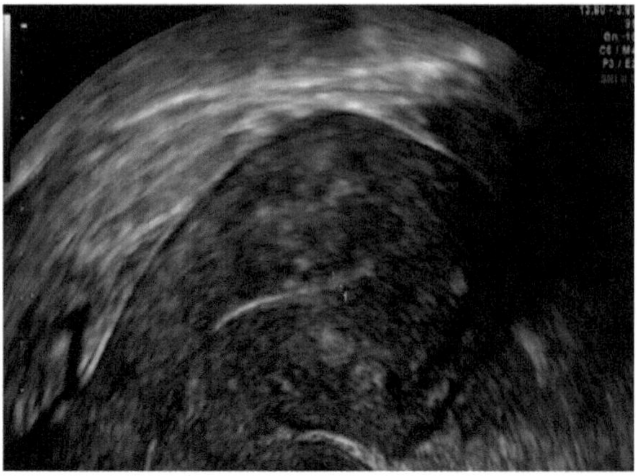

Fig. 21.1 Transvaginal ultrasound showing postmenopausal atrophic uterus (anteverted) with thin endometrium [5]

Table 21.1 Causes of postmenopausal bleeding [3]

(A) **Malignant lesions**
Endometrial cancer
Cervical cancer
Vulval cancer
Vaginal cancer
Cancer of ovaries or fallopian tube
Cancer adjacent organs (bladder, bowel)
(B) **Pre-malignant**
Endometrial hyperplasia
(C) **Benign lesions**
Atrophy (atrophy of vaginal mucosa or endometrium)
Endometrial polyps
Endometritis
(D) **Iatrogenic**
Hormone replacement therapy
Anticoagulants
Radiation
(E) Bleeding from GI tract (anus, rectum, bladder) or urinary tract (urethra, bladder)
(F) No identifiable cause

21.2 Causes of Postmenopausal Bleeding

Postmenopausal bleeding has several benign and malignant etiologies (Table 21.1). Endometrial atrophy, endometrial hyperplasia, endometrial polyps, endometrial carcinoma are common causes of PMB. The commonest cause of PMB is atrophy of endometrium or vaginal mucosa but the most concerning cause is endometrial cancer. Although endometrial cancer accounts for only 10% cases of PMB, 90% of postmenopausal women with endometrial cancer present with vaginal bleeding. About 85% of endometrial cancers occur in women of age 55 years and above. Evaluation of causes of PMB is aimed to detect presence of endometrial cancer or endometrial hyperplasia. Bleeding can arise from pathology in uterus, vulva, vagina, cervix, ovary or fallopian tube. Bleeding from GI tract (anus, rectum, bladder) or urinary tract (urethra, bladder) could be mistaken for postmenopausal bleeding (non-gynecological causes of bleeding).

21.3 Pathophysiology

1. Atrophy of vagina and endometrium occurs due to lack of estrogen, scant fluid in tissues leads to friction which causes micro erosions of epithelium leading to inflammation (endometritis). Chronic endometritis causes spotting.
2. Genetic predisposition—Lynch syndrome and Cowden disease.
3. Unopposed estrogen—PCOS, anovulation, estrogen secreting tumors, HRT (hormone replacement therapy).

21.4 Diagnosis

All cases of postmenopausal bleeding should be thoroughly evaluated as endometrial cancers account for up to 10% cases of PMB.

21.4.1 History and Examination

- Details of bleeding episodes—onset, duration, frequency, amount, pain, history of trauma, time since menopause, timing of bleeding (postcoital or after wiping etc).
- History of change in bowel and bladder habit, loss of appetite, weight loss, bloating.
- Whether on HRT—details of HRT, duration, regime, use of herbal supplements for menopausal symptoms.
- Past history—chronic medical conditions like Diabetes mellitus, Hypertension, Polycystic ovarian disease, bleeding disorder, previous Papanicolaou test (PAP) smear report, radiation exposure.
- Family history of breast, uterine, ovarian or colon cancer.
- Menopause secondary to oophorectomy, if patient has undergone hysterectomy indication of hysterectomy is important.
- Previous history of Abnormal uterine bleeding (AUB).

During physical examination general appearance and Body mass index (BMI) is important as obesity is high-risk factor for endometrial cancer. Rule out abdominal masses on palpation. Per speculum examination needs to be done to rule out vaginal and cervical pathology, e.g., polyp, ulcer, cancer, foreign body in vagina. Bimanual examination for size, mobility of uterus and adnexal evaluation. If required rectal examination has to be performed. Look for lesions on cervix, vagina, vulva, urethra, and anus. Atrophic vaginal mucosa appears dry, pale, shiny, smooth and shows absence of rugae. Obesity is an important factor as every 5 kg/m^2 increase in weight is associated with 50% increase risk of endometrial cancer [4].

21.4.2 Investigations

21.4.2.1 TVS (Transvaginal Sonography)

TVS in a normal postmenopausal woman shows small uterus, small ovaries, and thin endometrial stripe. In postmenopausal female thickness of endometrium correlates with the risk for endometrial cancer. ACOG recommends TVS as first-line investigation for PMB [5].

The risk of endometrial cancer increases with the increase in endometrial thickness. The endometrial thickness is measured at the area of maximal thickness of endometrial echo on long axis of uterus in anterior-posterior direction. ET less than or equal to 4 mm has 99% negative predictive value [5].

The number of cases of endometrial cancer missed by TVS using different ET thresholds is as follows:

5/1915 [1 in 383], 12/4073 [1 in 339], and 15/3587 [1 in 239] cases of endometrial cancer are missed when threshold of less than or equal to 3 mm, less than or equal to 4 mm and less than or equal to 5 mm are used respectively [5].

In postmenopausal female taking HRT endometrial thickness 8 mm and above need evaluation even if patient is asymptomatic, but in symptomatic patient cutoff of 4 mm needs further evaluation using hysteroscopy [6]. When endometrial fluid is present it should not be included in measuring ET. For incidentally diagnosed ET more than 4 mm without bleeding individualized assessment should be based on patient profile and high-risk factors. High-risk factors for endometrial cancer are mentioned in Table 21.2.

21.4.2.2 Endometrial Biopsy

Endometrial biopsy is indicated when ET is more than 4 mm, presence of increased echogenicity or heterogeneity (diffuse or focal), inability to visualize endometrium or recurrent and persistent postmenopausal bleeding [7]. Endometrial biopsy should be the first-line investigation for women with high-risk factors for endometrial cancer as it is a major cause of morbidity and mortality.

Type 2 endometrial cancer can present with ET less than 3 mm hence persistent or recurrent uterine bleeding should be evaluated by histology.

Endometrial biopsy can be performed using an endometrial pipelle (outpatient setting), hysteroscopy guided biopsy or curettage in either an outpatient (office

Table 21.2 Risk factors for endometrial cancer

Unopposed estrogen exposure, estrogen secreting tumors, early menarche, late menopause
Obesity
Diabetes
Endometrial hyperplasia
Lynch syndrome, Cowden syndrome, BRCA carriers
Tamoxifen

hysteroscopy) or inpatient setting. The pipelle endometrial sampling has a high sensitivity of 99.6% for detecting endometrial hyperplasia in postmenopausal women, while its sensitivity for cancer detection is 81% [8].

However, it is essential to note that sampling with a pipelle may not always detect pathology as less than 50% of the endometrium is sampled. Pipelle biopsy is most useful when pathology occupies more than 50% of the endometrium. Complications of endometrial pipelle biopsy procedure include uterine perforation, infection or further evaluation for insufficient or nondiagnostic sampling. Hysteroscopy ensures direct inspection of uterine cavity and helps identify and treat pathology [9].

Although hysteroscopy and curettage provide a more in-depth assessment of the endometrium, they are more invasive procedures associated with a higher risk of complications such as bleeding, infection, and uterine perforation [10].

Therefore, the choice of endometrial biopsy method should be based on the patient's individual characteristics, suspected pathology, and be discussed with the patient before the procedure.

21.4.2.3 Hysteroscopy

Hysteroscopy guided biopsy is considered the most reliable method for diagnosing endometrial polyps having a sensitivity of 100% and specificity of 97%. The overall accuracy of hysteroscopy is 91%. This procedure can be used as diagnostic as well as therapeutic tool. It offers added advantage of polypectomy for therapeutic purpose along with its use for diagnosis [10].

21.4.3 Histopathology

Glands and stroma are present in 1:1 ratio with regularly spaced glands in normal proliferative endometrium. Atrophic endometrial cells appear small and cuboidal with no mitotic cells. Glands appear cystic with inactive stroma. Chronic endometritis is characterized by plasma cell infiltration. Crowding of endometrial glands is seen in endometrial hyperplasia. Abnormal gland nuclei is seen in atypia. Endometrioid adenocarcinoma (type 1 endometrial cancer) is the most common histologic type (75%) which is low grade and confined to uterus. Solid areas, maze or cribriform patterns are seen in type 2 cancers. Though rare (10% uterine cancers) type 2 account for 40% deaths. These are high-grade lesions clear cell, papillary serous or carcinosarcoma [11].

21.4.4 Treatment

Once a diagnosis has been established after a comprehensive evaluation for postmenopausal bleeding (PMB), the next step is to determine the appropriate action to take. Women who are diagnosed with cervical or endometrial malignancy must be promptly referred to a gynecological oncology service for further management, as the situation demands urgency. Patient education is crucial, as it is important that patients are informed that any subsequent episodes of PMB need to be assessed again.

21.4.4.1 Urogenital Atrophy

Vulvovaginal atrophy can cause symptoms such as vaginal dryness, bleeding, burning, pruritis, and dyspareunia, in addition to vaginal bleeding or spotting. Management of atrophy typically involves the use of vaginal moisturizers, lubricants, and topical vaginal estrogens.

However, topical vaginal estrogens are generally more effective than moisturizers and lubricants. Treatment with these products typically involves daily use for 2 weeks, followed by twice-weekly use thereafter. Vaginal estrogen (topical use) is preferred over systemic hormone replacement therapy (HRT) for women with predominantly atrophic symptoms [12].

21.4.4.2 Postmenopausal Women with Thick Endometrium (Asymptomatic)

Schmidt et al. recommend for investigating postmenopausal women with thickened endometrium who are asymptomatic. They concluded that endometrial polyps were the most common pathology, only a small percentage of cases were with endometrial cancer. These findings have significant implications for managing women with increased endometrial thickness discovered during pelvic scans done for reasons other than vaginal bleeding [13].

21.4.4.3 Endometrial Fluid Detected by Transvaginal sonography

Endometrial fluid can be detected by transvaginal sonography (TVS) in postmenopausal women if their endometrial thickness is greater than 4 mm [5].

Presence of endometrial fluid in the absence of thickened endometrium does not require further investigation. TVS is thus useful in evaluation of PMB.

21.4.4.4 Endometrial Polyp

The treatment of endometrial polyps (Fig. 21.2) in postmenopausal women may vary based on the size, location, and potential for malignancy. However, the standard approach is to perform a hysteroscopic resection to remove the polyp and send it for histopathological examination. A study by Yu et al. (2018) found that hysteroscopic resection of endometrial polyps in postmenopausal women had a high success rate and low complication rate. Additionally, there was a low recurrence rate over a 2-year follow-up period [14]. It has been reported that hysteroscopic resection was an effective treatment for endometrial polyps in postmenopausal women (high cure rate and low complication rate) [15].

In summary, hysteroscopic resection of endometrial polyps in postmenopausal women should be done when required as it is a safe procedure.

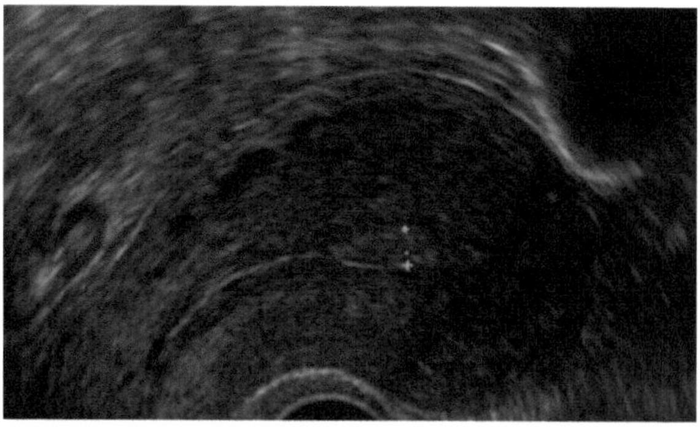

Fig. 21.2 TVS showing thickened endometrium with presence of endometrial polyp [5]

21.4.4.5 Treatment for Unscheduled Bleeding (When Patient Is on Hormone Replacement Therapy)

Breakthrough bleeding commonly occurs in women who are on cyclical HRT. Bleeding is also noted in some women on continuous combined HRT. Unscheduled bleeding is the term used to describe such type of bleeding [16].

There are various treatment options available to treat such type of bleeding in PMB. If sequential HRT is being administered to the patient, changing the type or dose of progestogen or estrogen may help relieve such type of bleeding. If there is prolonged or heavy withdrawal bleeding, the type of progesterone may be changed or the dose may be increased. Alternatively, the estrogen dose may be reduced. The type and dose of progestogen may be changed or increased if woman experience bleeding early in the progestogen phase. If spotting occurs before withdrawal, the estrogen dose may be increased. The regimen of progestogen or dose of progesterone may be changed if irregular bleeding occurs. Changing the type of progestogen may prove useful for women experiencing painful bleeding.

Continuous combined HRT using lower estrogen doses have also proven to be useful for treatment of unscheduled bleeding. If bleeding persists despite altering type and dose of progesterone, sequential HRT can ensure regular bleeding in postmenopausal women.

Options for managing postmenopausal bleeding in women receiving HRT include stopping HRT, switching to non-oral HRT, considering Mirena, or surgical interventions like endometrial ablation, endometrial resection, or hysterectomy in refractory cases.

21.4.4.6 Endometrial Hyperplasia or Malignancy

Multidisciplinary gynecology oncology services should manage cases of endometrial hyperplasia or malignancy in postmenopausal women due to the associated morbidity and mortality of endometrial carcinoma. Hysterectomy is generally the preferred treatment in this age group because of the high risk of malignancy in hyperplasia with atypia (risk of endometrial cancer for simple or complex hyperplasia with or without atypia is 1, 3, 8, and 29% respectively). However, in cases of hyperplasia without atypia, the use of a levonorgestrel intrauterine device (IUD) or medical management (progesterone preparations) has been suggested as a safe and effective alternative treatment. The new classification, WHO 2014, accepted by the International Society of Gynecological Pathologists has divided hyperplasia into two groups: benign hyperplasia and atypical hyperplasia/endometrial intraepithelial neoplasia (EIN) [17].

Staging laparotomy with total abdominal hysterectomy, bilateral salpingo-oophorectomy, pelvic washing, pelvic and para-aortic lymphadenectomy is indicated in cases of endometrial adenocarcinoma.

It is important to identify the underlying cause of postmenopausal bleeding before deciding on a management strategy for each individual woman. Proper management of postmenopausal bleeding is essential to ensure that women receive timely and appropriate treatment if necessary.

21.5 Conclusion

1. Postmenopausal bleeding (PMB) is an important symptom that should not be ignored, as it can be a sign of serious underlying conditions such as cervical or endometrial cancer.
2. A prompt referral to a gynecological oncology department for definitive management is crucial for women diagnosed with cervical or endometrial cancer.
3. Patient education plays a significant role in managing PMB. Patients need to understand that all episodes of PMB require evaluation.
4. Management of vulvovaginal atrophy, one of the common noncancerous causes of PMB, typically involves the use of vaginal moisturizers, lubricants, and topical vaginal estrogens.
5. Topical vaginal estrogen is preferred over systemic hormone replacement therapy (HRT) for women with predominantly atrophic symptoms.
6. Staging laparotomy with total abdominal hysterectomy with, bilateral salpingo-oophorectomy, pelvic washing, pelvic and para-aortic lymphadenectomy is indicated in cases of endometrial adenocarcinoma.
7. It is important to identify the underlying cause of postmenopausal bleeding before deciding on a management strategy for each individual woman. Proper management of postmenopausal bleeding is essential to ensure that women receive timely and appropriate treatment if necessary.

References

1. Goodman A. Postmenopausal uterine bleeding. UpToDate. Accessed online June 2023.
2. Sung S, Abramovitz A. Postmenopausal bleeding. [Updated 2022 Sep 18]. In: In: Stat Pearls [Internet]. Treasure Island, FL: Stat Pearls Publishing. p. 2023. https://www.ncbi.nlm.nih.gov/books/NBK562188/.
3. Jones ER, O'Flynn H, Njoku K, Crosbie EJ. Detecting endometrial cancer. Obstetr Gynaecol. 2021;23:103–12. https://doi.org/10.1111/tog.12722.

4. https://www.cancer.org/cancer/types/endometrial-cancer/causes-risks-prevention/risk-factors.html.
5. The role of transvaginal ultrasonography in evaluating the endometrium of women with post-menopausal bleeding. ACOG Committee Opinion No. 734. American College of Obstetricians and Gynecologists. Obstet Gynecol. 2018;131:e124–9.
6. Giri SK, Nayak BL, Mohapatra J. Thickened endometrium: when to intervene? A clinical conundrum. J Obstet Gynaecol India. 2021;71(3):216–25. https://doi.org/10.1007/s13224-020-01415-4. Epub 2021 Feb 2. PMID: 34408340; PMCID: PMC8310815.
7. Sung S, Abramovitz A. Postmenopausal bleeding. [Updated 2022 Sep 18]. In: StatPearls [Internet]. Treasure Island, FL: StatPearls Publishing; 2023. https://www.ncbi.nlm.nih.gov/books/NBK562188/.
8. Terzic MM, Aimagambetova G, Terzic S, Norton M, Bapayeva G, Garzon S. Current role of Pipelle endometrial sampling in early diagnosis of endometrial cancer. Transl Cancer Res. 2020;9(12):7716–24. https://doi.org/10.21037/tcr.2020.04.20. PMID: 35117374; PMCID: PMC8798375.
9. Ilavarasi CR, Jyothi GS, Alva NK. Study of the efficacy of pipelle biopsy technique to diagnose endometrial diseases in abnormal uterine bleeding. J Midlife Health. 2019;10(2):75–80. https://doi.org/10.4103/jmh.JMH_109_18. PMID: 31391756; PMCID: PMC6643712.
10. Moore JF, Carugno J. Hysteroscopy. [Updated 2023 Jul 18]. In: StatPearls [Internet]. Treasure Island, FL: StatPearls Publishing. p. 2023. https://www.ncbi.nlm.nih.gov/books/NBK564345/.
11. Mahdy H, Casey MJ, Crotzer D. Endometrial cancer. [Updated 2022 Sep 26]. In: StatPearls [Internet]. Treasure Island, FL: StatPearls Publishing; 2023. https://www.ncbi.nlm.nih.gov/books/NBK525981/.
12. Bachmann G, Santen R. Treatment of vaginal atrophy. UpToDate. Accessed online July 2023.
13. Schmidt T, Breidenbach M, Nawroth F, Mallmann P, Beyer IM, Fleisch MC, Rein DT. Hysteroscopy for asymptomatic postmenopausal women with sonographically thickened endometrium. Maturitas. 2009;62:176–8.
14. Yu T, Ye K, Wu K, et al. Hysteroscopic resection of endometrial polyps in postmenopausal women. Arch Gynecol Obstet. 2018;297(6):1471–6.
15. Nijkang NP, Anderson L, Markham R, Manconi F. Endometrial polyps: pathogenesis, sequelae and treatment. SAGE Open Med. 2019;7:2050312119848247. https://doi.org/10.1177/2050312119848247. PMID: 31105939; PMCID: PMC6501471.
16. chromeextension://efaidnbmnnnibpcajpcglclefindmkaj. https://www.hse.ie/eng/about/who/acute-hospitals-division/woman-infants/clinical-guidelines/assessment-and-management-of-postmenopausal-bleeding.pdf. Accessed July 2023.
17. Sobczuk K, Sobczuk A. New classification system of endometrial hyperplasia WHO 2014 and its clinical implications. Prz Menopauzalny. 2017;16(3):107–11. https://doi.org/10.5114/pm.2017.70589. Epub 2017 Oct 12. PMID: 29507578; PMCID: PMC5834925.

Premature Ovarian Insufficiency

22

Mohamed Rishard and Gayani Tissera

22.1 Introduction

Premature ovarian insufficiency (POI) is a syndrome that results from diminished ovarian activity before the age of 40 years. This condition can lead to many consequences in a woman's life, such as issues with women's reproductive potential, general medical health and psychosexual quality of life [1–3].

The prevalence of POI is estimated at around 1% of the population of which 0.1% are likely to be <30 years of age [4, 5]. It is estimated that 20–30% of women presenting with primary amenorrhoea and 5–20% of women presenting with secondary amenorrhoea may be due to POI [6, 7].

The first case of primary ovarian insufficiency was described in 1942 [8]. Subsequently, many terminologies such as primary ovarian failure, premature ovarian failure, premature ovarian insufficiency and premature menopause were introduced to name the entity.

However, as there is an entity called secondary causes for ovarian failure, many experts disagree with the term "primary ovarian failure". In addition to this, terms such as ovarian failure can be negative, demeaning and definite. Hence, many authorities propose the term "premature ovarian insufficiency" to describe this condition [1].

Although a myriad of aetiological factors are implicated, the pathophysiology of this complex condition is still poorly understood.

M. Rishard (✉)
Department of Obstetrics and Gynecology,Faculty of Medicine, Colombo, Sri Lanka

De Soysa Hospital for Women, Colombo, Sri Lanka
e-mail: mrishard@obg.cmb.ac.lk

G. Tissera
De Soysa Hospital for Women, Colombo, Sri Lanka

R. Garg (ed.), *Management of Menopause*,
https://doi.org/10.1007/978-981-96-0239-1_22

Irrespective of the aetiology, timely diagnosis, educating the patients and targeted interventions with the help of a multidisciplinary team can improve the outcomes.

22.2 Pathophysiology and Aetiology

It is understood that a gradual cessation of ovarian activity leading to a reduction in oestrogen levels and fertility results in menopause in healthy women. As a result of reduced ovarian function, low oestrogen levels and lack of response to gonadotrophins, and circulating gonadotrophins would rise. This hormonal milieu leads to irregular ovulation, anovulatory cycles or menstrual irregularities followed by a permanent cessation of the menstrual cycle. Menopause is diagnosed after amenorrhoea for 12 consecutive months and the average age of menopause is 50–51 years [9].

The reason for the majority of POI is unknown but the understanding of this clinical entity has improved over the decades.

Theories explain that despite the aetiology, premature cessation of ovarian activity may occur either due to the decline of the follicular pool or dysfunction of follicular maturation. An array of aetiological factors such as chromosomal, genetic, autoimmune, metabolic causes, infections like mumps, drugs and iatrogenic causes are implicated in the development of this complex condition [6].

22.2.1 Chromosomal Abnormalities and Genetic Causes

Chromosomal abnormalities, genetic polymorphisms and single-gene mutations have been implicated in the aetiology of many cases of POI [10].

It is estimated that the age of menopause is inheritable in about 30–85% and POI is inherited in around 30% of cases [5]. Moreover, it is reported that at least 10–30% of patients with idiopathic POI are first-degree relatives.

Chromosomal abnormalities are found in about one-third of cases of POI [11]. The X chromosome is essential for maintaining normal ovarian function and the functions of hypothalamic-pituitary-ovarian (HPO) axis depend on the integrity of genetic material. Hence, the absence or multiplication of the X chromosome will lead to menstrual abnormalities.

If the X chromosome is absent in women with Turner syndrome, they will experience primary amenorrhoea whereas women with Turner mosaic karyotype will experience menstrual cycles, However, about 4–5% of women with Turner mosaics will eventually develop POI [5, 12].

In Turners, complete or partial deletion of the q arm will lead to gonadal dysgenesis [13]. Similarly, women with XXX also have the risk of developing POI.

Autosomal gene mutations causing galactosemia are also associated with POI although the exact mechanism is not well known. In these cases, early-onset ovarian insufficiency is believed to occur secondary to ovarian hypo-glycosylation [14].

Fragile X syndrome is the most common cause of familial mental retardation. In these patients, the presence of a fragile X mental retardation 1 (*FMR 1*) gene in the q arm of the X chromosome leads to the development of POI. Hence, it is recommended to exclude fragile X syndrome in women with POI [15, 16].

In addition to this, there can be minor aberrant changes in the genes that play a role in the follicular genesis and normal ovarian functions that can lead to POI.

22.2.2 Chemotherapy and Radiotherapy

Chemotherapy and radiotherapy can be gonadotoxic leading to POI depending on the type, dosage, duration and mechanism of action of the treatment modality. Those who receive alkylating agents and procarbazine appear to be highly vulnerable. Radiation that mostly targets the pelvic area is also known to cause POI [2].

22.2.3 Autoimmune Conditions

It is believed that around 30% of POI occur due to autoimmune causes [5]. In addition, one in five women with POI due to autoimmune causes will eventually develop multiple autoimmune disorders [17].

The commonest cause for autoimmune disorders is thyroid disorders such as Graves' disease or Hushimoto's disease (20–30%). Autoimmune adrenal disorders such as Addison's disease is the next leading cause of autoimmune POI [15].

Interestingly many other autoimmune conditions also show the presence of circulating anti-ovarian antibodies. However, the prognostic benefit or diagnostic relevance of this phenomenon has not been established.

22.2.4 Infections

Infections are an aetiological factor in developing POI, even though the incidence and pathophysiology are uncertain. An array of microorganisms such as mumps, tuberculosis, cytomegalovirus, malarial parasites, varicella and shigella are implicated in this process [18].

22.2.5 Iatrogenic Causes

Bilateral oophorectomy is one of the most common iatrogenic causes of POI. Even in the absence of an oophorectomy, a disruption of blood flow to the ovaries can lead to POI. Similarly, data show that hysterectomy alone or hysterectomy with bilateral salpingectomy can also lead to earlier menopause [19, 20].

Box 22.1 Aetiologies for POI

Idiopathic—majority
Chromosomal and Genetic causes
X chromosomal abnormalities
Turner syndrome (45XO) or mosaic Turner (45X/46XX)
Trisomy X (47XXX or mosaic)
Fragile X Syndrome
Galactosemia
Autoimmune polyglandular syndrome (both types)
Follicle-stimulating hormone receptor mutations
17α-hydroxylase deficiency
Aromatase deficiency
Blepharophimosis, ptosis, epicanthus inversus syndrome
Bloom syndrome
Ataxia telangiectasia
Fanconi anaemia
Autoimmune disorders
Infections
Mumps, tuberculosis, malaria, cytomegalovirus, varicella and shigella
Drugs—chemotherapy and radiotherapy
Iatrogenic
Bilateral oophorectomy
Ovarian cystectomy
Pelvic vessel embolisation
Smoking

22.3 Sequelae

Sequelae can be subtle or gradual onset depending on the aetiology.

These are predominantly caused by the withdrawal of oestrogen and can lead to short-term and long-term effects. Prompt oestrogen deficiency will lead to hot flashes, night sweats, insomnia and headache. Infertility is the main concern since these women are young and of reproductive age.

However, 50% of the women with POI are known to have a fluctuating ovarian follicular function. Among those women, 5–10% eventually get pregnant [3].

Osteoporosis is another long-term health consequence of POI, which affects around 50%. Cardiovascular and neurological disease risk will increase. Most importantly, there is an increased risk of premature death. The main causes of premature death are cardiovascular, osteoporosis and fractures [21].

Further, there is an associated increased risk of other autoimmune disorders and thyroid disorders [22].

Iatrogenic POI patients develop more abrupt oestrogen deficiency compared to other aetiologies, where they have some time to adapt according to the disease course.

22.4 Clinical Presentation, History and Examination

Most patients present with a history of cessation of menstruation and some may present with menstrual irregularities before the age of 40 years.

The presence of associated symptoms such as hot flashes, night sweats, and insomnia should raise suspicion.

In addition, women may also complain of symptoms of oestrogen deficiency such as vaginal dryness, lack of libido, dyspareunia, urinary frequency and urinary tract infection [7].

It is estimated that about 10% of patients may present with primary amenorrhoea.

Although the commonest cause is idiopathic a detailed history should also be obtained focussing on various possible aetiologies mentioned in Box 22.1.

Medical history should include a history of infections like mumps and other endocrine disorders like thyroid diseases, adrenal disorders or diabetes. Also, history of autoimmune diseases like systemic lupus erythematosus, Crohn's disease, vitiligo, rheumatoid arthritis and Sjögren's syndrome.

History of previous ovarian surgeries, malignancies, history of chemotherapy and radiotherapy is important. Family history of similar conditions and diagnosis are needed to identify familial conditions.

Since low socioeconomic status has an association with POI, the patient's socioeconomic status and smoking history should be evaluated.

Severe bone pain or chronic back pain due to pathological fractures due to osteoporosis should not be ignored. Her psychological and psychosexual well-being and her fertility wishes should be assessed when planning the care pathway.

A targeted physical examination to identify possible aetiology and consequences is advised.

This includes looking for Turner's syndrome patients who will have short stature, neck webbing, lymphoma, oedema, low hairline, shield-like chest, wide apart nipples, small spoon-shaped nails, etc.

Observing for dysmorphic features of all possible syndromes is crucial.

A thorough neck examination of thyroid goitres and features of Graves' disease including eye signs should be performed.

Similarly, women with Addison's disease may present hyperpigmented lesions in the gum and skin folds.

Hair loss leading to alopecia, hypopigmentation, vasculitis rash and molar rash may be suggestive of the autoimmune condition systemic lupus erythematosus [7].

A pelvic examination may reveal features of atrophic vaginitis and oestrogen deficiency.

22.5 Diagnosis

Diagnosis is made based on the results of hormonal assay and clinical features. When a woman with amenorrhoea presents, investigations should be performed to confirm the diagnosis, establish aetiology, and identify complications. Further investigations should also be performed for follow-up.

When a patient <40 years of age presents with a history of amenorrhoea at least 4 months duration, establishing the diagnosis of POI requires two FSH assays more than or equal to 25 IU/L (mIU/ml) on two occasions at 4–6 weeks apart [23, 24].

Authorities recommend that there is no diagnostic value in performing additional tests such as AMH, USS, Laparoscopy or ovarian biopsy [1]. The involvement of a geneticist and organising investigations to rule out chromosomal and genetic abnormalities is important.

Although karyotype is considered the gold standard method of diagnosing Turner's syndrome, FISH (fluorescence in situ hybridisation), microarray base test and other novel methods can be performed depending on the availability.

Fragile X permutation testing can be performed in indicated POI women after pre-testing genetic counselling.

Testing for autosomal gene mutation or studies for copy number variants or testing for follicle-stimulating-receptor and other novel tests should not be performed without a clear indication.

Since the most prevalent autoimmune POI is adrenal autoimmune (60–80%) investigation to rule out Addison's disease should also be organised. This should be performed after the initial pre-test counselling [25].

In addition to this, thyroid peroxidase autoantibodies (TPO Ab) should also be performed in indicated cases. If TPO Ab is positive, serum TSH (thyroid stimulating hormone) levels should be assessed annually [26].

Although mumps oophoritis is a known association with POI, universal screening to look for the infective agent is not recommended [1].

Finally, a diagnosis of unexplained or idiopathic POI should only be made when the investigations and evaluation fail to rule out any specific aetiology.

22.6 Management

Breaking the bad news of POI should be done by a trained person. Patient-centred communication techniques and methods can be used to deliver sensitive information [27].

Since this condition is a complex and sensitive matter for the patient and their family members, improper way of breaking the bad news not only affects their view of the future negatively, but also makes it difficult for the caregivers to develop and sustain a therapeutic relationship with the patient.

Successful management of POI requires inputs from experts in many disciplines such as gynaecologists, endocrinologists, psychologists and geneticists inclusive of consultants from other specialities depending on the aetiology and complications. It is also important to note that the plan of management should be tailor-made and patient-centric.

22.6.1 Psychological Management

POI is a condition that can lead to significant psychological morbidity and mental health issues due to many reasons.

Most of the time POI is diagnosed at unexpected times and that can devastate their mental well-being. Sometimes, they may have been suffering from other conditions such as cancer or autoimmune conditions. Thus, additionally, a new diagnosis may make matters worse for them.

It is well known that these groups of women are prone to suffer from mental health issues such as depression [15]. Hence, it is crucial that caregivers involved in the management of women with POI should be responsive enough to handle them with a lot of empathy and support. Providing appropriate psychological support at the onset would not only reduce the psychological trauma but also increase their compliance with future treatment.

Sudden and gradual oestrogen deficiency will cause urogenital atrophy, and decrease libido and sexual desire, which will affect their future psychosexual relationships as well as psychological well-being.

Psychosexual counselling should include all these aspects into consideration and the psychologist along with gynaecologists and psychiatrists should play an integral role in optimising her psychological well-being through education and empowerment.

22.6.2 Hormone Replacement Therapy (HRT)

As oestrogen deficiency is the major factor that gives rise to all these consequences. Thus, replacing oestrogen with other necessary hormones is a crucial step.

A range of hormonal treatment options are available for them. Local oestrogen will improve vaginal dryness, dyspareunia and urinary symptoms. A small dose of testosterone will improve sexual desire and libido.

HRT along with lifestyle modification will improve their cognitive impairment.

There are multiple preparations of HRT available with different routes including oral, implants, skin patches and local applications. Caregivers should help the patients to select a suitable and culturally appropriate option for them.

Patients with a uterus require oestrogen and progesterone whereas patients without a uterus require only oestrogen. This is simply because that endometrium principally needs progesterone to contract the effect of oestrogen as exposure to unopposed oestrogen leads to endometrial hyperplasia and malignancy.

It is evident that supplementation of hormones up until the natural age of menopause (50–51 years) can reduce morbidity and mortality significantly in women with POI.

However, it has been noted that more than 52% of POI patients do not take HRT [15] despite the recommendations. Before commencing HRT, women should be informed that it won't increase the risk of breast cancer before the age of natural menopause. A clear explanation of the health benefits in simple language may help them to understand and comply with the treatment.

There is evidence to show that oestrogen replacement is better with 17β-oestradiol when compared to ethinyl oestradiol or conjugated equine oestrogen and endometrial protection is better with cyclical treatment than micronised natural progesterone [1].

Once the patient is on HRT, it is a good practice to organise an annual clinical review.

22.6.3 Reproduction and Contraception

As patients with POI belong to the reproductive age group, their main concern can be fertility. Even if they have been diagnosed with POI, about a 5–10% of them can conceive naturally. Patients should be educated regarding this and they should be advised to use proper contraception to avoid unwanted pregnancies if they do not intend to conceive.

Despite recent advances in reproductive medicine, there is no proven treatment modality to improve fertility or ovarian reserve in women with POI except by using a donor egg.

It is important to counsel women with POI and fertility wishes that identified familial conditions and chromosomal abnormalities can be potentially transmitted if their eggs fertilise and considering donor ovum can help to overcome this problem. However, the option is to consider in vitro fertilisation and preimplantation genetic testing to prevent generational transmission of such conditions.

Women who are vulnerable to POI should be identified and encouraged to opt for fertility preservation methods. An array of options ranging from preserving ovarian tissue, ovum or embryo can be considered. Although ovarian tissue preservation is a viable option it is still not considered an established method in clinical practices. Hence, the gold standard remains embryo cryopreservation.

Some couples may prefer adoption as an option and they need to be directed and supported according to their local policies.

However, gynaecologists should play a central role and direct them to choose their preferred method sensitively.

22.6.4 Management of Other Comorbidities

Bone health is largely dependent on oestrogen and women with POI may experience the consequences of poor bone mineral density (BMD) such as an increased risk of osteoporosis and fracture in later life. Many modalities exist to prevent and treat this issue and are patient-friendly to women with POI.

Lifestyle modification with weight-bearing exercise is a simple and effective non-medical approach that should be encouraged.

Pharmacological agents like bisphosphonates, selective oestrogen receptor modulators and multiple other agents are available to improve the outcomes. This complication can be prescribed along with HRT.

Calcium and vitamin D supplementation have been shown to improve bone health.

Dexa scans to assess BMD should be conducted to make a diagnosis every 5 years thereafter.

There are enough studies to show POI patients are prone to cardiovascular diseases. Modification of risk factors such as weight reduction, smoking cessation and regular exercise play a key role in minimising the burden of cardiovascular diseases. Research has confirmed that HRT also can improve cardiovascular health.

Patients with POI should also check their blood pressure levels, sugar levels, lipid levels and smoking status annually to optimise their overall health.

Key Points

- POI is menopause before 40 years of age.
- It is diagnosed when a woman is amenorrhoeic for 4 months with FSH > 25 IU/l on two occasions 4–6 weeks apart.
- There are multiple aetiologies involving genetic, autoimmune, infections and iatrogenic causes. But in the majority of cases, the aetiology is unknown.
- Acute and gradual oestrogen withdrawal cause clinical sequelae of the disease.
- POI will affect fertility and reproductive health, psychosexual health, cardiovascular well-being, bone density, urogenital issues and cognition.
- Above all, POI will significantly increase morbidity due to any reasons.
- Multidisciplinary involvement is necessary for successful management.
- The patient-centred approach should be adopted when caring for women with POI.
- HRT with lifestyle modification is the mainstay of management.
- An assisted reproductive technique with a donor ovum is a viable option for women who want to conceive. However, 5–10% of women with POI conceive naturally.

References

1. Eshre Guideline Group on POI, Webber L, Davies M, Anderson R, Bartlett J, Braat D, Cartwright B, Cifkova R, de Muinck K-SS, Hogervorst E, Janse F. ESHRE guideline: management of women with premature ovarian insufficiency. Hum Reprod. 2016;31(5):926–37.
2. American College of Obstetricians and Gynecologists. Primary ovarian insufficiency in adolescents and young women. Committee Opinion No. 605. Obstet Gynecol. 2014;124(1):193–7.
3. Arora P, Polson DW. Diagnosis and management of premature ovarian failure. Obstet Gynaecol. 2011;13(2):67–72.
4. Coulam CB, Adamson SC, Annegers JF. Incidence of premature ovarian failure. Obstet Gynecol. 1986;67(4):604–6.
5. Fenton AJ. Premature ovarian insufficiency: pathogenesis and management. J Mid-life Health. 2015;6(4):147.
6. Goswami D, Conway GS. Premature ovarian failure. Hum Reprod Update. 2005;11(4):391–410.
7. Anasti JN. Premature ovarian failure: an update. Fertil Steril. 1998;70(1):1–5.
8. Albright F, Smith PH, Fraser R. A syndrome characterized by primary ovarian insufficiency and decreased stature: report of 11 cases with a digression on hormonal control of axillary and pubic hair. Am J Med Sci. 1942;204(5):625–48.
9. Dave FG, Adedipe T, Disu S, Laiyemo R. Unscheduled bleeding with hormone replacement therapy. Obstet Gynaecol. 2019;21(2):95–101.
10. Wesevich V, Kellen AN, Pal L. Recent advances in understanding primary ovarian insufficiency. F1000Research. 2020;9

11. Bione S, Toniolo D. X chromosome genes and premature ovarian failure. In: Seminars in reproductive medicine 2000 (vol. 18, No. 01). New York, NY: Copyright© 2000 by Thieme Medical Publishers, Inc.; 2000. p. 051–8.
12. Cox L, Liu JH. Primary ovarian insufficiency: an update. Int J Women's Health. 2014:235–43.
13. Bondy CA, Turner Syndrome Consensus Study Group. Care of girls and women with Turner syndrome: a guideline of the Turner Syndrome Study Group. J Clin Endocrinol Metab. 2007;92(1):10–25.
14. Gubbels CS, Land JA, Evers JL, Bierau J, Menheere PP, Robben SG, Rubio-Gozalbo ME. Primary ovarian insufficiency in classic galactosemia: role of FSH dysfunction and timing of the lesion. J Inherit Metab Dis. 2013;36:29–34.
15. Murray A, Schoemaker MJ, Bennett CE, Ennis S, Macpherson JN, Jones M, Morris DH, Orr N, Ashworth A, Jacobs PA, Swerdlow AJ. Population-based estimates of the prevalence of FMR1 expansion mutations in women with early menopause and primary ovarian insufficiency. Genet Med. 2014;16(1):19–24.
16. Torrealday S, Kodaman P, Pal L. Premature Ovarian Insufficiency-an update on recent advances in understanding and management. F1000Research. 2017;6:F1000-aculty.
17. Labarbera AR, Miller MM, Ober C, Rebar RW. Autoimmune etiology in premature ovarian failure. Am J Reprod Immunol Microbiol. 1988;16(3):115–22.
18. Ebrahimi M, Asbagh FA. Pathogenesis and causes of premature ovarian failure: an update. Int J Fertil Steril. 2011;5(2):54.
19. Parker WH, Broder MS, Chang E, Feskanich D, Farquhar C, Liu Z, Shoupe D, Berek JS, Hankinson S, Manson JE. Ovarian conservation at the time of hysterectomy and long-term health outcomes in the nurses' health study. Obstet Gynecol. 2009;113(5):1027.
20. Jacoby VL, Grady D, Wactawski-Wende J, Manson JE, Allison MA, Kuppermann M, Sarto GE, Robbins J, Phillips L, Martin LW, O'Sullivan MJ. Oophorectomy vs ovarian conservation with hysterectomy: cardiovascular disease, hip fracture, and cancer in the Women's Health Initiative Observational Study. Arch Internal Med. 2011;171(8):760–8.
21. Wu X, Cai H, Kallianpur A, Li H, Yang G, Gao J, Xiang YB, Ji BT, Zheng W, Shu XO. Impact of premature ovarian failure on mortality and morbidity among Chinese women. PLoS One. 2014;9(3):e89597.
22. Podfigurna-Stopa A, Czyzyk A, Grymowicz M, Smolarczyk R, Katulski K, Czajkowski K, Meczekalski B. Premature ovarian insufficiency: the context of long-term effects. J Endocrinol Investig. 2016;39:983–90.
23. Vujovic S, Brincat M, Erel T, Gambacciani M, Lambrinoudaki I, Moen MH, Schenck-Gustafsson K, Tremollieres F, Rozenberg S, Rees M. EMAS position statement: managing women with premature ovarian failure. Maturitas. 2010;67(1):91–3.
24. Lumsden MA. The NICE Guideline–Menopause: diagnosis and management. Climacteric. 2016;19(5):426–9.
25. Silva CA, Yamakami LY, Aikawa NE, Araujo DB, Carvalho JF, Bonfá E. Autoimmune primary ovarian insufficiency. Autoimmun Rev. 2014;13(4–5):427–30.
26. Welt CK. Autoimmune oophoritis in the adolescent. Ann N Y Acad Sci. 2008;1135(1):118–22.
27. Rosenzweig MQ. Breaking bad news: a guide for effective and empathetic communication. Nurse Pract. 2012;37(2):1.

Primary Ovarian Insufficiency

23

C. Savitha and G. S. Anitha

23.1 Introduction

Natural menopause is defined as the permanent cessation of menstrual periods, determined retrospectively after a woman has experienced 12 months of amenorrhea without any other obvious pathological or physiological cause. It occurs at a median age of 51.4 years in normal women. Primary ovarian insufficiency is the depletion or dysfunction of ovarian follicles with cessation of menses before age 40 years [1]. The term premature menopause, premature ovarian failure is no longer preferred because ovarian function is intermittent or unpredictable in many cases. POI (premature ovarian insufficiency) is characterized by menstrual disturbance (amenorrhea or oligomenorrhea) with raised gonadotropins and low estradiol. The prevalence is affected by population characteristics like ethnicity [2]. The incidence of POI is approximately 1% of women under 40 years old and 0.1% of women under 30 years old [3]. POI is a result of deficiency of ovarian sex hormones and decreased ovarian follicles which leads to early onset of menopausal symptoms [4]. There is hypoestrogenism which causes subfertility, infertility, menstrual irregularities, and pregnancy failures. There are myriad of menopausal symptoms like hot flashes, night sweats, insomnia and the long-term risk of skeletal fragility, cardiovascular, and neurocognitive disorders. In spontaneous POI with XX karyotype, there may be intermittent resumption of ovarian activity in approximately 25% of women [5]. The diagnosis of POI in a young woman has potentially life-changing physical and emotional consequences for the

C. Savitha (✉) · G. S. Anitha
Department of Obstetrics & Gynecology, Bangalore Medical College & Research Institute, Bangalore, Karnataka, India

R. Garg (ed.), *Management of Menopause*,
https://doi.org/10.1007/978-981-96-0239-1_23

sufferer and her family. The diagnosis must be correct and in a timely manner for not only effective treatment of POI, but it is also vitally important that such a profound diagnosis is not made erroneously as this can also have a devastating impact on the woman's emotional well-being [6].

23.2 Etiology

Premature ovarian insufficiency is a heterogeneous disorder caused by genetic factors, autoimmune diseases, mitochondrial abnormalities, iatrogenic factors (including chemotherapy, radiotherapy, and surgical procedures), and environmental factors [7]. There is an understanding that POI is caused by early follicular depletion, blockage of follicular maturation or destruction of the oocyte pool, and resistant ovarian syndrome. At least 90% of cases of primary ovarian insufficiency are idiopathic [1].

The identified causes of POI have been grouped into two categories: genetic and nongenetic causes. In genetic causes, the most notable ones are where X chromosome is damaged (isochromosome X), lost (Turner syndrome and Turner mosaics), or altered (*FMR1* permutation carriers) [8].

A number of autoimmune disorders and single-gene defects also are associated with POI. Approximately 4% of women with POI will have adrenal or ovarian antibodies. Young women with cancer who have undergone chemotherapy or pelvic radiation are at risk because these agents may cause profound and rapid follicular atresia (Table 23.1).

Table 23.1 Causes of premature ovarian insufficiency (POI)

Genetic causes	Nongenetic causes
Trisomy X (47 XXX or mosaic)	Autoimmune polyglandular syndrome (1 and 2)
Deletion of X chromosome	Blepharophimosis-Epicanthus inversus syndrome
Turner mosaic (45XO/46XX)	Ataxia telangiectasia
Turner syndrome	Fanconi anemia
Fragile X premature	Fanconi anemia
	Infectious diseases: Shigelosis, Chickenpox, Mumps oophoritis, Tuberculosis, Malaria, Cytomegalovirus
	Enzyme deficiency: Galactosemia, 17α-hydroxylase deficiency, Aromatase deficiency
	Chemotherapy: Alkylating agents, Cyclophosphamide, Dacarbazine, Chlorambucil, Melphalan, Busulphan, Nitrogen mustard, Anthracyclines (doxorubicin), Substituted hydrazine (procarbazine)
	Iatrogenic: Bilateral oophorectomy, Bilateral ovarian cystectomy, Radiation, Pelvic vessel embolization
	Environmental toxins

23.3 Pathogenesis

There are many potential etiologies for POI because normal ovarian development is dependent on a carefully timed cascade of events. Pathophysiologically, these defects can be divided into two major categories:

- Accelerated follicle depletion.
- Decreased steroid production without oocyte loss.

The genetic, autoimmune, and environmental or toxic causes of POI often result in accelerated follicle depletion.

Genetic Causes: Whole exome or whole genome sequencing can identify the cause of POI in approximately 30–35% of patients [9, 10]. X chromosome disorders are the most common genetic cause for POI [11].

Turner syndrome XO is the most common chromosomal defect in humans, occurring in up to 1.5% of conceptions, 10% of spontaneous abortions, and 1 of 2500 live births. It is caused by X monosomy and deletions in the short arm of the X chromosome. The ovaries in Turner syndrome characteristically consist of small amounts of connective tissue and no follicles or only a few atretic follicles ("streak gonads"). There were studies of histology of ovaries of fetuses with Turner syndrome that gave us an understanding of the gonadal failure. When compared with age-matched normal fetuses, the ovaries of XO fetuses contained apparently normal numbers of primordial germ cells up to at least 12 weeks of gestation, but at later gestational ages, the numbers of germ cells were decreased and connective tissue was increased. This indicates that accelerated atresia caused the ovarian failure rather than abnormal germ cell formation.

Other X chromosome deletions/translocation/inversions/duplications and balanced X chromosome-to-autosome translocations can cause POI [11].

There is a strong relationship between age at menopause, including POI, and premutations for the fragile X syndrome (the fragile X messenger ribonucleoprotein 1 [FMR1] gene) [12]. Fragile X syndrome is an X-linked form of intellectual disability that is one of the most common causes of developmental delay worldwide [13]. The term premutation is defined based on the ability of the repeat to expand to a full mutation in one generation. Individuals with premutations appear to have increased FMR1 mRNA expression and decreased but not absent FMR1 protein. In comparison, full mutations in subjects with intellectual disability are associated with methylation of the FMR1 gene and lack of transcription and protein production. There is no association between POI and full FMR1 mutations. The increased levels of mRNA are postulated to cause a toxic effect since there is normal amount of protein. The prevalence of FMR1 premutations ranges from 2% to 5% in women with sporadic POI and from 12% to 14% in women with POI with at least one family member who also had menopause before age 40 years [14]. The frequency of fragile X premutations in normal women is estimated to be approximately 1 in 259. Thus, the American College of Obstetricians and Gynecologists (ACOG) now recommends that women with POI or an elevated FSH level before age 40 years without known cause be screened for FMR1 premutations [15]. This is especially necessary to help women who are trying to conceive with their own oocytes and identification of carrier status can also prompt screening of sisters and cousins in fertile age group.

POI is common in women with galactosemia due to by the toxic effects of galactose metabolites.

A number of new genes like STAG3, SYCE1, MCM8, MCM9, SPIDR, MARF1, PSMC3IP, BRCA2, and ESR2 have been discovered using whole exome sequencing in consanguineous families [16]. These mutations, which appear to be rare, cause primary amenorrhea associated with POI (XX gonadal dysgenesis). These genes are important for meiosis, homologous recombination, and DNA damage and repair. There are other genes like FIGLA, NOBOX, eIF4ENIF1, and BMP15 which are under study in the pathogenesis of POI.

Some rare syndromic defects can also present with POI. They include blepharophimosis/ptosis/epicanthus inversus syndrome (BPES), ataxia telangiectasia, Bloom syndrome, Perrault syndrome, and mitochondrial disorder like progressive external ophthalmoplegia.

The autoimmune diseases which can be associated with POI are commonly hypothyroidism, autoimmune adrenal insufficiency, autoimmune polyglandular syndrome, and autoimmune Addison's disease. In addition, smoking can generate POI through polycyclic hydrocarbons in smoke. There is an association between myasthenia gravis and POI. When POI is associated association with adrenal autoimmunity, there is intense lymphocytic infiltration of thecal cells proven by histologic evidence [17].

Chemotherapeutic drugs and radiation therapy are the most common causes of toxin-induced ovarian failure. Acute ovarian failure is the immediate loss of ovarian function after chemotherapy or radiation. The age, type of medication, number of doses can have an effect on gonadotoxicity which is greater after use of alkylating agents/procarbazine, younger age of patients at the time of chemo/radiotherapy, site of irradiation (whole body, whole brain, pelvis and spinal) and combination of chemotherapy & radiotherapy. It should be noted that even females who menstruate after chemotherapy have an increased lifetime risk of primary ovarian insufficiency [1].

Viruses such as mumps, cytomegalovirus has been presumed to cause oophoritis and ovarian failure in women. Pelvic tuberculosis has been found to cause POI in 3% of patients.

Other toxins may have more subtle effects on ovarian function like cigarette smoking [18] and endogenous factors that correlate with age at menopause include weight and socioeconomic status, which increase it, and parity, which decreases it.

Endogenous mediators of gonadotropin receptor activation defects, abnormal production of intraovarian modulators and steroidogenic enzyme defects (StAR, CYP17, Aromatase, and NR5A1) that prevent estradiol production can cause POI without follicular depletion. Mutations of the gene for the FSH (or LH) receptor and Gs alpha subunit gene mutations are also implicated in the pathogenesis of POI.

23.4 Histology of Ovary [3]

Ovarian morphology and histology are different in POI and gonadal dysgenesis. The main difference is that the follicles in gonadal dysgenesis deplete during embryogenesis or early life with only stroma left as fibrous streaks while ovaries of women with POI contain follicles. Ovarian histology is different in various phenotypes of POI but most antral follicles are histologically abnormal. There is stroma and corpora albicantia in ovaries which is an eosinophilic mass and surrounding connective tissue capsule rich in collagen. There can be lymphoplasmacytic infiltration around the primordial follicle. There is no clear demarcation between the inner medulla and outer cortex under light microscopy. The fibrillar elements and cells are distributed heterogeneously.

23.5 Clinical Features

The characteristic features of POI are menstrual irregularities (oligomenorrhea and/or amenorrhea), increased levels of serum gonadotropins, low serum estradiol and estrogen deficiency symptoms. However, there can be intermittent ovarian function in approximately 50–75% [19] and this can explain the absence of estrogen deficiency symptoms like hot flushes or vaginal dryness in many cases of POI. Many women with POI can present with infertility, subfertility or pregnancy failures. Most of the women with POI with 46XX experience normal puberty and regular menstruation and they present commonly with disturbance in menstrual pattern which may be amenorrhea or a prolonged oligomenorrhea. In women who present with amenorrhoea, the incidence of POI ranges from 2% to 10%. In women using oral contraceptives (OCs) or following pregnancy, POI can become first apparent when there is failure of return of menstruation. There is an increased risk for symptoms and complications which are consequences of estrogen deficiency in women with POI. Estrogen deficiency in POI can lead to vasomotor symptoms, typically hot flushes and night sweats, vulvovaginal atrophy; vaginal dryness, dyspareunia, insomnia, mood disturbances, cognitive problems, e.g., memory issues, tiredness, loss of libido, weight gain and subfertility which can have devastating consequences in a young woman. Over prolonged period of hypoestrogenism, decreased bone density and increased risk of cardiovascular disease (CVD) are debilitating. The most common symptoms are hot flushes and vaginal dryness. The vasomotor symptoms (hot flushes) usually start before menstrual irregularities especially just prior to menstruation when the estrogen levels are lowest or during pill free duration in women taking OCs. Symptoms of atrophic vaginitis like vaginal dryness and dyspareunia are prominent when there is progression to amenorrhea. This is due to profound estrogen deficiency. POI is a significant risk factor for osteoporosis, [20] especially in young women with POI before attainment of peak adult bone mass. The incidence of osteoporotic fractures is higher in women with POI [21]. They have lower bone density especially in lumbar spine, femoral neck and hip and there is evidence of vitamin D deficiency also. There is an increase in cardiovascular morbidity and mortality in women with POI which may be due to endothelial dysfunction. [22] Early menopause may be associated with ischemic heart disease [23] and ischemic stroke but there is insufficient evidence to recommend hormone replacement therapy only for the prevention. Diminished sexual well-being is one of the potential consequences of estrogen deficiency in POI [24]. Dementia and cognitive decline is seen in women less than 43 years who have undergone bilateral oophorectomy and without estrogen replacement in some studies [25]. Emotional health is adversely affected on diagnosis of POI and it is traumatic for most women. There is disruption of family life and life plans with regard to procreation. Depression and anxiety disorders are seen in women with POI [26]. Women with 46, XX POI score adversely in the domains of physical and emotional health on the World Health Organization Quality of Life (WHOQOL)-BREF instrument. Most women with 46, XX POI have no abnormalities on physical examination, but occasionally, the following may be found:

- Evidence of Hashimoto's thyroiditis or Graves' disease.
- Increased skin pigmentation or vitiligo, anorexia, weight loss, salt craving, fatigue related to autoimmune primary adrenal insufficiency. In this case, orthostatic hypotension may also be present.
- Signs of atrophic vaginitis.
- Ovarian enlargement associated with autoimmune lymphocytic oophoritis or a steroidogenic enzyme defect on pelvic ultrasound.
- Ptosis, which has been associated with a rare familial form of POI (blepharophimosis/ptosis/epicanthus inversus syndrome [BPES]).
- Features of Turner syndrome include short stature, low posterior hairline, low hairline, high arched palate, shield chest with widely spaced nipples, a wide carrying angle, and short fourth and fifth metacarpals.

23.6 Diagnosis

The diagnosis of POI is life altering and hence should be made carefully. Early diagnosis is vital for planning of pregnancy, osteoporosis prevention, and possibly preventing coronary heart disease. It can be made definitively in women aged less than 40 years with irregular cycles/amenorrhea and serum with follicle-stimulating hormone (FSH) levels in the postmenopausal range. Amenorrhea may not be present always and is not necessary for diagnosis as many women can have intermittent ovarian function and menstruation spontaneously. Menstrual irregularity for 3 or more consecutive months in young women with previous regular cycles may require evaluation. Low serum estradiol (50 pg/mL) and increased serum follicle-stimulating hormone (FSH) (30–40 mIU/mL) concentrations are the typical biochemical features of POI except in women who have intermittent ovarian function may have normal laboratory findings. FSH is ideally measured on day 3 in women with menstrual cycles and can be done on a random day for women with amenorrhea. At least two FSH tests > 25I U/L are needed to confirm the diagnosis which is done 4 weeks apart. In approximately 75% of women with 46, XX POI, active antral follicles can be seen in transvaginal ultrasound. In autoimmune oophoritis, ultrasound characteristically shows enlarged cystic ovaries. For evaluation of diminished ovarian reserve, day 3 FSH and estradiol levels, serum anti-mullerian hormone concentration, transvaginal ultrasound for antral follicle count are used. Some other causes of menstrual cycle dysfunction may be required to not wrongly the diagnose POI like pregnancy test, serum prolactin and thyroid-stimulating hormone (TSH).

After making a diagnosis of POI, there are other evaluations and investigations required to determine the underlying cause and also any coexisting disorders [1]. Detailed history must be collected. All relevant history of prior ovarian surgery, cancer treatment like chemotherapy or radiation therapy, symptoms of primary adrenal insufficiency, personal or family history of autoimmune diseases, infections (mumps, TB) must be elaborate. All patients with POI must be asked about family history of POI (about 10% of cases are familial), family history of fragile X syndrome, intellectual disability, developmental delay, Parkinsonism, intension tremor, ataxia, or dementia (about 6% of cases of POI are associated with premutations in the fragile X messenger ribonucleoprotein 1 (FMR1) gene), deafness (familial autosomal recessive Perrault syndrome). Asymptomatic autoimmune adrenal insufficiency can be detected by serum adrenal cortical and 21-hydroxylase antibodies. If positive, then adrenal insufficiency can be evaluated by an 8 AM serum cortisol and plasma corticotropin (ACTH). Thyroid disorders, as a part of polyglandular autoimmune syndromes, can be evaluated by thyroid-stimulating hormone (TSH) and thyroid-peroxidase autoantibodies.

A karyotype should be done for all patients with POI, with or without stigmata of Turner syndrome. The age of onset of symptoms or prior parity may not rule out chromosomal abnormality. This is very important in women with idiopathic or unexplained POI (approximately 70%). Tests for FMR1 premutation can be offered. The risk of osteoporosis and bone loss necessitates a bone density test (dual-energy x-ray absorptiometry [DEXA]).

The most important steps after diagnosis are to counsel the patient of the diagnosis in a sensitive manner, age-appropriate manner, provide accurate information, and offer referral to appropriate resources for emotional support. The issues that are of paramount importance are emotional health, fertility, sexual function, bone health, cardiovascular health, and the risk for developing primary adrenal insufficiency (Table 23.2).

Table 23.2 Investigations in POI

Tests	Relevance
Serum hormones	
Follicle-stimulating hormone, luteinizing hormone, estradiol	Hypergonadotropic hypogonadism is a diagnostic criterion for primary ovarian insufficiency (POI)
Anti-Müllerian hormone Inhibin B	Marker of ovarian reserve-undetectable in POI
Prolactin level Thyroid-stimulating hormone	To diagnose hyperprolactemia To assess thyroid function
Genetic testing	
Karyotype	Aneuploidy/mosaicism/deletion/duplications
Fragile X premutation carrier screening	Fragility, mental retardation (FMR)
Autoimmunity screening	
Thyroid autoantibodies, thyroid peroxidase antibody, thyroglobulin antibody	Risk for thyroid dysfunction
21-hydroxylase antibodies—immunoprecipitation or indirect immunofluorescence	Risk for adrenal insufficiency
Imaging studies	
Ultrasound: Ovarian antral follicle count	Ovarian reserve assessment
Dual x-ray absorptiometry: Bone mineral density	Quantify lifetime risk for fracture

23.7 Turner Syndrome [27]

After diagnosis, a comprehensive initial evaluation is recommended, preferably, by a multidisciplinary team. In 23–50% of Turner syndrome patients, there can be congenital heart defects which are the most common cause of early mortality. An approach by American Heart Association [28] includes measurements of blood pressure in all extremities, electrocardiography—conduction abnormalities (e.g., prolonged QTc interval), echocardiography—structural abnormalities (coarctation of the aorta, bicuspid aortic valve) & cardiac magnetic resonance can be done as soon as the patient can tolerate the procedure without general anesthesia (typically around 12 years of age) to detect abnormalities such as dilated ascending aorta, elongated transverse aortic arch, aortic arch hypoplasia and partial anomalous pulmonary venous return. Any abnormality must be managed by a cardiologist or vascular specialist. There must be integration of multiple specialties like neuropsychology and allied behavioral health services, serial audiology evaluations every 5 years, renal ultrasonography, ophthalmologic evaluations every 3 years, screening for celiac disease by measuring tissue transglutaminase immunoglobulin A antibodies (tTG-IgA; usually combined with total IgA), liver disease by measuring alanine aminotransferase (ALT), aspartate aminotransferase (AST), gamma-glutamyl transpeptidase (GGTP), and alkaline phosphatase annually, screening for hyperglycemia by measuring hemoglobin A1c, with or without fasting glucose, annually, screening for dyslipidemia by measuring a lipid panel annually and screening for vitamin D deficiency by measuring serum 25-hydroxyvitamin D every

2–3 years. Height is monitored on growth curves specific for this disorder. Growth hormone therapy is given to patients with Turner syndrome to maximize their adult height and improve body composition. Induction of puberty in primary hypogonadism with Turner syndrome is with estradiol replacement therapy. AMH measurements can be used as a sensitive marker of ovarian function. Estradiol initiated at around 11–12 years of age can mimic the normal progression of puberty and cyclic progestins are added later to induce cyclic uterine bleeding and endometrial hyperplasia prevention. For girls with ovarian function, consultation with a fertility expert (reproductive endocrinologist) may be helpful to discuss prognosis and fertility options. Early referral would be needed for consideration of ovarian tissue cryopreservation. Parents should be aware that even if the cryopreservation procedure is successful, future pregnancy may not be advisable, because of the excess risk of mortality due to aortic complications such as dilatation and dissection. However, use of a gestational carrier allows a woman the option of using her own oocytes.

23.8 Management

After diagnosis of POI, women must be communicated with empathy and patience. She should be provided with information and adequate information on POI. The clinician must develop a personalized management plan using the woman's opinion and plans. POI should be treated as any other endocrine deficiency and treatment should include physiological replacement of ovarian steroid hormones (estrogens and progestogens) up to the age of natural menopause. There should be an individualized hormone replacement therapy (HRT) according to age, patient characteristics and patient needs and preferences. The route of administration depends upon the patient and her symptoms. Higher estrogens dose is required in women with younger onset of POI. Adolescents presenting with primary amenorrhea require a multidisciplinary approach with pediatric endocrinologist for proper induction of puberty with emphasis on secondary sexual characteristics. Initiating with low dose of estrogen and adding progesterone for withdrawal bleed on follow-up later is an effective strategy. In reproductive age, HRT with standard or low doses of oral or transdermal estrogens and progestogens should be used initially. The titration of dose must alleviate the symptoms and aim to maintain physiological estrogen levels in a premenopausal woman. Body identical hormone like 17β estradiol (E2) 2–4 mg is preferred or transdermal 17β-E2 50–100 μg (patches or gels) in cases where oral estrogens are not ideal like obesity or risk of thromboembolic disorders. Transdermal estradiol has many advantages compared to oral estrogens like bypassing hepatic first pass metabolism, lower risk of venous thromboembolism, dose adjustment by measuring serum estradiol, improved metabolism due to increase in IGF-1, lesser activation of rennin-angiotensin system with decreased risk of hypertension and increased bone mineral accrual. Topical vaginal estrogens like creams/tablets/vaginal rings may be used as an adjunct to systemic therapy in vulvovaginal atrophy (VVA). Conjugated equine estrogens (CEE) 0.625–1.25 mg is used less since there is greater risk of hypertension and thrombosis.

In cases of primary amenorrhea, progestin therapy should begin after a maximum of approximately 2 years of estradiol monotherapy (typically around 13 or 14 years of age) or when vaginal breakthrough bleeding first occurs. In patients after hysterectomy, estrogen only therapy is enough since progestogen is added in HRT to prevent endometrial hyperplasia. Oral progestogens are administered once or twice daily sequentially for 10–14 days per month, leading to regular monthly menstrual bleeding. Cyclical therapy can lower the risk of venothrombotic complications. Transdermal norethisterone is administered twice weekly for 14 days per month. In patients who want to increase their chances of spontaneous conception or planning oocyte donation IVF, cyclic regimens are preferable.

Androgen therapy is indicated in women with persistent sexual dysfunction despite optimized HRT.

HRT provides many benefits for women with POI like improvement in body fat composition, increase insulin sensitivity, decrease cardiovascular disease (CVD) risk, improve vascular function, improves bone mineral density (BMD), and decreases fracture risk in later life. Some studies show that HRT increases the risk of breast cancer and thrombosis. However, these results are mainly derived from studies involving older, postmenopausal women.

HRT should be continued in women with POI up to the age of normal natural menopause, approximately 51 years (Tables 23.3, 23.4 and 23.5).

One of the devastating adverse effects of POI is fertility impairment and early inevitable cessation of fertility. In the early course of the disease, there can be intermittent ovarian activity in up to 25% of women with POI and spontaneous natural conception (1.5–10%) may occur. The positive predictors for ovarian activity are serum estradiol, inhibin B, presence of follicles on ultrasound, secondary amenorrhea, and positive family history of POI. Women with POI should be advised for not delaying efforts for pregnancy. If pregnancy is undesirable, then use of contraceptive methods is advised since HRT doesn't provide contraceptive protection unless levonorgestrel intrauterine system is used.

If fertility interventions are needed, then she can be offered techniques of assisted conception (ovulation induction and/or autologous in vitro fertilization, daily administration of oral estradiol for 6 months, oral ethinyl estradiol for 2 weeks before and during gonadotrophin administration, treatment with GnRH analogue

Table 23.3 HRT drugs for POI [6]

Estrogens	Progestogens (for women with intact uterus only)
17β-E2 2–4 mg orally	Natural progesterone orally 200 mg cyclically or 100 mg continuously
CEE 0.625–1.25 mg orally	Norethisterone 1–5 mg orally
17β-E2 50–100 μg transdermally	Norethisterone 0.25 mg transdermally
Topical vaginal estrogens when VVA/GSM is diagnosed	Dihydrogesterone 10–20 mg orally

E2 estradiol, *CEE* conjugated equine estrogens, *VVA* vulvovaginal atrophy, *GS* genitourinary syndrome

Table 23.4 Bioequivalent hormonal dosages for hormone therapy for primary ovarian insufficiency [8]

Estrogen	Progestogen[a]	
Continuous	Continuous	Sequential
1–2 mg micronized 17β-estradiol (oral)	2.5–5 mg medroxyprogesterone acetate daily (oral)	10 mg medroxyprogesterone acetate daily (oral) for 12 days each month
100 μg 17β-estradiol (transdermal)	100 mg micronized progesterone daily (oral)	200 mg micronized progesterone daily (oral) for 12 days each month
0.625–1.25 mg conjugated equine estrogen (oral)		

[a]Select one of the estrogen options to be combined with one of the progestogen options

Table 23.5 Monitoring of women with POI on HRT [6]

Baseline
• Body weight and height
• Body mass index
• Renal function
• Liver function
• Thyroid function
• Fasting glucose and HbA1c
• Lipids levels
• Calcium and vitamin D
• Blood pressure
• Cardiovascular disease risk estimation
• Bone mineral density (if normal, repeat in 2–3 years)
• Fracture risk estimation
• Mammography (as per national guidelines, no additional breast screening is required in women on HRT for POI unless clinically indicated)
• Cervical cancer screening (as per national guidelines)
Follow-up
• Body weight and height
• BMI
• Blood pressure
• Thyroid function (depending on baseline evaluation)
• CVD risk estimation
• Fracture risk estimation
• Mammography (as per national guidelines, no additional breast screening is required in women on HRT for POI unless clinically indicated)
• Cervical cancer screening (as per national guidelines)

and gonadotrophins with co-administration of dexamethasone, and treatment with azathioprine in cases of autoimmune POI, oocyte donation).

Women at risk for imminent POI (women with idiopathic low ovarian reserve, women with a history of extensive ovarian surgery, women with a strong family history of POI, some women with Turner syndrome showing ovarian activity for an

Table 23.6 Recommendations for long-term follow-up of women with POI [6]

Assess quality of life
Mental health
• Screen for mood disorders regularly
• Antidepressants and psychotherapy are proven strategies for management of depression
• Estrogen therapy may have positive effects on mood sexual health
• Screen for sexual dysfunction regularly
• Use a multidisciplinary approach to the management of sexual dysfunction
Treat VVA/GSM with systemic and/or local vaginal estrogen therapy
Androgen therapy is not routinely recommended
Lifestyle changes: Balanced diet, Exercise (weekly aerobic), No smoking, Reduced salt intake, Reduced alcohol consumption
Investigate and treat dyslipidemia, diabetes or hypertension
Adequate intake of calcium and vitamin D

unpredictable period after menarche, survivors of childhood or adolescent cancer, and patients who will receive gonadotoxic chemotherapy or radiotherapy) should be counseled about the necessity of not delaying efforts for spontaneous conception (if applicable), and to offer some type of fertility preservation (if possible). Fertility preservation techniques include embryo, oocyte or ovarian tissue cryopreservation. Ovarian tissue cryopreservation (and later auto-transplantation) is may be the only option for patients requiring immediate gonadotoxic treatment or for prepubertal girls but this is still experimental.

Women with POI require long-term follow-up, especially for, quality of life, mental health and depressive symptoms. This follow-up must continue for lifelong. Many studies report that women with POI have better mental health, social functioning if they are satisfied with medical care. Healthy lifestyle including balanced nutrition, exercise, and avoidance of smoking, alcohol consumption in moderation, maintaining healthy body weight, adequate calcium and vitamin D intake should be an integral part of each session of counseling and follow-up. These lifestyle interventions are the cornerstone for prevention of CVD risk factors and osteoporosis. Appropriate screening for diabetes, dyslipidemia, and hypertension should be done (Table 23.6).

23.9 Recent Advances

One of the latest advances in treatment of POI is stem cell therapy and residual follicle rescue. [4] The stem cells can be bone marrow derived, peripheral blood mononuclear cells and endometrial mesenchymal cells. Platelet-rich plasma (PRP) which is prepared from autologous plasma can be injected intraovarian and this increases the viability and growth of preantral follicles. This mechanism can increase concentration of local growth factors like platelet-derived growth factor (PDGF), epidermal growth factor (EGF), insulin-like growth factor (IGF), transforming growth factor b-I (TGFb-I), vascular endothelial growth factor (VEGF), hepatocyte growth factor (HGF), and basic fibroblast growth factor (bFGF).

ASCOT (autologous stem cell ovarian transplant) improves ovarian reserve and IVF outcomes in women significantly. ROSE trial showed improved estrogen levels and ovarian reserve and thereby rejuvenation of ovaries in POI with stem cells [29]. In experimental studies, targeting the gene expression pathways regulating the activation of primordial follicle growth and involved in causation of POI (c-Kit/Kit ligand signaling pathway, FOXO3, phosphatase and tensin homolog, protein kinase A, rapamycin, Hippo signaling pathway and FOXO3) has been shown to halt the progress and reverse POI. The use of exogenous AMH has been explored as an innovative new preventative strategy and treatment option for gonadotoxin-induced follicle loss.

References

1. American College of Obstetricians and Gynecologists. Primary ovarian insufficiency in adolescents and young women. Committee Opinion No. 605. Obstet Gynecol. 2014;123:193–7.
2. ESHRE guideline-POI 2015.
3. Chon SJ, Umair Z, Yoon M-S. Premature ovarian insufficiency: past, present, and future. Front Cell Dev Biol. 2021;9:672890.
4. Wesevich V, Kellen AN, Pal L. Recent advances in understanding primary ovarian insufficiency. F1000 Res. 2020;9:1101.
5. Lambrinoudaki I, et al. Maturitas. 2021;147:53–63.
6. Panay N, Anderson RA, Nappi RE, Vincent AJ, Vujovic S, Webber L, Wolfman W. Premature ovarian insufficiency: an international menopause society white paper. Climacteric. 2020;23(5):1–21.
7. Rudnicka E, Kruszewska J, Klicka K, Kowalczyk J, Grymowicz M, Skórska J, et al. Premature ovarian insufficiency—aetiopathology, epidemiology, and diagnostic evaluation. Prz Menopauzalny. 2018;17:105–8.
8. American College of Obstetricians and Gynecologists. Hormone therapy in primary ovarian insufficiency. Committee Opinion No. 698. Obstet Gynecol. 2017;129:e134–41.
9. Gorsi B, Hernandez E, Moore MB, et al. Causal and candidate gene variants in a large cohort of women with primary ovarian insufficiency. J Clin Endocrinol Metab. 2022;107:685.
10. Heddar A, Ogur C, Da Costa S, et al. Genetic landscape of a large cohort of primary ovarian insufficiency: new genes and pathways and implications for personalized medicine. EBioMedicine. 2022;84:104246.
11. Eskenazi S, Bachelot A, Hugon-Rodin J, et al. Next generation sequencing should be proposed to every woman with "Idiopathic" primary ovarian insufficiency. J Endocr Soc. 2021;5:bvab032.
12. Allingham-Hawkins DJ, Babul-Hirji R, Chitayat D, et al. Fragile X premutation is a significant risk factor for premature ovarian failure: the International Collaborative POF in Fragile X study—preliminary data. Am J Med Genet. 1999;83:322.
13. De Vries BB, Halley DJ, Oostra BA, Niermeijer MF. The fragile X syndrome. J Med Genet. 1998;35:579.
14. Gersak K, Meden-Vrtovec H, Peterlin B. Fragile X premutation in women with sporadic premature ovarian failure in Slovenia. Hum Reprod. 2003;18:1637.
15. American College of Obstetricians and Gynecologists Committee on Genetics. ACOG committee opinion. No. 338: Screening for fragile X syndrome. Obstet Gynecol. 2006;107:1483.
16. Wood-Trageser MA, Gurbuz F, Yatsenko SA, et al. MCM9 mutations are associated with ovarian failure, short stature, and chromosomal instability. Am J Hum Genet. 2014;95:754.
17. Hoek A, Schoemaker J, Drexhage HA. Premature ovarian failure and ovarian autoimmunity. Endocr Rev. 1997;18:107.

18. Willett W, Stampfer MJ, Bain C, et al. Cigarette smoking, relative weight, and menopause. Am J Epidemiol. 1983;117:651.
19. Hubayter ZR, Popat V, Vanderhoof VH, et al. A prospective evaluation of antral follicle function in women with 46, XX spontaneous primary ovarian insufficiency. Fertil Steril. 2010;94:1769.
20. Leite-Silva P, Bedone A, Pinto-Neto AM, et al. Factors associated with bone density in young women with karyotypically normal spontaneous premature ovarian failure. Arch Gynecol Obstet. 2009;280:177.
21. De Vos M, Devroey P, Fauser BC. Primary ovarian insufficiency. Lancet. 2010;376:911.
22. Honigberg MC, Zekavat SM, Aragam K, et al. Association of premature natural and surgical menopause with incident cardiovascular disease. JAMA. 2019;322:2411.
23. Blümel JE, Mezones-Holguín E, Chedraui P, et al. Is premature ovarian insufficiency associated with mortality? A three-decade follow-up cohort Maturitas. 2022;163:82.
24. De Almeida DM, Benetti-Pinto CL, Makuch MY. Sexual function of women with premature ovarian failure. Menopause. 2011;18:262.
25. Ryan J, Scali J, Carrière I, et al. Impact of a premature menopause on cognitive function in later life. BJOG. 2014;121:1729.
26. Schmidt PJ, Luff JA, Haq NA, et al. Depression in women with spontaneous 46, XX primary ovarian insufficiency. J Clin Endocrinol Metab. 2011;96:E278.
27. Gravholt CH, Andersen NH, Conway GS, et al. Clinical practice guidelines for the care of girls and women with Turner syndrome: proceedings from the 2016 Cincinnati International Turner Syndrome Meeting. Eur J Endocrinol. 2017;177:G1.
28. Silberbach M, Roos-Hesselink JW, Andersen NH, et al. Cardiovascular health in turner syndrome: a scientific statement from the American Heart Association. Circ Genom Precis Med. 2018;11:e000048.
29. Herraiz S, et al. Autologous stem cell ovarian transplantation to increase reproductive potential in patients who are poor responders. Fertil Steril. 2018;110(3):496–505.

Management of Menopause 24

Poonam Yadav and Abhilasha Yadav

Every phase of life is beautiful and needs specialized and individualized care. Menopause is a normal phase of life and not a disease. The goal of menopausal management is to enforce preventive health care, which includes physical, mental, and emotional domains.

Treatment includes:

1. Natural—live a healthy lifestyle—enhance and accept what nature has given you.
2. Medical treatment—treat specific symptoms.
3. Hormonal treatment—if indicated.

Dietary management—maintenance of normal body functions, physical activity, and health—requires a well-balanced, nutritious diet that varies with age, physiological status, and level of activity. The nutrients must be obtained from a variety of food items from various food groups.

24.1 Factors Affecting the Nutritional Status at Menopause

1. Cessation of menstruation leads to changes in metabolic needs after menopause. Weight gain is common due to a decrease in basal metabolic rate and the redistribution of fat to the abdomen. Overall, this decreases the need for calories.
2. Nutritional needs may be altered by illness and medical status.
3. Intake of various medications may affect her nutritional needs by affecting her appetite, absorption, and metabolism of various nutrients.
4. Social factors may have an important role.

P. Yadav (✉) · A. Yadav
Department of Obstetrics and Gynaecology, S N Medical College, Agra, Uttar Pradesh, India

R. Garg (ed.), *Management of Menopause*,
https://doi.org/10.1007/978-981-96-0239-1_24

24.2 A Balanced, Healthy Menopausal Diet (Table 24.1)

24.2.1 Daily Calorie Requirement

- 2000 calories—sedentary work
- 2230 calories—moderate work
- 2800 calories—heavy work.

50–60% from complex carbohydrates and high fiber
30% from fats (saturated fat should be <10%)
15% from proteins
A good breakfast is important.
Whole grains, beans, and lentils should be included daily.
Mixed proteins should be included around 1 g per kg per day.
1–3 servings per week of fish like salmon, etc.
Powered flax seeds, fenugreek, saunf, and cinnamon can be added to salads and curd.
Phytoestrogen-rich foods are lentils, kidney beans, Bengal dal, and soybeans.
Cooking oil should be limited to 0.5 L per person per month or 2 tablespoons per person per day.
Use a combination of two cooking oils: MUFA-rich oils (rice bran oil, groundnut oil, and olive oil) and omega-3-rich oils (soybean oil and mustard oil).
Coffee and tea, not more than 3 cups per day.
Milk and curd (low-fat) 500–600 ml.
Lots of vitamin C-rich fruits and vegetables enhance calcium absorption.
Limit your consumption of sugar.
Use iodized salt: 1.5 teaspoons per day (3.5 g).

24.2.2 In a Nutshell

2 tablespoons of oil, 1 teaspoon of salt, 100 g of fruits, and 300 g of vegetables.
Avoid visible sugar—not more than 6 teaspoons.
High-fiber diet (25–40 g/day).

Table 24.1 Nutritional requirement for an adult sedentary women

S. No.	Type of food	Gram per day
1.	Millets and cereals	270
2.	Pulses	60
3.	Nonvegetarian food	30
4.	Vegetables	300
5.	Fruits	100
6.	Dairy products	300
7.	Fats and oils	20
8.	Sugar	20
9.	Salt	5
10.	Water	8–10 glass

8–10 glasses of water
Handfuls of nuts more than 5 times per week.

24.2.2.1 Exercise Management

In India, the mean age of menopause is 46 years, which is lower than that of Caucasians. The early age of menopause predisposes Indian women to chronic health disorders a decade earlier than Caucasian women, like osteoporotic fractures, myocardial infarction, and type 2 diabetes mellitus. As compared to the Western population, the mean bone mineral density (BMD) in Indian women is <2 standard deviations.

All the above facts point toward the need for an effective management plan to promote health in the aging population.

24.2.3 Benefits of Regular Exercise

- Maintain cardiovascular health.
- Maintain lipid levels in the body (HDL).
- Maintain body weight, body strength, muscle mass, and bone density.
- Pelvic floor exercise maintains urogenital health.

A well-balanced exercise program comprising aerobics, resistance, endurance yoga, flexibility, balance, and posture as per the health status of the woman is of great benefit at menopause.

24.2.4 Global Recommendation for Physical Activity in Middle-Aged and Older Adults

- 30 min or more of moderate physical activity on most days, preferably all days of the week.
- Weight-bearing exercise such as walking.
- Strength training is done 2–3 times per week.
- Balanced training for fall prevention.

Take activities that can be consistently done. Joining a group helps maintain consistency.

Exercise plays an important role in healthy aging. As the saying goes, "Aging happens, but good health is planned."

24.2.5 Recommendations for Physical Activity and Exercise

- Exercise should include aerobics, muscle strengthening, breathing, and balance.
- 30 min of moderate-to-intense physical activity for 5 days per week.

- Muscle-strengthening activities should be included at least twice a week.

30 min per day—for fitness and reduced risk of chronic diseases.
60 min per day—for prevention of weight loss.
60–90 min per day—to avoid regain of weight loss.

24.3 Immunization

Adult vaccination is challenging to implement when target goals for childhood vaccination are not up to par. Clinicians in India have to develop a system for adult vaccination that helps reduce morbidity and mortality from vaccine-preventable diseases (Table 24.2).

Aging leads to changes in the innate and adaptive immune systems and a less-than-ideal immune response. This is known as immune sensing, and clinicians have to be aware of this suboptimal response after vaccination in adults.

In 2009, the Association of Physicians of India published consensus recommendations on adult immunization in India [1]. By using these recommendations along with those from the WHO, clinicians have to identify adult populations most likely to benefit from immunization [2].

24.3.1 Special Considerations

Cholera for Kumbh Mela attendees

Meningococcal for Hajj attendees

*Recommended for all vaccinated adults at risk of hepatitis B virus and adults seeking post-exposure prophylaxis.

Table 24.2 Summary of adult vaccination recommendation by WHO, ACIP

Routine vaccination	WHO	ACIP
Hepatitis A	–	✓
Hepatitis B	✓	✓
Herpes Zoster	–	✓
HPV	–	✓
Influenza >50 years	✓	✓
MMR	✓	✓
Meningococcal	✓	✓
Pneumococcal >65 years	–	✓
Tdap	✓	✓
Varicella	–	✓

24.4 Hormonal Therapy

The term hormonal therapy includes the use of various estrogens, progesterone, combined formulations, androgen, and tibolone.

Hormonal therapy also includes:

- Different routes of administration
- Effects or benefits
- Risk or side effect

Various studies indicate that benefits and risks can be different for the same individual over a different time span.

24.4.1 Standard Abbreviation

MHT: Menopausal hormonal therapy

HT: Hormonal therapy (MHT and HT are interchangeable)

HRT: Hormone replacement therapy (when used as replacement therapy for premature ovarian insufficiency)

ET: Estrogen therapy

EPT: Estrogen-progesterone therapy

AP: Androgen therapy

SERM: Selective estrogen receptor modulator

OCP: Oral contraceptive pills

CC: Combined contraceptive

POP: Progesterone-only pill.

The current concept of MHT:

MHT should be selectively used for symptom relief within 10 years of menopause.

The use of MHT for the prevention of chronic diseases is controversial.

The MHD dose should be tailored according to the needs of women.

The transdermal route is preferable to the oral route for MHT.

The use of dydrogesterone and micronized progesterone appears to be safer options for progesterone in MHT.

24.4.2 Contraindications for MHT

1. Menopause onset >10 years or age > 60 years.
2. Undiagnosed abnormal uterine bleeding.
3. History of active endometrial and gynecological hormone-dependent cancer.
4. High risk for breast cancer or active breast cancer.
5. High risk of cardiovascular diseases (CVD) or established CVD.
6. Diabetes is an end-organ disease.
7. Severe active liver disease.
8. Systemic lupus erythematous.

24.4.3 Relative Contraindications

1. Hypertriglyceridemia
2. Active gallbladder disease
3. Obesity
4. Smokers
5. Migraine with aura
6. Moderate risk for CVD; history of deep vein thrombosis
7. Uterine fibroids and endometriosis
8. Moderate risk for breast cancer

24.4.4 Indications for MHT

1. MHT is the most effective treatment for vasomotor symptoms.
2. Bone-MHT may be useful as a first-line treatment for the prevention and treatment of osteoporosis in early menopause in symptomatic women, if not contraindicated.
3. Depression: estrogen can be used to treat symptoms of depression when other causes of depression have been ruled out.
4. Premature menopause: MHT is recommended until at least the median age of menopause.
5. Urogenital symptoms: recurrent UTI and urinary incontinence, dyspnea, and vaginal dryness.
6. General somatic symptoms: frequent headaches, dizziness, back pain, and joint pain.

24.4.5 Investigations

Menopause is a clinical diagnosis that is made 12 months after the cessation of menses. Elevated serum FSH and decreased serum estradiol levels aid in the diagnosis of menopause.

24.4.6 General Management

Avoid stress, caffeine, alcohol, and spicy food, and reduce the trigger of hot flushes.

Calcium: 1 g daily.

Vitamin D: 1000–2000 IU/day, or 60,000 IU per month.

24.4.7 Counseling for MHT

1. Indications and risks of MHD
2. Pre-MHT tests

3. Types of MHT available
4. Follow-up of MHT
5. How long to continue
6. Other available options

24.4.8 Pre-assessment of Women for MHT

1. Detailed history, clinical examination, and investigations
2. Evaluate the preferences and needs of women
3. Type and stage of menopause
   - Menopause transitions: cyclical progesterone, OCP, and cyclical MHT
   - Earle menopause <12 months-sequential EPT
   - Late menopause >12 months: continuous-combined EPT/tibolone
   - Surgical menopause: estrogen only or tibolone
   - Premature ovarian insufficiency/early menopause (OCP/MHT): sequential
   - Urogenital atrophy: local estrogens

   All symptomatic menopausal women should be screened for:

- Diabetes
- CVD
- Osteoporosis
- Sarcopenia
- Cancer
- Oral health
- Eye check-up
- Nutritional health

24.4.9 Essential Investigations

- A complete blood picture
- Urine R/M
- Fasting blood sugar, HbA1C
- Lipid profile
- Serum TSH
- Pap smear, vaginal pH
- TVS
- Mammogram/ultrasound
- Eye check-up for refraction, retinal, and intraocular pressure

  Investigations based on indications:

- Serum FSH, AMH
- Serum estradiol

Tests to assess the increased risk of thrombosis:

- Antithrombin III
- Tissue factor pathway inhibitor activity
- Protein C and protein S activity
- Stool for occult blood
- Lupus anticoagulant
- Anticardiolipin
- Endometrial biopsy
- Bone mass measurement
- LFT
- Urodynamic study
- 25 OH vitamin D3
- Ultrasound liver

24.4.10 The Preferred Route of Administration of MHT

Transdermal ET lowers the risk of DVT, stroke, and MI.

Oral estrogen increases lipid metabolism and, hence, cardiovascular protection.

Estrogen vaginal therapy for urogenital symptoms as blood levels are well below the postmenopausal range, there is a need for progesterone (Tables 24.3 and 24.4).

Table 24.3 Types of estrogen progestogen therapy (EPT) regimens

Regimen	Estrogen	Progestogen
Cyclic	Day 1–25	Last 10–14 days of the month
Cyclic-combined	Day 1–25	Days 1–25
Continuous-cyclic (sequential)	Daily	10–14 days every month
Continuous long cyclical	Daily	14 days every 3–6 months
Continuous-combined	Daily	Daily
Intermittent-combined (pulsed-progestogen; continuous pulsed)	Daily	Repeated cycles of 3 days on, 3 days off

Table 24.4 Dosage and types of systemic estrogens used in MHT

Estrogens	Ultra-low	Low	Standard	High
Conjugated equine estrogens (mg, CEE) oral	0.15	0.3, 0.45	0.625	1.25
17β-estradiol (mg) oral	0.5	1	2	4
17β-estradiol (mg) oral transdermal patch	0.014	0.025	0.05	0.1
17β-estradiol (mg) oral transdermal gel	0.375	0.75	1.5	3
Estradiol valerate (mg) oral		1	2	4S

24.4.11 Indications of the Transdermal Route

1. Trigylceridemia, hyperlipidemia, and increased CRP
2. Migraine
3. Controlled hypertension
4. Existing GB diseases
5. Obesity
6. Smoking.
7. Previous VTE
8. Varicose vein
9. Bowel disorders such as irritable bowel syndrome
10. Sexual dysfunction

24.4.12 Various Regimes of EPT

- Use of low-dose estrogen with low-dose progesterone.
- Natural progesterones like micronized progesterone and dydrogestrone are preferred.
- Progesterone in an adequate dose should be supplemented with oral estrogen in women.
- Estrogen alone is given to hysterectomized women.

  Progesterone is required even after hysterectomy in women with:

- Residual endometriosis.
- Who has had stage II/III adenocarcinoma of the endometrium.
- Previously treated endometrioid tumor of the ovary.
- Patients undergoing supracervical hysterectomy and endometrial ablation should be treated with an estrogen-progesterone combination.

24.4.13 Follow-Up

- Review after 1 month for efficacy and side effects (Table 24.5).

  Check your weight and blood pressure.

- After 3 months, assess the effect and compliance.
- Annually: physical examination.

  Update medical and family history.
  Relevant laboratory and imaging investigations.
  Discussion on lifestyle.
  Strategies to prevent or reduce chronic disease.

Table 24.5 Side effects of ET/EPT and their management

Side effects	Management
Fluid retention	Restrict salt intake, maintain adequate water intake, exercise, and herbal or mild prescription diuretics
Bloating	Switch to low-dose transdermal estrogen; lower the progesterone dose to a level that still protects the uterus; switch to another progestin or to micronized progestin
Breast tenderness	Lower the estrogen dose; switch to another estrogen; restrict salt intake; switch to another progestin; cut down on caffeine and chocolate
Headaches	Switch to transdermal estrogen; lower the dose of estrogen and/or progestogen; switch to a continuous-combined regimen; ensure adequate water intake; restrict salt; caffeine and alcohol, add tibolone
Mood changes	Lower the progestogen dose; switch progestogen; switch from systemic progestin to the progestin intra uterine system (IUS); change to a continuous-combined EPT regimen; ensure adequate water intake; restrict intake of salt, caffeine, and alcohol, add tibolone
Nausea	Take oral estrogen tablets with meals or before bed; switch to another oral estrogen; switch to transdermal estrogen; lower the estrogen or progestogen dose
Chloasma	Use sun screen lotion

24.5 Role of Progesterone in MHT

The primary role of progesterone in MHT is the inhibition of estrogen-induced proliferation of the endometrium. Hysterectomized women should be given estrogen alone. Some special conditions have indications for the use of a combined EP regimen even after a hysterectomy.

Patients with endometriosis: NMP and dydrogesterone are both effective in treating endometriosis-related symptoms. Tibolone can also be used.

Patients who have been treated with stage I and II adenocarcinoma of the endometrium need an EP-combined regimen.

24.5.1 Ideal Progesterone for MHT

Induces endometrial atrophy.

Should not blunt the beneficial effect of estrogen on bones, vessels, and the CNS.

NMP (200 mg/day) and dydrogestrone (10–20 mg/day) as oral and LNG IUS are the choices in today's practice.

Dienogest can also be a suitable option for MHT. It has a strong progestational effect on endometrium and also does not interfere with lipid or carbohydrate metabolism.

24.6 Role of Androgen in Postmenopausal Women

Examples of symptoms and physical signs indicative of perimenopausal and postmenopausal women include a depressed mood, diminished energy, depression, and impaired sexuality. These women are at increased risk of "hypoactive sexual desire disorder" (HSDD).

Physiological menopause is not associated with a sudden loss of androgen synthesis, so routinely, postmenopausal women do not require androgen replacement.

Indication: Severe androgen deficiency, as in patients with bilateral oophorectomy and adrenal insufficiency.

Route of administration: Recently, a female androgen patch was launched in the USA for the treatment of HSDD. No testosterone preparation is available in India.

24.6.1 Absolute Contraindication

- Presence of risk factors for breast cancer, endometrial cancer, the risk of VTE, and CVD.

24.6.2 Relative Contraindications

- Androgen alopecia.
- Acne.
- Hirsutism.
- Hypolipidemia.
- Liver dysfunction.

Current guidelines are not in favor of the widespread role of androgen therapy in postmenopausal women.

24.6.3 Tibolone

Tibolone is related to the 19-nortestosterone group and is a synthetic steroid. It selectively regulates estrogenic activity and is grouped under STEAR (selective tissue estrogenic activity regulator) (Fig. 24.1).

Estrogenic effects on tissues like the brain, bone, and vagina (not on the endometrium and breast) [3, 4].

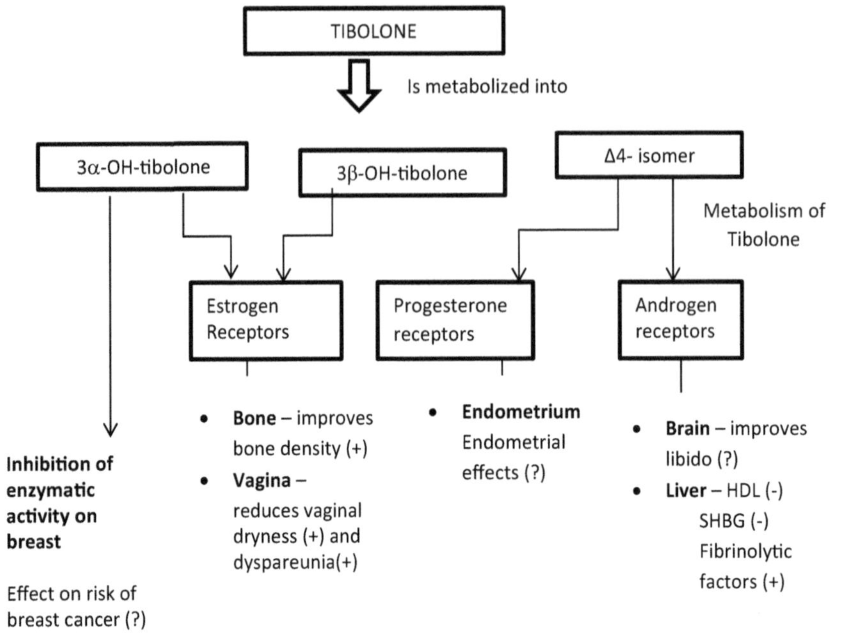

Fig. 24.1 Metabolism of tibolone

Dosing schedule: Tibolone can be started when women experience natural menopause (12 months after menopause) and immediately in cases of artificial menopause.

It is given in doses of 1.5–2.5 mg/day, preferably at the same time of day. Improvement in symptoms can be observed in a few weeks, and it can be used uninterrupted for longer periods, but not beyond 65 years of age.

In the case of switching from conventional hormonal therapy, the endometrium is already stimulated, so tibolone is to be given after withdrawal bleeding.

24.6.3.1 Contraindications of Tibolone

1. Acute liver disease with or without abnormal liver functions.
2. Hypertension, smoking, diabetes, and atrial fibrillation.
3. Suspected estrogen-dependent malignant tumor.
4. Previous and current thromboembolic diseases.
5. Porphyria.
6. Patients with a high risk for stroke.

24.6.3.2 Pros and Cons of the Use of Tibolone

- Tibolone reduces the risk of vertebral and non-vertebral fractures in osteoporotic women.
- It increases the BMD to statistically significant levels.
- It does not increase the risk of CVD and VTE events.
- It does not cause endometrial hyperplasia or carcinoma.

- Tibolone can be used as an add-back therapy with GnRH analogs.
- It can be used in women with myomas and endometriosis.
- It should not be used by breast cancer survivors, as it may increase the recurrence risk.

24.7 Selective Estrogen Receptor Modulators

These are nonhormonal compounds that bond to estrogen receptors but induce different estrogen responses in various tissues (Table 24.6).

24.7.1 Raloxifene

It is the only SERM approved for the prevention and treatment of osteoporosis in postmenopausal women [5]. The MORE (Multiple Outcomes of Raloxifene Evaluation) trial on 7705 postmenopausal women showed a 68% reduction in vertebral fractures, but no significant decrease was observed in non-vertebral fractures at the end of 4 years. This trail has also shown a 65% reduction in RR in all breast cancers.

Hot flushes and leg cramps are side effects of raloxifene, although the incidence is low.

24.7.2 Tamoxifen

The US FDA has approved the use of tamoxifen for breast cancer chemotherapy protection in premenopausal and postmenopausal women. The use of tamoxifen causes a two to threefold higher risk of endometrial carcinoma. Tamoxifen causes

Table 24.6 Types of SERMs and their clinical effects

Name	Uses	Effects/location
Clomiphene	Anovulation	Antagonist at hypothalamus
Famarelle	Menopausal symptoms, osteoporosis	Agonist breast and bone
Ormeloxifine	Contraceptive	Agonist bone, antagonist breast and uterus
Raloxifene	Osteoporosis, breast cancer prevention	Agonist bone, antagonist breast and uterus
Tamoxifen	Breast cancer	Agonist bone, antagonist breast and uterus
Toremifene	Breast cancer	Agonist bone, antagonist breast and uterus
Lasofoxifene	Osteoporosis, breast cancer, vaginal atrophy	Agonist bone, antagonist breast and uterus
Bazedoxifene	Osteoporosis	Agonist bone, antagonist breast and uterus

subepithelial sonoluscent changes along with atrophic endometrium. Levonorgestrel IUS is effective against these types of changes where oral progesterone preparations are not effective. It improves the lipid profile, reduces fractures, and is less effective than raloxifene.

24.7.3 Ormeloxifene

It is used for perimenopausal abnormal uterine bleeding (AUB). It controls the bleeding by regularizing the estrogen expression. Lasofoxifene 0.5 mg/day reduces the risk of vertebral and non-vertebral fractures.

24.7.4 Bazedoxifene

It reduces bone marrow turnover by 20–25% in doses of 20–40 mg daily. It binds both α and β estrogen receptors and antagonists in breast tissue and uterine tissue.

24.7.5 Phytoestrogens

Three main classes:

- Isoflavones.
- Coumestans.
- Lignans.

These are plant derivatives with more affinity for estrogen beta receptors. All have shown to reduce hot flushes [6].

24.8 Nonhormonal Management of Menopausal Symptoms (Tables 24.7 and 24.8)

Isoflavones: 70–80 mg per day for 6 weeks–3 months.

Lycopene: 18–24 mg per day.

Table 24.7 Choice of medication depends on prominent symptom

Medicine	VMS	Sleep	Mood
Gabapentin or pregabalin	++	+++	
SSRI/SNRI	++	±	+++
CBT or hypnosis			+

Table 24.8 Doses of SSRIs & SNRIS

Medications	Dosage
Paroxetine	10–20 mg/day
Venlafaxine	37.5–150 mg/day
Desvenlafaxine	25–150 mg/day
Fluoxetine	10–20 mg/day

24.9 SSRIs and SNRIs

Common side effects of SSRIs/SNRIs are nausea, drowsiness, and sexual dysfunction.

Symptoms of menopause are varied, customized tests should be conducted for each risk factor based on the basic examination conducted according to the life cycle necessary for women. Before initiating any treatment indications and contra-indications must be check listed which requires detailed history, physical examination, and other tests.

References

1. Expert group of the Association of Physicians of India on Adult Immunization in India. The Association of Physicians of India evidence-based clinical practice guidelines on adult immunization. JAPI. 2009;57:345–56.
2. World Health Organization. Recommendation for routine immunization [online] available from https://www.who.int/teams/immunization-vaccines-and-biologicals/policies/who-recommendations-for-routine-immunization%2D%2D-summary-tables.
3. Pinto-Almazán R, Segura-Uribe JJ, Farfán-García ED, Guerra-Araiza C. Effects of Tibolone on the central nervous system: clinical and experimental approaches. Biomed Res Int. 2017;2017(1):8630764. 9 pages. https://doi.org/10.1155/2017/8630764.
4. Del Río JP, Molina S, Hidalgo-Lanussa O, Garcia-Segura LM, Barreto GE. Tibolone as hormonal therapy and neuroprotective agent. Trends Endocrinol Metab. 2020;31(10):742–59. https://doi.org/10.1016/j.tem.2020.04.007.
5. Barrett-Connor E, Grady D, Sashegyi A, Anderson PW, Cox DA, Hoszowski K, Rautaharju P, Harper KD. MORE Investigators (Multiple Outcomes of Raloxifene Evaluation). Raloxifene and cardiovascular events in osteoporotic postmenopausal women: four-year results from the MORE (Multiple Outcomes of Raloxifene Evaluation) randomized trial. JAMA. 2002;287(7):847–57. https://doi.org/10.1001/jama.287.7.847.
6. Chen LR, Ko NY, Chen KH. Isoflavone supplements for menopausal women: a systematic review. Nutrients. 2019;11(11):2649. https://doi.org/10.3390/nu11112649.

Alternative Therapies at Menopause 25

Piyusha Milani Atapattu

25.1 Introduction

Menopause is a physiological phase in the life of women. However, the associated negative outcomes such as vasomotor symptoms, genitourinary dysfunction and increase in the risk of noncommunicable diseases (e.g., osteoporosis and cardiovascular disease) warrant the use of medical and surgical management in a significant proportion of women [1, 2]. Though menopausal hormone therapy is the mainstay of treatment, many women are hesitant to use hormonal therapy due to the fear of adverse effects. Furthermore hormonal treatment is contraindicated in some women due to concurrent medical problems, and some women refuse hormonal treatment due to other varied reasons. For the management of vasomotor symptoms, the commonest troublesome symptom in postmenopausal women, studies report the use of non-hormonal therapies in the majority of menopausal women ranging from 50–80% [3, 4].

Complementary and alternative therapies span a range of varied management options. They include dietary modifications and supplements using plant-based products, lifestyle modifications, mind-body techniques, as well as non-hormonal pharmacological treatments [1, 2, 5].

25.2 Dietary Supplements and Herbal Preparations

Numerous herbal preparations and dietary supplements have been used by women of different cultures over the years to alleviate troublesome menopausal symptoms, especially vasomotor symptoms. Though there are many trials on the different types of supplementary products, the evidence for their use is conflicting especially as

P. M. Atapattu (✉)
Faculty of Medicine, Department of Physiology, University of Colombo, Colombo, Sri Lanka

R. Garg (ed.), *Management of Menopause*,
https://doi.org/10.1007/978-981-96-0239-1_25

trials are nonhomogeneous. These preparations include phytoestrogens, black cohosh, evening primrose oil, Chinese herbal products, St John's wort, vitamin E, and other products [1, 2, 5].

25.2.1 Phytoestrogens

These are plant-based compounds that have estrogenic properties. Among the phytoestrogens, isoflavone- and lignin-containing supplements are commonly used for improving menopausal symptoms. Isoflavones or their precursors are found in soy beans, red clover, and legumes such as beans, peas, alfalfa and chick peas, and lignans or their precursors are found in foods such as flaxseed, cereals, legumes, and some fruits and vegetables [5]. Coumestans are plant phenols having estrogenic properties which are found in sprouts of alfalfa, mung bean, and soy [5]. Hops and beer contain a potent phytoestrogen 8-prenylnaringenin [2]. Soy foods contain isoflavone, which bind to both ERα and ERβ, with a greater affinity to ERβ causing both estrogenic and anti-estrogenic effects [1].

As estrogen deficiency is a main cause of menopause-related symptoms, phytoestrogens are likely to be a logical management option especially for vasomotor symptoms. However conflicting results are found among the many studies conducted on the efficacy of phytoestrogens for management of menopausal symptoms [6].

The use of phytoestrogens has been shown to significantly reduce the frequency of vasomotor symptoms with no difference in adverse effects compared to placebo users, in a systematic review and meta-analysis of 15 high-quality randomized controlled trials (RCTs) [6]. A systematic review and meta-analysis of 23 randomized controlled trials including 1880 postmenopausal women found supplementary phytoestrogen followed by usual diet did not contribute to a significant changes in body weight [7]. The estrogenic properties of phytoestrogens is a cause for concern of developing adverse effects especially on estrogen sensitive tissues such as breasts and ovaries, and interference with the actions of selective estrogen receptor modulators [5]. There is no evidence to recommend phytoestrogens for vasomotor symptoms [1, 6, 7].

25.2.2 Black Cohosh (Actaea racemosa or Black Snakeroot)

Black cohosh is a plant from North America used over years as an indigenous herb for managing symptoms of menopause [1, 2, 5]. Currently it is a popular plant-based product for alleviating menopausal symptoms [2]. Neither its active ingredients nor its mechanism of action are clearly elucidated [1, 5].

Though its effect on many aspects of menopause (e.g., vasomotor symptoms, genitourinary syndrome of menopause, osteoporosis and quality of life) have been studied in many RCTs, in a Cochrane Database systematic review of 16 RCTs with 2027 participants, there was inconclusive evidence to show a significant benefit of any of the aspects studied [8]. Furthermore, black cohosh carries a risk of causing adverse effects such as gastrointestinal problems, skin rashes, and acute hepatitis [1, 2]. The risk of hepatotoxicity emphasizes the need for caution when using this product, warning the patients to discontinue its use if they develop abdominal pain, dark urine, or jaundice [1, 5].

25.2.3 Evening Primrose Oil (EPO)

EPO derived from the seeds of the flowering plant *Oenothera biennis* contains essential omega-6 fatty acids. It has been used to treat a variety of inflammatory diseases as well as menopausal symptoms [1, 2]. Though there are few studies including RCTs evaluating the effects of EPO on vasomotor symptoms and bone mineral density, the results of different studies are conflicting [1, 2]. Currently there is inadequate evidence for recommending EPO to alleviate menopausal symptoms [1, 2].

25.2.4 Chinese Herbal Products

Traditional Chinese products have been used for over 2000 years, and are usually given as mixed decoctions using multiple routes of administration [9]. Among the many Chinese herbs used, dong quai and ginseng are well known for their effects on improving menopausal symptoms [1, 5].

Dong quai (*Angelica sinensis*) is extracted from the root of the plant, and is used in combination with other herbs to treat gynecological problems. There are only a few studies on its use which have found no consistence results on the improvement of vaginal and endometrial tissues or alleviation of vasomotor symptoms over placebo [1, 2]. Furthermore, dong quai has been associated with drug interactions (e.g., warfarin), photosensitization, and possible carcinogenicity [2].

Ginseng is used to describe products of several species of plants, e.g., *Panax* (e.g., *P. ginseng, P. qinquefolium*), and Siberian ginseng (*Acanthopanax senticosus* or *Eleutherococcus senticosis*) [1]. It is a favorite herbal product used in eastern Asia. Studies show no significant association of ginseng with improvement of vasomotor symptoms, quality of life, mood, reproductive hormones or integrity of vagina or endometrium in postmenopausal women [1]. It is not recommended for managing menopausal symptoms [1].

25.2.5 Vitamins and Nutrient Supplements

Vitamin E, a vitamin with antioxidant properties and omega-3 fatty acids, contains polyunsaturated fatty acids such as α-linolenic acid, docosahexaenoic acid (DHA), and eicosapentaenoic acid (EPA) [1, 2]. They are nutrient supplements used for a variety of diseases including menopausal symptoms. The trials studying these supplements show inconsistent results and insufficient evidence on their effectiveness in improving vasomotor symptoms [1, 2, 5].

25.2.6 Other Dietary Supplements

Wild yam (*Diascorea spp.*), St John's wort (*Hypericum perforatum)*, sage leaf, maca (*Lepidium meyenii*), pollen extract, valerian root, kwao krua, (*Pueraria mirifica*), Siberian rhubarb (*Rheum rhaponticum*), pine bark from the Mediterranean pine (*Pinus pinaster*), *Lactobacillus acidophilus*, ammonium succinate, and chasteberry (*V. agnus-castus*) are some other products used or studied in the management of menopausal symptoms [1, 2, 5]. However there is insufficient evidence on their benefits, doses and dose frequency to recommend their use for the relief of menopausal symptoms [1, 2, 5]. Furthermore some products contain adulterants and lack data on long-term safety (e.g., wild yam cream) and cannot be recommended for managing vasomotor symptoms [1, 2]. Kava kava (*Piper methysticum*) has more serious safety concerns and is banned in the UK due to hepatotoxicity [5].

25.3 Lifestyle Measures

Unhealthy lifestyle practices such as smoking, alcohol consumption, and sedentary behaviour are associated with many noncommunicable diseases and are also linked to vasomotor symptoms [5]. Lifestyle changes are advocated in most noncommunicable disorders as initial measures in their management. They have the advantage of being simple, cheap, and usually with no serious adverse effects. Though extensively studied, many lifestyle measures practiced for the management of menopausal symptoms reveal inconsistent results [1, 2, 5].

25.3.1 Cooling Techniques

As the commonest menopausal symptom hot flushes is triggered by the changes in the temperature regulating mechanisms, cooling techniques are commonly practiced by affected women. They include common measures such as wearing cotton or linen clothing, wearing less clothes, using fans or cooling packs, air conditioning and other measures such as forehead cooling devices [1]. However, there is no consistent evidence to support the use of cooling interventions to manage vasomotor symptoms [1].

25.3.2 Avoiding Triggers

Some food and beverages such as coffee, spicy or hot foods, and alcohol are thought to worsen hot flushes, and so women are advised to limit their use. However, there are no good trials showing evidence for the use of these measures [1].

25.3.3 Exercise and Yoga

Physical exercise has shown to have multiple benefits on bodily functions and is recommended for many disorders. They include aerobic exercise, strength training exercise, and yoga as popular forms of exercise and specific types such as pelvic floor exercises.

A systematic review and meta-analysis of 9 RCTs with 882 women, found a positive effect of exercise on physical and psychological quality of life (QoL) scores on postmenopausal women, with yoga having a significant positive effect on physical QoL [10]. In another systematic review of 21 RCTs with 2884 participants on the impact of aerobic exercise on vasomotor symptoms (VMS), a significant improvement in severity of vasomotor symptoms were found though with no effect on their frequency [11]. Systematic reviews and meta-analyses of RCTs on the benefits of yoga on menopausal symptoms too are inconsistent; one with 10 RCTs showing a significant reduction in insomnia severity and improving sleep problems [12], a more recent one of 13 RCTs with 1306 participants revealing only a significant improvement of vasomotor symptom when compared with exercise controls [13] and another of 5 RCTs with 582 participants showing only moderate evidence for short-term improvement of psychological symptoms, with no effects on vasomotor symptoms [14].

Although there are numerous benefits of exercise on health, there is no consistence high level evidence from RCTs, to recommend exercise as a means of improving vasomotor symptoms in menopause [10–14].

25.3.4 Weight Loss

Weight gain in perimenopause and menopause are linked to increase in cardiovascular disease, malignancies and in some studies vasomotor symptoms, and so women are likely to benefit from weight loss [15, 16]. Physical exercise and healthy diet are lifestyle measures that lead to weight loss, with no serious adverse effects, and with important positive effects of healthy weight loss such as improvement in cardio-metabolic and cancer risk, sexual dysfunction, mood, self-esteem, and body image [15, 16]. Some studies have found a higher incidence of vasomotor symptoms in obese women, and RCTs have revealed an improvement in vasomotor symptoms with weight loss [1]. The cumulative findings of multiple studies suggest that loss of weight might be useful in alleviating vasomotor symptoms in some women [1].

25.4 Mind-Body Techniques

Mind-body techniques include a variety of techniques including cognitive behavioral therapy (CBT), mindfulness-based interventions, clinical hypnosis, paced respiration, and relaxation methods [1]. Studies have found a positive outcome on menopausal symptoms, especially vasomotor symptoms and psychological disturbances by the practice of different mind-body techniques [1, 17]. The mechanism of action of these techniques is likely to be through stress reduction, as stress is thought to trigger hot flushes via reducing the threshold for heat dissipation response [17].

25.4.1 Cognitive Behavioral Therapy (CBT)

CBT has been extensively studied for many menopause-related symptoms including vasomotor symptoms, mood disorders, insomnia, and stress [1, 2, 18]. Since the initial randomized double blind clinical trials MENOS 1 and MENOS 2 found that CBT is useful in the management of vasomotor symptoms in menopausal women with or without a history of breast cancer, many studies have confirmed the findings [1]. The methods of administration of CBT in studies range from physical group therapy, online delivery, by telephone or as self-help books, where most of them show a positive effect on the management of menopausal symptoms [18]. A systematic review and meta-analysis of cognitive therapy and behavior therapy in 14 RCTs including 1618 participants found a significant improvement in vasomotor symptoms, fatigue, mood disturbances such as depression and anxiety and quality of life [19]. Another systematic review and meta-analysis which pooled the findings of 12 RCTs with 1016 postmenopausal women on CBT, mindfulness and behavior-based therapy revealed that psychological interventions resulted in a statistically significant short-term improvement in vasomotor and other menopausal symptoms as well as medium-term improvement in vasomotor symptoms, especially in breast cancer survivors [20]. Based on the available evidence, several professional bodies have recommended CBT as an effective treatment of vasomotor symptoms in both menopausal women including breast cancer survivors [1, 2, 20].

25.4.2 Clinical Hypnosis

Clinical hypnosis is a low-risk procedure, and has been widely used in the management of many chronic diseases [1, 2]. Several randomized clinical trials in postmenopausal women including group of women with a history of breast cancer have shown that hypnosis significantly improves the frequency and severity of vasomotor symptoms when compared with controls using pharmacological interventions, placebo or structured attention control [1, 2, 21]. Studies have further reported a significant improvement in sleep, sexual functions and mood in menopausal women practicing clinical hypnosis over controls [1, 2]. The delivery of hypnosis can be by trained persons on site or via applications over smartphones [21]. Clinical hypnosis is recommended for the management of vasomotor symptoms [1, 2].

25.4.3 Mindfulness-Based Interventions (MBI)

MBI mainly use approaches incorporating meditation, and getting the participants to accept thoughts, physical sensations and feelings, as they are, in a nonreactive manner [1]. They are psychological interventions frequently practiced by menopausal women which also include yoga together with these mind-based practices [1, 22]. These interventions are thought to act via stress reduction and are safe without any serious adverse effects [2]. Studies have observed the effects of mindfulness-based interventions on vasomotor symptoms, mood disturbances and sleep quality, and have some have found beneficial effects on each of these menopause-related problems [1, 2]. A systematic review and meta-analysis of 13 studies in 1138 postmenopausal women found that mindfulness-based interventions caused a significant reduction in stress but had no significant improvement in anxiety and depression [22]. As at present there is no conclusive evidence that MBI can be recommended for the management of menopausal symptoms [1, 2].

25.5 Other Techniques

25.5.1 Biofeedback and Relaxation Techniques

These approaches use a variety of relaxation techniques including progressive muscle relaxation, audiotape relaxation as well as respiratory techniques such as paced respiration. The participants receive feedback from bodily physiological parameters such as skin temperature, heart-rate and muscle tension using sensors placed on the body, so that these could be used as indicators of controlling the stress response [2]. There are many small studies and a few RCTs comparing the different biofeedback and relaxation techniques, with some showing positive effects on menopausal symptoms. However the study designs are heterogeneous, the studies are limited and there is inconsistent evidence to recommend the use of relaxation techniques including paced respiration for the management of vasomotor symptoms [1, 2].

25.5.2 Aromatherapy

Aromatic oil from various herbs such as lavender are used in the treatment of many diseases, and are thought to act via relieving anxiety and stress reduction while promoting relaxation of the body [2]. A few trials studying the effects of aromatherapy have found beneficial effects on relieving vasomotor symptoms, but the this low-risk techniques still does not have adequate evidence to be recommended as a treatment method for alleviating menopausal symptoms [2].

25.5.3 Reflexology

This is a technique aimed at massaging specific sites on the hands and feet thought to be reflex points corresponding to certain of body organs which are relieved by diseases when stimulated by the massage [2]. As there are only a few RCTs with inconclusive findings, reflexology cannot be recommended for managing menopausal symptoms [2].

25.5.4 Homeopathy

Homeopathy is practiced by millions of patients for a range of diseases. Specific herbal preparation such as sepia, lachesis, and pulsatilla are administered to patients requiring a "cure". There are insufficient studies to recommend homeopathy as a treatment modality for menopausal symptoms [2].

25.5.5 Acupuncture

Acupuncture, a traditional Chinese technique where small needles are inserted into skin at certain "acupoints", is used for treating a variety of bodily dysfunctions [2]. A newer modification is électroacupunture, where small electrical currents are passed between acupuncture needles. There are few studies to show that vasomotor symptoms, somatic symptoms, mood and sleep show beneficial effects with acupuncture, but as their results are inconsistent acupuncture cannot be recommended for menopausal symptoms without further evidence [2, 5].

25.6 Pharmacotherapy

Nonhormonal pharmacotherapy is emerging as a promising means of alleviating menopausal symptoms. Among the many medications available United states Food and Drug Administration (FDA) has approved only two medications; paroxetine mesylate 7.5 mg daily and fezolinetant 45 mg daily for the relief of vasomotor symptoms [1]. Medications such as selective serotonin reuptake inhibitors (SSRIs), serotonin-norepinephrine reuptake inhibitors (SNRIs), gabapentin, and oxybutynin, have level I or level II evidence from RCTs to support their use for the management of VMS in menopausal women [1].

25.6.1 Selective Serotonin Reuptake Inhibitors (SSRI)/Serotonin-Norepinephrine Reuptake Inhibitors (SNRI)

SSRIs and SNRIs are both recommended for the use alleviation of vasomotor symptoms [1]. A systematic review and meta-analysis of 11 RCTs with 2069 menopausal women revealed a significant reduction in the frequency and severity of hot flashes without an increase in adverse effects with SSRI compared to the placebo [23]. It was also noted that the efficacy of escitalopram was greater than other SSRIs [23]. A recent systematic review of 36 clinical trials including 7347 menopausal women, both SSRI (escitalopram, paroxetine, and fluoxetine) and SNRI (venlafaxine and desvenlafaxine) revealed a significant efficacy in the alleviation of vasomotor symptoms. However, there were insufficient and inconsistent study findings to show effectiveness of sertraline, citalopram, fluvoxamine, and duloxetine for the management of vasomotor symptoms [24]. Several meta-analyses, a Cochrane review, a pooled review and a review of cancer survivors all show the beneficial effects of SSRIs and SNRIs on improving vasomotor symptoms [1]. Low-dose paroxetine 7.5 mg/day was the first nonhormonal prescription medicine approved by FDA for the treatment of moderate to severe vasomotor symptoms with concomitant improvement in sleep and without significant negative effects on libido or weight gain [1].

SSRIs and SNRIs are contraindicated in menopausal women with history of neuroleptic malignant syndrome, serotonin syndrome, and those on monoamine oxidase inhibitors [1]. They should be used with caution in women with uncontrolled seizures, bipolar disorder, renal or hepatic disorders, uncontrolled hypernatremia, poorly controlled hypertension, and those on other SSRIs or SNRIs [1]. SSRIs, especially paroxetine and fluoxetine decrease tamoxifen activity by inhibition of CYP2D6 enzyme, so SSRIs with less CYP2D6 inhibition (e.g., venlafaxine, desvenlafaxine, escitalopram, or citalopram) are better for women using tamoxifen [1]. Nausea or dizziness are expected adverse effects, usually improving within 2 weeks [1].

25.6.2 Gabapentin

The antiepileptic gabapentin in daily doses ranging from 900 to 2400 mg has been found to improve the frequency and severity of vasomotor symptoms in several trials, with higher doses found to have similar efficacy to estrogen [1]. A systematic review and meta-analysis of 19 RCTs and 2 randomized crossover trials with 3519 women, analyzed the efficacy and safety of gabapentin and pregabalin for vasomotor symptoms [25]. It was revealed that gabapentin was effective in relieving vasomotor symptoms compared to controls, but less than estrogen [25]. The reported adverse effects include dizziness, impaired balance or coordination, headache and drowsiness but somnolence maybe an added benefit in women with poor sleep due to vasomotor symptoms, where a bed-time dose of gabapentin will improve both vasomotor symptoms and sleep [1].

25.6.3 Fezolinetatnt

This is a selective neurokinin-3 receptor antagonist approved by the FDA for the treatment of vasomotor symptoms [1]. A recent double-blind, placebo-controlled, phase 3 trial showed that fezolinetant in daily doses of 30–45 mg were safe, resulting in significant reduction in the frequency and severity of moderate to severe vasomotor symptoms associated with menopause [26].

25.6.4 Oxybutynin

The antimuscarinic, anticholinergic agent oxybutynin is used in the management of urinary incontinence. Few studies have shown that oxybutynin at doses ranging from 2.5 mg or 5 mg bid, up to 15 mg extended-release daily, significantly improved moderate to severe vasomotor symptoms [1, 27]. It is shown to be beneficial for both women with or without breast cancer as shown in a recent randomized, multicenter, double-blind study [27]. Its adverse effects include dry mouth, urinary retention, abdominal pain, and cognitive decline in long-term users, especially in older adults [1, 27]. The 2023 position statement of North American Menopause Society (NAMS) on nonhormonal therapies for menopausal symptoms recommends the use of oxybutynin for the management of vasomotor symptoms [1].

25.6.5 Other Medications

Pregablin is a product structurally similar to gabapentin which has shown to be beneficial in alleviating hot flushes. However, the unavailability of sufficient evidence on its efficacy, presence of adverse effects, and its potential for abuse have resulted it not being recommended for the management of menopausal symptoms [1].

Clonidine is an alpha-2 adrenergic receptor agonist which has shown some effect on improving vasomotor symptoms. However it is less efficient than SSRIs and SNRIs and has several troublesome adverse effects such as hypotension, dizziness, headache, sedation, and the risk of developing high blood pressure on sudden cessation of the medication [1]. Clonidine is not recommended for the management of vasomotor symptoms as there are more efficient medications with less side effects and the lack of recent trials showing its efficacy [1].

Other interventions such as administering suvorexant (an orexin-receptor antagonist), cannabinoids and chiropractic interventions have been studies for the management of vasomotor symptoms. However there is insufficient evidence to recommend their use for this indication [1].

25.7 Stellate Ganglion Blockade

Blockage of the sympathetic stellate ganglion by injection of local anesthetics and steroids, interferes with the transmission of nerve impulses along the cervical sympathetic chain and is used in the treatment of a variety of medical disorders [28]. A review of stellate ganglion block as an adjunctive treatment modality revealed a significant decrease in vasomotor symptoms [28]. A scoping review of 24 trials on non-pain indications for stellate ganglion blockade found similar results [29]. Multiple studies have shown the benefit of this procedure in improving the severity and frequency of vasomotor symptoms in menopausal women including women with breast cancer [1]. As stellate ganglion blockade is a procedure associated with potential risk, it could be used for alleviation of menopausal symptoms in carefully evaluated women [1].

25.8 Other Options

For vulvovaginal complaints such as dryness, dyspareunia and burning, simple non-pharmacological alternatives to estrogen such as vaginal moisturizers can be effective to rehydrate vaginal tissues. They are available as bioadhesive moisturizers, and gels and resemble the action of vaginal secretions, especially when they have similar pH and osmolality to vaginal secretions [30]. Studies reveal that laser therapy is emerging as an effective and safe technique for the management of vulvovaginal symptoms, including urinary dysfunction [30].

Key Points

- Menopause is a physiological phase in the life of a woman, and is associated with the development of unpleasant symptoms, especially vasomotor symptoms.
- The most effective treatment for menopausal symptoms is menopausal hormone therapy.
- Alternative and complementary nonhormonal treatment is sought by women who are unable or unwilling to use hormone therapy.
- A wide variety of nonhormonal treatment options are available, both traditional methods and newer techniques.
- Current evidence supports the recommendation of pharmacological options such as selective serotonin reuptake inhibitors and serotonin-norepinephrine reuptake inhibitors, gabapentin, fezolinetant and oxybutynin, cognitive behavioral therapy, clinical hypnosis, weight loss, and stellate ganglion blockade for the management of menopausal symptoms (mainly vasomotor symptoms).
- Other methods such as cooling techniques, avoiding triggers, exercise including yoga, dietary modifications and supplements, mindfulness-based intervention, relaxation techniques including paced respiration, acupuncture, and pharmacological treatment such as clonidine and pregabalin are not recommended due to insufficient evidence.
- Awareness of the current recommendations, indications, risks and benefits of nonhormonal therapies for menopausal symptoms will enable healthcare workers to deliver optimal care for menopausal women.

References

1. Advisory Panel. The 2023 nonhormone therapy position statement of The North American Menopause Society. Menopause. 2023;30(6):573–90. https://doi.org/10.1097/gme.0000000000002200.
2. Johnson A, Roberts L, Elkins G. Complementary and alternative medicine for menopause. J Evid Based Integr Med. 2019;24:2515690X19829380. https://doi.org/10.1177/2515690X19829380.
3. Bair YA, Gold EB, Zhang G, Rasor N, Utts J, Upchurch DM, et al. Use of complementary and alternative medicine during the menopause transition: longitudinal results from the Study of Women's Health Across the Nation: longitudinal results from the Study of Women's Health Across the Nation. Menopause. 2008;15(1):32–43. https://doi.org/10.1097/gme.0b013e31813429d6.
4. Peng W, Adams J, Hickman L, Sibbritt DW. Longitudinal analysis of associations between women's consultations with complementary and alternative medicine practitioners/use of self-prescribed complementary and alternative medicine and menopause-related symptoms, 2007-2010. Menopause. 2016;23(1):74–80. https://doi.org/10.1097/GME.0000000000000479.
5. Alternatives to HRT for the management of symptoms of the menopause. Org.uk. [cited 2023 Aug 1]. https://www.rcog.org.uk/media/gwbntgdu/sip_6.pdf.
6. Chen M-N, Lin C-C, Liu C-F. Efficacy of phytoestrogens for menopausal symptoms: a meta-analysis and systematic review. Climacteric. 2015;18(2):260–9. https://doi.org/10.3109/13697137.2014.966241.
7. Glisic M, Kastrati N, Musa J, Milic J, Asllanaj E, Portilla Fernandez E, et al. Phytoestrogen supplementation and body composition in postmenopausal women: a systematic review and meta-analysis of randomized controlled trials. Maturitas. 2018;115:74–83. https://doi.org/10.1016/j.maturitas.2018.06.012.
8. Leach MJ, Moore V. Black cohosh (Cimicifuga spp.) for menopausal symptoms. Cochrane Database Syst Rev. 2012:(9):CD007244. https://doi.org/10.1002/14651858.CD007244.pub2.
9. Cano A, editor. Menopause. Cham: Springer International Publishing; 2017.
10. Nguyen TM, Do TTT, Tran TN, Kim JH. Exercise and quality of life in women with menopausal symptoms: a systematic review and meta-analysis of randomized controlled trials. Int J Environ Res Public Health. 2020;17(19):7049. https://doi.org/10.3390/ijerph17197049.
11. Liu T, Chen S, Mielke GI, McCarthy AL, Bailey TG. Effects of exercise on vasomotor symptoms in menopausal women: a systematic review and meta-analysis. Climacteric. 2022;25(6):552–61. https://doi.org/10.1080/13697137.2022.2097865.
12. Qian J, Sun S, Wang M, Sun Y, Sun X, Jevitt C, et al. The effect of exercise intervention on improving sleep in menopausal women: a systematic review and meta-analysis. Front Med (Lausanne). 2023;10:1092294. https://doi.org/10.3389/fmed.2023.1092294.
13. Cramer H, Peng W, Lauche R. Yoga for menopausal symptoms—a systematic review and meta-analysis. Maturitas. 2018;109:13–25. https://doi.org/10.1016/j.maturitas.2017.12.005.
14. Cramer H, Lauche R, Langhorst J, Dobos G. Effectiveness of yoga for menopausal symptoms: a systematic review and meta-analysis of randomized controlled trials. Evid Based Complement Alternat Med. 2012;2012:863905. https://doi.org/10.1155/2012/863905.
15. Ranjan P, Chopra S, Sharma KA, Malhotra A, Vikram N, Kumari A. Weight management module for perimenopausal women: a practical guide for gynecologists. J Midlife Health. 2019;10(4):165. https://doi.org/10.4103/jmh.jmh_155_19.
16. Fenton A. Weight, shape, and body composition changes at menopause. J Midlife Health. 2021;12(3):187. https://doi.org/10.4103/jmh.jmh_123_21.
17. van Driel CM, Stuursma A, Schroevers MJ, Mourits MJ, de Bock GH. Mindfulness, cognitive behavioural and behaviour-based therapy for natural and treatment-induced menopausal symptoms: a systematic review and meta-analysis. BJOG. 2019;126(3):330–9. https://doi.org/10.1111/1471-0528.15153.

18. Hunter MS. Cognitive behavioral therapy for menopausal symptoms. Climacteric. 2021;24(1):51–6. https://doi.org/10.1080/13697137.2020.1777965.
19. Ye M, Shou M, Zhang J, Hu B, Liu C, Bi C, et al. Efficacy of cognitive therapy and behavior therapy for menopausal symptoms: a systematic review and meta-analysis. Psychol Med. 2022;52(3):433–45. https://doi.org/10.1017/s0033291721005407.
20. Sarri G, Davies M, Lumsden MA, on behalf of the Guideline Development Group. Diagnosis and management of menopause: summary of NICE guidance. BMJ. 2015;351:h5746. https://doi.org/10.1136/bmj.h5746.
21. Elkins GR, Fisher WI, Johnson AK, Carpenter JS, Keith TZ. Clinical hypnosis in the treatment of postmenopausal hot flashes: a randomized controlled trial. Menopause. 2013;20(3):291–8. https://doi.org/10.1097/gme.0b013e31826ce3ed.
22. Liu H, Cai K, Wang J, Zhang H. The effects of mindfulness-based interventions on anxiety, depression, stress, and mindfulness in menopausal women: a systematic review and meta-analysis. Front Public Health. 2022;10:1045642. https://doi.org/10.3389/fpubh.2022.1045642.
23. Shams T, Firwana B, Habib F, Alshahrani A, AlNouh B, Murad MH, et al. SSRIs for hot flashes: a systematic review and meta-analysis of randomized trials. J Gen Intern Med. 2014;29(1):204–13. https://doi.org/10.1007/s11606-013-2535-9.
24. Azizi M, Khani S, Kamali M, Elyasi F. The efficacy and safety of selective serotonin reuptake inhibitors and serotonin-norepinephrine reuptake inhibitors in the treatment of menopausal hot flashes: a systematic review of clinical trials. Iran J Med Sci. 2022;47(3):173–93. https://ijms.sums.ac.ir/article_47540.html
25. Shan D, Zou L, Liu X, Shen Y, Cai Y, Zhang J. Efficacy and safety of gabapentin and pregabalin in patients with vasomotor symptoms: a systematic review and meta-analysis. Am J Obstet Gynecol. 2020;222(6):564–579.e12. https://doi.org/10.1016/j.ajog.2019.12.011.
26. Johnson KA, Martin N, Nappi RE, Neal-Perry G, Shapiro M, Stute P, et al. Efficacy and safety of fezolinetant in moderate to severe vasomotor symptoms associated with menopause: a phase 3 RCT. J Clin Endocrinol Metab. 2023;108(8):1981–97. https://doi.org/10.1210/clinem/dgad058.
27. Leon-Ferre RA, Novotny PJ, Wolfe EG, Faubion SS, Ruddy KJ, Flora D, et al. Oxybutynin vs placebo for hot flashes in women with or without breast cancer: a randomized, double-blind clinical trial (ACCRU SC-1603). JNCI Cancer Spectr. 2020;4(1) https://doi.org/10.1093/jncics/pkz088.
28. Kirkpatrick K, Khan MH, Deng Y, Shah KB. A review of stellate ganglion block as an adjunctive treatment modality. Cureus. 2023; https://doi.org/10.7759/cureus.35174.
29. Feigin G, Velasco Figueroa S, Englesakis MF, D'Souza R, Hoydonckx Y, Bhatia A. Stellate ganglion block for non-pain indications: a scoping review. Pain Med. 2023;24(7):775–81. https://doi.org/10.1093/pm/pnad011.
30. Hamoda H, Panay N, Pedder H, Arya R, Savvas M. The British Menopause Society & Women's Health Concern 2020 recommendations on hormone replacement therapy in menopausal women. Post Reprod Health. 2020;26(4):181–209. https://doi.org/10.1177/2053369120957514.

Prescribing Menopausal Hormone Therapy

26

Asna Beg Ashraf

26.1 Introduction

Menopause is a state of permanent cessation of menses due to the loss of ovarian function. It can occur spontaneously as a consequence of the depletion of ovarian follicles due to ageing (natural menopause) or, can be induced by bilateral oophorectomy, or cancer treatments (chemotherapy, radiotherapy or endocrine therapy). Menopause is said to have occurred when 12 months have passed since the last menses. Perimenopause also known as menopause transition is the phase immediately before menopause, and begins with the onset of menstrual irregularity, and continues for 12 months after the final menstrual period [1]. The mean age of natural menopause is considered to be 51 years and the majority of women enter menopause between 45 and 55 years, but there can be ethnic variations. In Indian women, menopause occurs at an estimated mean age of 46 years [2]. Menopause is referred to as "early" if it occurs between 40 and 45 years. Primary ovarian insufficiency (POI) or premature menopause is said to occur when menses ends before the age of 40 years.

At birth, a female new-born has about 300,000 ovarian follicles. By age 37 ovarian follicles decline to about 25,000, and finally, at menopause, only a few follicles remain in the ovaries [1]. Depletion of follicles is associated with decreased production of the ovarian hormones estradiol (E2) and inhibin B, and increased production of follicle-stimulating hormone (FSH) from the pituitary gland. There is also a resultant fall in the production of anti-müllerian hormone (AMH) [1]. The deficiency of estrogen can have significant short- and long-term effects and women usually experience a unique set of symptoms, both in perimenopause and menopause. Clinical manifestations include vasomotor symptoms (VMS) (including hot flushes, night sweats and sleep disturbances), genitourinary symptoms, mood swings, and depression. Many chronic diseases such as hypertension, diabetes

A. B. Ashraf (✉)
Ujala Medical Center, Indiranagar, Lucknow, Uttar Pradesh, India

R. Garg (ed.), *Management of Menopause*,
https://doi.org/10.1007/978-981-96-0239-1_26

mellitus, coronary artery disease, and osteoporosis are also associated with menopause and may affect the quality of life.

The occurrence and severity of menopausal symptoms ranges from mild to no symptoms in some women, to debilitating symptoms continuing for several years, and impacting the quality of life in others. Menopausal hormone therapy (MHT) earlier known as hormone replacement therapy (HRT) can be prescribed during or after the menopause transition to alleviate the symptoms associated with menopause and improve a woman's quality of life. MHT is a broad term that covers a range of hormonal treatments and includes various types and combinations of estrogen and progesterone, estrogen + selective estrogen receptor modulator (Bazedoxifene) and Tibolone. Estrogen alone therapy is referred to as ET, combined estrogen-progestogen therapy as EPT, and the broader term hormone therapy (HT) is also sometimes used.

26.2 Controversy Surrounding MHT

The Women's Health Initiative (WHI) was a set of two trials (ET alone, and continuous combined EPT versus placebo) in about 27,000 postmenopausal women (average age 63 years), that studied the effect of hormone therapy on healthy women with special focus on cardiovascular disease outcomes. Preliminary analysis of WHI data (2002) reported an excess risk of coronary heart disease (CHD), venous thromboembolism (VTE), stroke and breast cancer with HT [3]. In 2003 the combined arm of the study was shutdown. Results from the WHI trials were contrary to the earlier belief that HT was protective for the heart. They reported an unfavorable balance of risks compared with benefits, in older postmenopausal women, but did not focus on the effect of HT in symptomatic younger postmenopausal women. The benefits of HT if given in the "window of opportunity", before ageing has set in, were not addressed. The reanalysis of the WHI study (2007) provided critical insights into the timing and safety of HT. The findings suggested that prescribing HT to women who are within 10 years of menopause was associated with fewer risks, and a decrease in cardiovascular events [4]. However, the damage had already been done, and it led to a paradigm shift in menopause management. The fear generated by the early WHI results led to a significant reduction in HT prescriptions. Even after the reanalysis many clinicians remain hesitant to prescribe HT, leaving menopausal women to suffer devastating symptoms without recourse.

26.3 Effects of MHT

Our knowledge of MHT has evolved over the last few decades leading to a better understanding of its beneficial effects, risks and side-effects profile. Choosing the right MHT is important because benefits and risks can vary depending on the type of formulation, dose of constituents, routes of administration, the stage at which therapy is initiated in the woman's lifespan, treatment duration, and co-prescription of progestogen. Taking stock of the available evidence the treatment should be individualized to augment the benefits and minimize the risks [5]. The potential benefits of MHT are many but all of them are not indications for initiating therapy.

- **Relief from vasomotor symptoms**: The chief indication for MHT is the relief of moderate to severe VMS estimated to occur in about 75% of women in perimenopause and menopause. A quarter of these women may have severe symptoms which may last up to 7 years or more, and one-third may experience long-term symptoms that may persist for up to 15 years [6]. Studies have proven that MHT remains the most effective treatment for alleviating VMS. By restoring hormone levels, MHT can significantly reduce hot flushes, night sweats, and sleep disturbances, improve overall well-being and quality of life [7].
- **Prevention and treatment of osteoporosis**: Estrogen plays a crucial role in preserving bone mineral density (BMD) and averting bone loss in women. During menopause, the fall in estrogen levels contributes to accelerated bone loss. ET has been shown to reduce the rate of bone loss and improve BMD, thus lowering the risk of osteoporosis and fractures in postmenopausal women [7]. MHT reduces the risk of all fractures and can be used for prevention of bone loss and osteoporosis in postmenopausal women [8].
- **Improved genitourinary health and sexual function**: The fall in estrogen can cause vaginal symptoms (dryness, burning, and irritation), urinary symptoms (urgency, dysuria, and recurrent urinary tract infections), and sexual symptoms (dyspareunia and impaired sexual function) that constitute a chronic progressive condition called the genitourinary syndrome of menopause (GSM) [9]. Local estrogen therapy can safely and effectively alleviate vaginal dryness and improve lubrication without the risks associated with systemic therapy [10]. In women with overactive bladder, local ET improves symptoms of frequency, nocturia, urgency, incontinent episodes, and bladder capacity [11]. Systemic ET relieves vaginal symptoms of GSM, and also positively impacts sexual function (including reduced libido) and quality of life [12].
- **Potential cardiovascular benefits in younger women**: The cardiovascular effects of MHT can vary depending on factors such as age, timing, and type of hormones used. MHT started at a younger age, i.e., before 60 years, or within 10 years of menopause, is associated with a limiting of atherosclerosis progression, beneficial effects on lipid profile, reduced risk of CHD, death from cardiovascular causes, and all-cause mortality [4, 13]. Thus, MHT may be cardioprotective, if started at the right time. This is known as the "timing hypothesis" or the concept of "window of opportunity" in a healthy woman [2, 14]. MHT is not currently approved for this indication.
- **Protection against colon cancer**: MHT has been linked to a reduced risk of colorectal cancer (CRC) and this benefit is predominantly seen for tumors arising through the adenoma-carcinoma pathway, distal colon and rectal tumors [15]. Research is still on, but initial data suggests that conjugated equine estrogen (CEE) + medroxyprogesterone acetate (MPA) therapy reduces the risk of colon cancer, while CEE alone does not [7].

- **Cognitive function**: Oral ET may have a beneficial effect on certain cognitive functions, and improve mood in recently postmenopausal women [16]. When MHT is initiated early or closer to the onset of menopause, it may have potential cognitive benefits, but MHT started later in postmenopause may not provide the same benefits or may even have detrimental effects [17, 18]. Women who had a surgical menopause are more likely to get cognitive benefits from MHT. Further research is needed to establish conclusive evidence [18].
- **Type 2 diabetes mellitus**: MHT may have a role in preventing or delaying the onset of type 2 diabetes, however, it is not currently approved for this indication. Both oral and transdermal estrogen reduce blood glucose and improve insulin sensitivity, but oral ET has a stronger effect [8].
- **Other possible benefits**: MHT may help decrease abdominal adipose tissue and weight gain associated with menopause transition, and thus help prevent metabolic syndrome [2]. Beneficial effects also include improvement of dry eye syndrome and preservation of collagen in the skin.

MHT also carries potential risks and side effects that need to be carefully considered.

- **Increased risk of breast cancer**: The connection between MHT and breast cancer has been controversial. A 2019 meta-analysis concluded that for a woman of average weight, MHT intake for 5 years beginning at 50 years would increase the 20-year probability of breast cancer as follows for different formulations [19]:
- Continuous combined EPT—1 extra case in 50 women.
- Sequential combined EPT—1 extra case in 70 women.
- ET alone—1 extra case in 200 women.
- For continuous combined EPT from a baseline risk of 3/50 in women not taking HT to 4/50 (1 extra case in 50 women), for sequential combined EPT from 4/70 in women not on HT to 5/70 (1 extra case in 70 women), and for ET alone, from 13/200 women to 14/200 (1 extra case in 200 women). There is either no increase, or a very small added risk of breast cancer when using estrogen only MHT in hysterectomized women. Long-term use of EPT has been linked to a small increase in the absolute risk of breast cancer. However, the overall benefits of MHT may outweigh the risks for many women. In this analysis majority of the women were using CEE and MPA [6, 19]. Regimens being used currently have lower doses of estrogen as well as different types and routes (transdermal 17-B estradiol) combined with natural progesterones, which are considered safer. Estrogen and micronized progesterone combination does not increase breast cancer risk for up to 5 years of use [2, 20].
- **Venous thromboembolism**: Oral ET (but not transdermal), is associated with a small increase in the risk of VTE including deep vein thrombosis (DVT) and pulmonary embolism (PE). The risk is greater in the first year of use [21, 22]. Women with a history of VTE or known thrombophilic conditions may be at higher risk, and should be evaluated carefully before initiating MHT. Alternative

routes of administration, such as transdermal gels or sprays, may be considered for high-risk women.

- **Stroke and coronary heart disease**: The use of EPT has been linked to a slightly increased risk of stroke and CHD, especially in older women. The risks may vary depending on the age, comorbidities, type of hormone used, the route of administration, and the timing of initiation [23]. MHT is considered safe for most women in their 50 s or for the first 10 years after the onset of menopause [8].
- **Endometrial cancer**: ET alone if given in women with a uterus increases the risk of endometrial cancer, which can be mitigated by adding progestogen [8].
- **Gallbladder disease**: Oral estrogen, has been associated with an increased risk of gallstones, cholecystitis, and cholecystectomy [2].
- **Effect on cognition**: Results of the WHI Memory Study (WHIMS) indicated that combination therapy (CEE + MPA) was associated with double the risk of dementia in women aged 65 and older, compared to women assigned placebo [23]. The Women's Health Initiative Memory Study of Younger Women (WHIMSY) found that in younger women (50–54 years) CEE with or without MPA had neutral effects on cognition after about 7 years of follow-up [24].
- **Other side effects**: may include bloating, breast tenderness, headache, nausea, mood changes, and vaginal bleeding. The side effects are temporary and, may resolve with time or with adjustments to the hormone regimen.

The benefit-risk ratio is favorable for the treatment of bothersome VMS and prevention of bone loss for most women in their 50 s, or who are within 10 years of onset of menopause and have no contraindications. If HT is initiated later than 10 years from menopause onset or in women older than 60, the benefit-risk ratio is discouraging because of the higher absolute risks of deleterious consequences like CHD, stroke, VTE, and dementia [5].

26.4 Current Guidelines and Recommendations of World Organizations

Various international and national organizations have published comprehensive clinical practice guidelines on the use of MHT. These include The Menopause Society formerly known as North American Menopause Society (NAMS), the International Menopause Society, the Endocrine Society, British Menopause Society, and the Indian Menopause Society. A few of them are briefly summarized here.

26.4.1 The 2022 Hormone Therapy Position Statement of the North American Menopause Society (NAMS) [5]

- MHT is a highly efficacious treatment for VMS and GSM and also protects against bone loss and fracture. Risks of MHT vary based on the dose, duration, type, route, timing of initiation, and use of progestogen. Treatment decisions should be taken after careful consideration of age, menopause stage, symptoms, risk factors, and individual preferences, thus aiming to minimize the risks and maximize the benefits of the therapy.

- Initiating MHT in women <60 years or within 10 years of menopause gives greater benefits and fewer risks. In women more than 10 years from menopause onset, or older than 60 years, the benefit-risk ratio is much less favorable with higher risks of CHD, VTE, stroke, and dementia.
- The duration of MHT should be individualized. If MHT is considered for a longer duration for persistent VMS, it should involve shared decision-making between the woman and her healthcare provider, with periodic re-evaluation and weighing the benefits and risks of continuing therapy.
- Women who do not have an indication for systemic HT but have troublesome GSM symptoms should be treated with low-dose local vaginal estrogen therapy or other therapies (e.g., oral ospemifene or vaginal DHEA).

26.4.2 The International Menopause Society (IMS) 2016 [7]

- MHT is the most efficacious treatment for vasomotor symptoms and urogenital atrophy. Joint and muscle pain, sleep disturbances, mood swings, sexual dysfunction, and quality of life may also improve on MHT.
- MHT should be a component of a comprehensive lifestyle approach including diet, exercise, and smoking cessation to conserve the health of peri- and postmenopausal women.
- MHT should be tailored to suit the woman's symptoms, medical history, investigations, expectations, and choices.
- Use of the term "class effect" for MHT is not appropriate because it includes many different hormonal products.
- Women who had POI or spontaneous or iatrogenic menopause before 45 years (early), should be advised MHT till at least the natural age of menopause to reduce the risk of CHD, osteoporosis, and dementia.
- Comprehensive counselling about the benefits and risks of MHT in simple language should be done to allow the woman to make an informed decision.
- MHT is not to be prescribed without a clear indication. An annual follow-up for women on MHT should include a physical examination, medical and family history, relevant investigations, and guidance on lifestyle and ways to prevent chronic diseases.
- MHT should not be stopped only because of age. Data supports safe use for 5 years in healthy postmenopausal women who start therapy before 60 years. Further continuation of therapy should be a shared decision between the woman and health professional based on individual factors. The dose should be the lowest effective dose.

26.4.3 Endocrine Society Guidelines 2015 [25]

- MHT is the most effective therapy for vasomotor and other symptoms related to menopause.
- For many symptomatic postmenopausal women who are <60 years or within 10 years of entering menopause, the benefits of MHT may exceed the risks.
- MHT should be individualized according to clinical factors and patient preferences. All women should be screened for cardiovascular and breast cancer risk factors prior to initiating MHT.
- Current evidence does not support the use of MHT for the primary prevention of CHD or dementia. MHT is contraindicated in breast cancer patients and other nonhormonal options for those with VMS should be considered.
- Treatment of GSM is low-dose vaginal estrogen and ospemifene. For those choosing not to use hormone therapy, vaginal moisturizers and lubricants are available.
- Lifestyle measures should be a part of the advice given to all postmenopausal women.

26.5 Formulations of MHT

26.5.1 Estrogen Therapy

The various types of estrogen can be categorized as follows:

- Human estrogens—17beta-estradiol (E2), estrone (E1), and estriol (E3).
- Animal-derived—conjugated equine estrogen (CEE).
- Synthetic—ethinyl estradiol (EE).

The human estrogen *17B-estradiol* or E2 is the primary estrogen produced by the ovaries and is biologically the most active. It is the only FDA-approved formulation [8]. *Estradiol hemihydrate* is the micronized form of E2 which is structurally identical to estradiol. *Estradiol valerate* is an estradiol ester or a prodrug. Most oral estrogens are derived from plant sources except CEE which is comprised of a mixture of estrogens derived from the urine of pregnant mares [8]. The synthetic estrogen *ethinyl estradiol* is used in combined oral contraceptive pills (OCP) and is more potent than natural estrogens.

26.5.1.1 Routes of Administration

The absorption of estrogens through the gastrointestinal (GI) tract, mucus membranes, and skin is good. The route of administration can be oral, vaginal (creams, tablets and rings), and transdermal (patches, spray, and gels). Women seeking treatment for VMS require systemic estrogen (oral or transdermal), while low-dose vaginal estrogens are sufficient for those with only symptoms of GSM [8]. Low oral doses sometimes may not be sufficient to relieve GSM symptoms and supplemental low-dose vaginal estrogen may be needed.

26.5.1.2 Oral Estrogen Therapy

Oral estrogen therapy in the most widely used formulation. When estrogen is administered orally it undergoes hepatic metabolism, the "first-pass effect," thereby increasing hepatic production of triglycerides, HDL cholesterol, sex hormone-binding globulin (SHBG), and coagulation factors. Hence, there is a potential elevated risk of VTE, and gallstones [8]. The different estrogen formulations along with their various doses are as follows [8, 25].

- 17 ß-estradiol (oral)—0.5 mg/1 mg/2 mg
- Estradiol valerate (oral)—1 mg/2 mg/4 mg
- Estradiol hemihydrate (oral)—0.5 mg/1 mg/2 mg/4 mg
- CEE (oral)—0.3 mg/0.45 mg/0.65 mg/1.25 mg

26.5.1.3 Transdermal and Topical Estrogens

When given by the transdermal route estrogen circulates systemically before reaching the liver so the first-pass metabolism in the liver is avoided, and lower doses of the drug are effective. The overproduction of triglycerides and coagulation factors is averted, hence it is associated with a lower risk of VTE and stroke [8]. Transdermal estrogen is as effective as oral ET for preserving bone density, therefore it is considered as the first choice in women with risk factors. It is preferable in women with obesity, hypertension, diabetes, hypertriglyceridemia, VTE risk, metabolic syndrome, or history of GB disease. The only absolute contraindications are estrogen-dependent gynecological malignancies [25].

The different transdermal estrogen formulations along with their various doses are listed here. There can be regional variations in the availability of different compositions [8, 25, 26].

- 17ß-estradiol patch (transdermal)—25 mcg/37.5 mcg/50 mcg/75 mcg/100 mcg
- Estradiol hemihydrate gel (transdermal)—0.5 mg/1 mg/1.5/2 mg.
- 17ß-estradiol gel 0.06% w/w (transdermal)—0.375 mg/0.75 mg/1.5 mg/3 mg
- Estradiol hemihydrate spray (EMDTS) (transdermal)—1.53 mg/spray.

Estradiol metered-dose transdermal spray (EMDTS) is the latest application method. Dosage is individualized as per symptoms—1/2/3 sprays of 1.53 mg each, per day are given on the inner aspect of the forearm or thigh. Maximum concentration is reached 18–20 h after use, and by 1 week of application a stable level is reached. Transdermal estrogen spray combines the advantages of safety of transdermal route with the prospect of precise dosing [26].

26.5.1.4 Vaginal Estrogen Therapy

Estrogens are used in very low doses locally in the vagina as creams, tablets, gels, pessaries, and vaginal rings for the management of symptoms of GSM. They do not increase the serum estrogen levels above the normal range for postmenopausal women ($\leq$20 pg/ml) and are not associated with any systemic effects. There is no risk of endometrial hyperplasia and progestogen is not required [6, 7, 8].

Vaginal tablets and creams are to be used every night for 2 weeks (3 weeks for pessary and gel) followed by twice weekly administration. The maintenance doses given twice weekly can be continued long-term to relieve symptoms. Symptoms of GSM frequently recur on stopping the therapy. The different vaginal estrogen formulations with doses are as follows [8, 25]:

- Conjugated estrogen cream—0.625 mg/g
- Estriol vaginal cream—0.1%/0.01%
- Estriol vaginal gel—50 mcg/g
- Estriol vaginal pessary—0.03 mg
- Estradiol vaginal tablets—10 mcg
- Estradiol vaginal ring—7.5 mcg

26.5.2 Progestogen Therapy

Unopposed systemic estrogen therapy can cause endometrial hyperplasia and cancer therefore progestogens should be given with estrogen in all women who have an intact uterus. Progestogens decrease estrogen receptors in target tissues, and inhibit the luteinizing hormone surge that results in increased estrogen production from ovaries, thus protecting against endometrial thickening [8]. Progestogens increase 17ß-hydroxysteroid dehydrogenase activity, which converts estradiol to estrone in the endometrium. Estrone has a weaker estrogen activity and results in less endometrial stimulation [8].

26.5.2.1 Oral Progestogens

Synthetic progestogens medroxyprogesterone acetate (MPA), norethindrone, and norethisterone acetate (NETA) had commonly been prescribed as part of MHT, until recently and have 10- to 100-fold greater activity compared to natural progestogens [8]. They are testosterone-derivatives and stimulate the androgen receptors causing side effects like acne and hirsutism [6]. They are effective for endometrial protection but negate the advantageous effects of estrogen on lipids, and increase the risk of CVD and breast cancer.

Dydrogesterone is also a synthetic progesterone but is metabolically neutral and has less effect on breast tissue.

Micronized progesterone (MP) is a natural progestogen and is more selective for progesterone receptors. It has less effect on androgenic and mineralocorticoid receptors resulting in less side effects. It is associated with a lesser risk of MHT-associated breast cancer than synthetic progestogens [6]. Micronized progesterone is bioidentical to the hormone produced in the body and has good oral absorption. Vaginal administration is also possible [8].

The different oral progestogen formulations along with their doses are as follows [25]:

- Dydrogesterone—2.5, 5, 10 mg/day.

- Micronized progesterone—100, 200 mg/day.
- MPA—2.5, 5, 10 mg/day.
- Norethindrone—0.35 mg/day.
- NETA—5 mg/day.
- Megestrol acetate—20–40 mg/day.

26.5.2.2 Levonorgestrel Intrauterine System (LNG-IUS)

The 52 mg levonorgestrel-releasing intrauterine system (LNG-IUS) creates a very high intrauterine but low systemic concentrations of levonorgestrel, resulting in an atrophic endometrium in almost all women [6]. It releases 20 mcg/24 h of levonorgestrel and is effective for 5 years. It is a good alternative for women who are unable to tolerate oral progestogens, and is especially useful in perimenopausal women who need contraception. It is also an important treatment modality for heavy menstrual bleeding (HMB) besides being used for endometrial protection in MHT.

26.5.2.3 Progestogenic Side Effects

An important reason for reduced compliance with HT is progestogenic side effects. Different progestogens have different side-effect profiles. If there is a problem with one oral progesterone, change to another. Reducing progesterone from 14 to 10 days/month can also be considered. Continuous progesterone therapy allows for a lower dosage to be given, and there are no cyclical fluctuations, resulting in less side effects. If oral progesterone is not tolerated well, switch to the vaginal or intrauterine route.

26.5.3 Combination Hormone Therapies

Fixed-dose oral combined EPT is a reasonable option for most women with an intact uterus due to its convenience of use, but it should be carefully chosen after consideration of both the components. The Postmenopausal Estrogen/Progestin Interventions (PEPIs) trial concluded that women with an intact uterus had a 34% increased risk of endometrial hyperplasia if they were given ET alone, whereas the risk reduced to 1% on combined therapy [27].

Combined oral formulations can be administered in two regimens—sequential and continuous [8, 25]. In sequential combined EPT estrogen is given daily with progestogen added cyclically for 12–14 days per month followed by withdrawal bleeding every month. In continuous combined EPT estrogen and progestogen are administered daily continuously and regular withdrawal bleeding is avoided [8]. A combined (E + P) transdermal patch is also an option.

The various combined (EPT) formulations along with their doses are as follows [8, 25]:

- Sequential combined EPT
  Oral
    17ß-estradiol 1 mg daily + Dydrogesterone 10 mg (last 14 days)

17ß-estradiol 2 mg daily + Dydrogesterone 10 mg (last 14 days)
CEE 0.625 mg daily + MPA 5 mg (last 14 days)

- Continuous combined EPT
  Oral
  17ß-estradiol 1 mg daily + Dydrogesterone 2.5–5 mg daily
  17ß-estradiol 1 mg daily + MP 100 mg daily
  CEE 0.625 mg daily + MPA 2.5–5 mg daily
  Transdermal
  17ß-estradiol 0.05 mg/day + NETA 0.14–0.25 mg/day—patch applied twice weekly
  17ß-estradiol 0.045 mg/day + LNG 0.15 mg/day—patch applied once a week

If there are problems with symptom control, or side effects develop, then the MHT should be broken down into its components—estrogen and progesterone, and the doses should be selected separately.

26.5.4 Tissue Selective Estrogen Complex (TSEC)

Tissue selective estrogen complex combines 20 mg Bazedoxifene, a selective estrogen-receptor modulator (SERM) with 0.45 mg of CEE. It is used in postmenopausal women with an intact uterus to treat moderate to severe VMS. It can also be prescribed for the prevention of osteoporosis. Bazedoxifene works as an estrogen receptor agonist in bone and an antagonist in the endometrium. TSEC prevents bone loss without increasing breast density, endometrial thickness, or risk of coronary artery disease, stroke, or VTE. Thus TSEC has an advantage over other formulations and can be regarded as a first-line treatment for postmenopausal women with severe symptoms. It causes amenorrhea in more than 83% of users. It provides an alternative to progesterone therapy for women who cannot tolerate the side effects of progesterone [25, 28].

26.5.5 Tibolone

Tibolone is a normethyltestosterone progestogen derivative and has estrogenic, progestogenic, and androgenic effects. It is a selective tissue estrogenic activity regulator (STEAR) and alleviates VMS, improves sleep, and urogenital atrophy. Due to its weak androgenic effect it can improve mood and libido. Tibolone has an estrogenic effect on bone, prevents bone loss and osteoporotic fractures. The dose is 1.25–2.5 mg per day. It should be prescribed 1 year after amenorrhea [2, 6, 25].

26.5.6 Ospemifene

Ospemifene is an oral drug which is effective for the treatment of symptoms of GSM. It is a selective estrogen receptor modulator (SERM). It can be a good alternative to local vaginal estrogen therapy. Older women who find using a vaginal preparation technically challenging may prefer it. The dose is 60 mg daily. It is contraindicated in women undergoing active treatment for breast cancer [6].

26.6 Prescribing Considerations

26.6.1 Evaluation Required Before Initiating MHT

When a woman presents for any complaint during the menopause transition phase, this opportunity should be used to address important issues like weight management, bone health, smoking cessation, cardiovascular risk assessment, and cancer screening and prevention. A full assessment of the woman needs to be done before initiating MHT and it should include the following [1]:

History: A thorough medical, gynecological, personal, treatment, family, and social history.

Physical examination: Height, weight, BMI, waist circumference, blood pressure, complete general and systemic examination including breast and thyroid.

Investigations: CBC, TSH, lipid profile, blood sugar, HbA1C, liver function tests, renal function tests, Vit. D level, mammogram, Pap LBC + HPVDNA, BMD test and endometrial biopsy if indicated according to individual risk factors [1].

26.6.2 How and What to Prescribe?

Individualized approach: Prior to initiating MHT the age of the woman and severity of symptoms should be considered. An individual baseline risk assessment for cardiovascular (CHD, stroke, and VTE) and breast cancer risk should be done [8, 25]. The decision to start MHT, the treatment goals, choice of formulation, the starting dose, route of administration, and the duration of therapy, should be decided on an individual basis after discussing the benefits and risks with the woman, to help her make an informed choice [6, 25].

- **Perimenopausal woman**: The most appropriate option would be continuous estrogen with sequential progesterone (in the second half of the cycle). Treatment should be started from day 1 of the natural cycle so that the HT cycle can coincide with the natural cycle. If MHT is started randomly the side effect of irregular bleeding is more pronounced. Combined OCPs can also be used if they are not contraindicated. OCPs provide the added advantage of contraception and cycle regulation along with the alleviation of symptoms. In a perimenopausal woman who is already using or wants to use LNG-IUS for contraception or HMB, continuous estrogen therapy can be added [1]. After a minimum of 1 year of HT, or 1 year after the last menstrual period, women who want to avoid a monthly withdrawal bleed can be put on a continuous combined regimen which is bleed-free. This will also minimize the risk of endometrial hyperplasia. Alternatively, Tibolone can be started [6].

- **Postmenopausal with an intact uterus**: If the last menstrual period was more than a year ago, a bleed-free regimen can be used right from the beginning if HT is being started [6]. The options are either oral continuous combined E + P or transdermal estrogen with oral progesterone or LNG-IUS. A combined (E + P) transdermal patch can also be used [1]. Transdermal estrogen plus Dydrogesterone or micronized progesterone may be associated with fewer progestogenic side effects and fewer adverse effects on the breast. Transdermal/oral estrogen plus LNG-IUS is a convenient no bleeding option, for women who are unable to tolerate oral progesterone.
- **At any stage posthysterectomy**: If the woman has undergone hysterectomy the options for her are oral estrogen, transdermal estrogen or Tibolone [1]. Progestogen may need to be given with estrogen even in hysterectomized women in certain conditions like endometriosis, or rarely after supracervical hysterectomy.

26.6.3 Follow-Up and Monitoring

- The first follow-up visit at 6–8 weeks is important to review the treatment, assess symptom relief, and any side effects, or other concerns that the patient may have. If the patient has adequate symptom relief the next visit can be after 6 months. If symptom relief is not adequate or side effects are there, then the dose or therapy should be reviewed. The next visit can be at 6–12 monthly intervals [1].
- The annual follow-up for women on MHT should include a general examination, an update of medical and family history, relevant investigations, and a counselling on lifestyle measures [7]. A re-evaluation of efficacy, side effects and risks and benefits of MHT should be done.

26.6.4 Dose and Duration of Use

- The most appropriate starting dose and duration of therapy should be decided according to the severity of symptoms and response to therapy. The accepted approach is to start with lower doses and increase as needed. Lower doses are better for older women and relatively higher doses for younger women. Duration of use of up to 3–5 years is the standard recommendation (usually up to the age of 60 years). There are no arbitrary limits to the duration of treatment as long as it can be safely assumed that the benefits of symptom control outweigh any risks. HT should not be discontinued solely based upon patient age [5].
- In women in whom hot flushes recur after stopping HT, initially nonhormonal options can be tried. If symptoms persist, HT can be resumed at the lowest possible dose in carefully selected women with persistent, severe hot flashes.

26.6.5 Special Patient Groups

26.6.5.1 Premature Ovarian Insufficiency (POI)

Premature ovarian insufficiency affects about 1% of women under the age of 40 years. It is diagnosed by elevated FSH levels (>40 IU/L) on at least two occasions 4–6 weeks apart [7]. Women with spontaneous or iatrogenic premature menopause suffer from severe menopausal symptoms, including sexual dysfunction. They are also at higher risk of cardiovascular disease, osteoporosis, and cognitive impairment [7].

Hormone replacement therapy or a combined OCP is strongly recommended in POI (unless contraindicated) [7]. Effect of HT in improving bone health and cardiovascular risk may be more beneficial compared to OCPs [6]. Standard (medium or high) doses of HT should be prescribed, and the woman should be counselled about the long-term goals of therapy to reduce the risk of CHD, stroke, dementia and osteoporosis. HT has to be continued until at least the age of natural menopause with periodic re-evaluation [7].

26.6.5.2 Breast Cancer

MHT is not recommended in women with active breast cancer or history of breast cancer. Although menopausal symptoms are an important issue for breast cancer survivors, nonhormonal options are considered to be first-line therapy for these women [26]. Recommended treatments include cognitive behavioral therapy, clinical hypnosis, weight loss, stellate ganglion block, and drugs like SSRIs, SNRIs, gabapentin, fezolinetant, and oxybutynin [29].

Key Points

- MHT is till date the most efficacious treatment for vasomotor symptoms of menopause, which are common, and can have an adverse impact on a woman's life.
- MHT is considered safe for healthy, symptomatic women who are within 10 years of menopause or <60 years and who do not have any contraindications.
- EPT is indicated in women with a uterus, and ET alone in those who are posthysterectomy. For women with urogenital symptoms vaginal estrogen should be used.
- MHT is not recommended solely for the prevention of chronic diseases such as cardiovascular or bone disease.
- Various types, formulations and routes are available, therefore MHT should be tailored to suit the individual.
- ET is not associated with a change in the risk of breast cancer. EPT can be associated with a slight increase in risk, which may vary with the type of progesterone used. Natural progesterone and SERMs optimize metabolic and breast effects.

References

1. Jane FM, Davis SR. A practitioner's tool kit for managing the menopause. Climacteric. 2014;17(5):564–79. https://doi.org/10.3109/13697137.2014.929651.
2. Meeta M, Digumarti L, Agarwal N, Vaze N, Shah R, Malik S. Clinical practice guidelines on menopause: *an executive summary and recommendations: Indian Menopause Society 2019-2020. J Midlife Health. 2020;11(2):55–95. https://doi.org/10.4103/jmh.JMH_137_20.
3. Rossouw JE, Anderson GL, Prentice RL, et al. Risks and benefits of estrogen plus progestin in healthy postmenopausal women: principal results from the Women's Health Initiative randomized controlled trial. JAMA. 2002;288:321–33.
4. Rossouw JE, Prentice RL, Manson JE, Wu L, Barad D, Barnabei VM, et al. Postmenopausal hormone therapy and risk of cardiovascular disease by age and years since menopause. JAMA. 2007;297:1465–77.
5. "The 2022 Hormone Therapy Position Statement of The North American Menopause Society" Advisory Panel. The 2022 hormone therapy position statement of The North American Menopause Society. Menopause. 2022;29(7):767–94. https://doi.org/10.1097/GME.0000000000002028.
6. Hamoda H, Panay N, Pedder H, Arya R, Savvas M. The British Menopause Society & Women's Health Concern 2020 recommendations on hormone replacement therapy in menopausal women. Post Reprod Health. 2020;26(4):181–209. https://doi.org/10.1177/2053369120957514.
7. Baber RJ, Panay N, Fenton A, IMS Writing Group. 2016 IMS Recommendations on women's midlife health and menopause hormone therapy. Climacteric. 2016;19(2):109–50. https://doi.org/10.3109/13697137.2015.1129166.
8. Mehta J, Kling JM, Manson JE. Risks, benefits, and treatment modalities of menopausal hormone therapy: current concepts. Front Endocrinol (Lausanne). 2021;12:564781. https://doi.org/10.3389/fendo.2021.564781.
9. Portman DJ, Gass ML, Vulvovaginal Atrophy Terminology Consensus Conference Panel. Genitourinary syndrome of menopause: new terminology for vulvovaginal atrophy from the International Society for the Study of Women's Sexual Health and the North American Menopause Society. Menopause. 2014;21(10):1063–8. https://doi.org/10.1097/GME.0000000000000329.
10. Simon JA, Maamari RV. Ultra-low-dose vaginal estrogen tablets for the treatment of postmenopausal vaginal atrophy. Climacteric. 2013;16(Suppl. 1):37–43. https://doi.org/10.3109/13697137.2013.807606.
11. Nappi RE, Cucinella L, Martella S, Rossi M, Tiranini L, Martini E. Female sexual dysfunction (FSD): prevalence and impact on quality of life (QoL). Maturitas. 2016;94:87–91. https://doi.org/10.1016/j.maturitas.2016.09.013.
12. Cardozo L, Lose G, McClish D, Versi E. A systematic review of the effects of estrogens for symptoms suggestive of overactive bladder. Acta Obstet Gynecol Scand. 2004;83(10):892–7. https://doi.org/10.1111/j.0001-6349.2004.00581.x.
13. Boardman HM, Hartley L, Eisinga A, et al. Hormone therapy for preventing cardiovascular disease in post-menopausal women. Cochrane Database Syst Rev. 2015;3:CD002229.
14. Hodis HN, CollinsP MWJ, SchierbeckLL. The timing hypothesis for coronary heart disease prevention with hormone therapy: past, present and future in perspective. Climacteric. 2012;15(3):217–28.
15. Labadie JD, Harrison TA, Banbury B, Amtay EL, Bernd S, Brenner H, Buchanan DD, Campbell PT, Cao Y, Chan AT, Chang-Claude J, English D, Figueiredo JC, Gallinger SJ, Giles GG, Gunter MJ, Hoffmeister M, Hsu L, Jenkins MA, Lin Y, Milne RL, Moreno V, Murphy N, Ogino S, Phipps AI, Sakoda LC, Slattery ML, Southey MC, Sun W, Thibodeau SN, Van Guelpen B, Zaidi SH, Peters U, Newcomb PA. Postmenopausal hormone therapy and colorectal cancer risk by molecularly defined subtypes and tumor location. JNCI Cancer Spectr. 2020;4(5):pkaa042. https://doi.org/10.1093/jncics/pkaa042.

16. Gleason CE, et al. Effects of hormone therapy on cognition and mood in recently postmenopausal women: findings from the randomized, controlled KEEPS-cognitive and affective study. PLoS Med. 2015;12(6):e1001833.; discussion e1001833. https://doi.org/10.1371/journal.pmed.1001833.
17. Henderson VW, St John JA, Hodis HN, McCleary CA, Stanczyk FZ, Shoupe D, Kono N, Dustin L, Allayee H, Mack WJ. Cognitive effects of estradiol after menopause: a randomized trial of the timing hypothesis. Neurology. 2016;87(7):699–708. https://doi.org/10.1212/WNL.0000000000002980.
18. Sharma A, Davies R, Kapoor A, Islam H, Webber L, Jayasena CN. The effect of hormone replacement therapy on cognition and mood. Clin Endocrinol. 2023;98(3):285–95. https://doi.org/10.1111/cen.14856.
19. Collaborative Group on Hormonal Factors in Breast Cancer. Type and timing of menopausal hormone therapy and breast cancer risk: individual participant meta-analysis of the worldwide epidemiological evidence. Lancet. 2019;394(10204):1159–68. https://doi.org/10.1016/S0140-6736(19)31709-X.
20. Stute P, Wildt L, Neulen J. The impact of micronized progesterone on breast cancer risk: a systematic review. Climacteric. 2018;21(2):111–22. https://doi.org/10.1080/13697137.2017.1421925.
21. Canonico M, Oger E, Plu-Bureau G, Conard J, Meyer G, Lévesque H, Trillot N, Barrellier MT, Wahl D, Emmerich J, Scarabin PY, Estrogen and Thromboembolism Risk (ESTHER) Study Group. Hormone therapy and venous thromboembolism among postmenopausal women: impact of the route of estrogen administration and progestogens: the ESTHER study. Circulation. 2007;115(7):840–5. https://doi.org/10.1161/CIRCULATIONAHA.106.642280.
22. Vinogradova Y, Coupland C, Hippisley-Cox J. Use of hormone replacement therapy and risk of venous thromboembolism: nested case-control studies using the QResearch and CPRD databases. BMJ. 2019;364:k4810. https://doi.org/10.1136/bmj.k4810. Erratum in: BMJ 2019 Jan 15;364:l162
23. Manson JE, et al. Menopausal hormone therapy and health outcomes during the intervention and extended poststopping phases of the Women's Health Initiative randomized trials. JAMA. 2013;310(13):1353–68. https://doi.org/10.1001/jama.2013.278040.
24. Espeland MA, Shumaker SA, Leng I, Manson JE, Brown CM, LeBlanc ES, et al. Long term effects on cognitive function of postmenopausal hormone therapy prescribed to women aged 50-55 years. JAMA Int Med. 2013;173(15):1429–36. https://doi.org/10.1001/jamainternmed.2013.7727.
25. Stuenkel CA, et al. Treatment of symptoms of the menopause: an Endocrine Society Clinical Practice Guideline. J Clin Endocrinol Metabol. 2015;100(11):3975–4011. https://doi.org/10.1210/jc.2015-2236.
26. Fait T, Fialova A, Pastor Z. The use of estradiol metered-dose transdermal spray in clinical practice. Climacteric. 2018;21(6):1–5. https://doi.org/10.1080/13697137.2018.1504916.
27. Judd HL, Mebane-Sims I, Legault C, Wasilauskas C, Johnson S, Merino M, Barrett-Connor E, Trabal J, Miller VT, Barnabei V, Levin G. Effects of hormone replacement therapy on endometrial histology in postmenopausal women The Postmenopausal Estrogen/Progestin Interventions (PEPI) Trial. The writing Group for the PEPI Trial. JAMA. 1996;275(5):370–5. https://doi.org/10.1001/jama.275.5.370.
28. Lello S, Capozzi A, Scambia G. The tissue-selective estrogen complex (bazedoxifene/conjugated estrogens) for the treatment of menopause. Int J Endocrinol. 2017;2017(1):5064725. 9 pages
29. Advisory Panel. The 2023 nonhormone therapy position statement of The North American Menopause Society. Menopause. 2023;30(6):573–90. https://doi.org/10.1097/GME.0000000000002200.

27 Menopause and Cancer Risk

Hemangi Jignesh Kansaria, Raksha Shetty,
and Prabhat Agrawal

27.1 Introduction

According to WHO, age at natural menopause is generally between 45 and 55 years, worldwide. The risk of having cancer increases as women age.

27.2 Menopause and Cervical Cancer

Cervical cancer shows bimodal distribution with second peak at 65–69 years of age [1]. Cancer progresses generally over 10–20 years duration [2].

Postmenopausal women tend to have persistent infection with human papillomavirus (HPV) which is a risk factor [3]. There is a substantial rate of infection with persistent oncogenic HPV in women, hence the need for continuous screening after menopause, to detect preneoplastic genital lesion [4].

Albeit there is no role of vaccination for primary prevention of cervical cancer in menopausal women, secondary prevention by Pap smear examination and HPV testing should be done [5].

HPV testing has improved sensitivity decreasing the incidence of both adenocarcinoma and squamous carcinoma of cervix compared to cytology screening alone. Postmenopausal women should be followed up every 3 years until 50 years of age, after which the follow-up frequency is every 5 years. Routine screening can be discontinued on or after 60 years of age.

Irregular bleeding per vaginum, usually bleeding after coitus, is the most common symptom of cervical cancer. Pyometra in cervical cancer is a frequent finding

H. J. Kansaria (✉) · R. Shetty
Seth G S Medical College and KEM Hospital, Mumbai, Maharashtra, India

P. Agrawal
PG Department of Medicine, SN Medical College, Agra, India

R. Garg (ed.), *Management of Menopause*,
https://doi.org/10.1007/978-981-96-0239-1_27

in menopausal women. Profuse watery cervicovaginal discharge, abnormal uterine bleeding and abdominal pain, bulky cervix on examination and a multicystic cervical lesion on MRI warrant a thorough assessment to rule out HPV-independent cervical cancer, even if a primary HPV screening is negative [6].

Invasive cervical cancer in menopausal women is complicated by osteoporosis.

27.3 Ovarian Cancer and Menopause

Ovarian cancer is predominantly a disease of postmenopausal women with the majority (50%) of ovarian cancer rates are highest in women 55–64 years of age [7].

Early menarche, late menopause pose a greater risk of ovarian cancer, while use of oral contraceptive pills, tubal ligation and breast feeding protect against it. Women with first-degree female relative have more than twofold increased risk of ovarian cancer compared with women with no family history [8]. Women with HNPCC (Lynch syndrome) are at greater risk of ovarian cancer. A total of 10% of ovarian cancer cases have an identifiable genetic mutation such as BRCA1 and BRCA2, therefore such patients should undergo prophylactic bilateral salpingo-oophorectomy [8, 9].

Epithelial origin forms majority cases of ovarian cancer (90%) [8]. Of these, invasive serous carcinomas are the most common histological type consisting up to 80% of advanced ovarian cancer (ESMO). Mucinous, endometroid and clear cell (5%), Brenner, undifferentiated cancer are less common types.

Ovarian cancer screening should be directed towards: (a) peri- and postmenopausal women, (b) women of age >50 years, (c) nulliparous women with history of PCOS, (d) women with family history of cancer of ovary, (e) women with personal or family history of breast and colon cancer and (f) women with BRCA 1 and BRCA 2 mutation. Women at high risk of ovarian cancer should be offered testing for BRCA 1 and BRCA 2 gene mutations and positive women with completed family should be advised prophylactic bilateral salpingo-oophorectomy [10].

Routine annual pelvic examination is suitable and should be done along with other transvaginal USG, serum CA125 and colour flow Doppler imaging [10]. ACOG recommends opportunistic (at the time of clinically indicated hysterectomy) and bilateral salpingectomy in women with genetic risk [11] who wish to retain their ovaries, as a way to reduce risk of later developing high-grade serous ovarian carcinoma [12].

Ovarian cysts are frequent in postmenopausal women; a simple cyst <5 cm in diameter without complex features can reliably be followed-up with repeat USG. Ovarian cyst of >5 cm who are either symptomatic with complex features such as multiloculated, bilateral, consider salpingo-oophorectomy. Risk of malignancy index (RMI) score of <25 suggest low risk of malignancy that is <3%, RMI score of 25–250 suggest 25% risk of malignancy and RMI score >350 suggest 75% risk of malignancy.

Patient should be referred for gynaecological oncology multidisciplinary review of malignancy [13]. Utilisation of RMI may make easier better triage of suspicious pelvic masses to gynaecological oncologist.

Postmenopausal women on oestrogen-only HRT are at increased risk of cancer of ovary, especially after greater than or equal to 10 years of use.

Surgery for early ovarian cancer aims at tumour resection and adequate staging. Accurate surgical staging is important as it may unmask occult advanced disease [7]. Adequate surgery should consist of peritoneal washings, ideally taken before manipulation of tumour, bilateral salpingo-oophorectomy, hysterectomy, multiple peritoneal biopsies of all abdominal fields, at least infracolic omentectomy, appendectomy in case of mucinous histology and pelvic and para-aortic lymph node dissection up to renal veins [7].

A recent Cochrane meta-analysis of five large prospective clinical trial showed that in patients with early stage ovarian cancer chemotherapy is more beneficial than observation, with better overall survival in those receiving platinum-based adjuvant chemotherapy [14].

Single-agent carboplatin to all women with intermediate and high-risk stage I disease is recommended. The risk of recurrence of disease spread beyond ovary is significant and chemotherapy is proposed after surgery for all patients with FIGO stage II–IV disease [7].

Standard chemotherapy consists of combination of paclitaxel 175 mg/m^2 and carboplatin AUC 6.5, intravenously every 3 weeks [7]. The combination of cisplatin and paclitaxel is equally effective but more toxic and less convenient to administer. Alternative schedule of administration of paclitaxel and platinum chemotherapy include intraperitoneal delivery of dose-dense regimens. The addition of bevacizumab is recommended for patients with advanced ovarian cancer with poor prognostic features such as stage IV or suboptimal debulking as defined in the ICON7 trial [7]. Bevacizumab should be given with paclitaxel or carboplatin for a duration of 1 year. CA 125 measurement is useful marker to assess response to chemotherapy as per GCIG criteria. CT should be performed before interval debulking or at the end of first-line chemotherapy [7].

Follow-up clinical evaluation with or without pelvic examination and measurement of CA125 is performed every 3 months for 2 years, then every 6 months during years 4 and 5 until progression occurs. For all patients with stage III–IV ovarian cancer who have responded to chemotherapy, niraparib monotherapy (PARP inhibitors) is licenced [7].

27.4 Menopause and Endometrial Cancer

The most common gynaecological malignancy in the USA and UK. Majority of cases in the UK occur between 65 and 75 years of age [15].

More than 90% of cases of endometrial cancer occur in women >50 years of age, with a median age at diagnosis of 63 years [16]. Risk factors for endometrial carcinoma include conditions associated with chronic elevation of endogenous oestrogen levels or increased oestrogen action at endometrium. These are age, obesity, early menarche and late menopause, nulliparity, PCOS, diabetes mellitus (DM), oestrogen secreting tumours, exogenous oestrogen unopposed by progesterone, tamoxifen use, family history of Lynch type 2 syndrome (hereditary non-polyposis colorectal, ovarian or endometrial cancer). Routine surveillance in asymptomatic women with obesity, PCOS, DM, nulliparity or late menopause is not recommended [16].

Ninety percent of women with endometrial carcinoma present with postmenopausal bleeding [15].

British Gynaecological Cancer Society (BGCS) recommends TVS as first-line investigation in postmenopausal bleeding followed by endometrial biopsy with or without hysteroscopy if endometrium is thickened. BGCS currently recommends ET cut-off of ≥4 mm.

Endometrial cancers have primarily been classified as endometrioid and non-endometrioid cancers. Majority of endometrial cancers are endometrioid, most commonly present at early stage grade 1–2 disease, are often hormone-dependent and have more favourable clinical course. Endometrial cancers grade 3 are a more mixed entity and have, in general, less favourable prognosis. Non-endometrioid cancers comprise the most aggressive serous cancers, clear cell cancers and choriocarcinomas and these have higher risk of early distant spread and presentation in more advanced stage.

Endometrial sampling by biopsy or dilatation & endometrial curettage are initial approaches to histological diagnosis of endometrial cancer. The preoperative workup should include clinical and gynaecological examination, TVS, pelvic MRI, full blood count and liver and renal function profile. Additional imaging test (e.g. thoracic and abdominal CT scan and/or FDG-PET-CT) may be considered in those at high risk of extra-pelvic disease.

Hysterectomy with bilateral salpingo-oophorectomy is the standard surgical procedure in early stage endometrial carcinoma. Minimal invasive surgery is the recommended approach in stage I, grade 1 & grade 2 endometrial cancer. Minimal invasive surgery may also be the preferred surgical approach in stage I, grade 3. Sentinel lymph node can be considered for nodal assessment in low risk-intermediate risk endometrial carcinoma (e.g. stage IA grade 1 to grade 3 and stage IB grade 1 to grade 2). It can be excluded in cases without myometrial invasion. Surgical lymph node (LN) staging should be carried out in patients with high-intermediate risk or high-risk disease. Sentinel LN biopsy is an acceptable alternative to systemic LN assessment for LN staging in high-intermediate risk or high-risk stage I and II.

In serous endometrial carcinoma and carcinosarcoma, full surgical staging including omentectomy, peritoneal biopsy and LN staging should be considered. When feasible and with acceptable morbidity, cytoreduction surgery to a maximum surgical extent should be considered in stage III and IV.

In intermediate risk endometrial carcinoma, i.e. stage IA grade 3, 1B G1-G3, stage IIGA endometrioid (DMMR and NSMP) and no or focal LVSI, adjuvant vaginal brachetherapy is recommended to decrease vaginal recurrence.

High-intermediate risk endometrial carcinoma with lymph node staging or without lymph node staging for patient with stage IA and IB with substantial LVSI stage IB3, stage II G1 with substantial LVIS and stage IIG2-G3 (mismatch repair Deficient (dMMR) and non-specific molecular profile (NSMO)). Adjuvant external beam radiation therapy (EBRT) is recommended, adding chemotherapy to EBRT could be considered, especially for G3 and/or substantial lymphovascular space invasion (LVSI).

For high-risk endometrial carcinoma, adjuvant EBRT with concurrent and adjuvant chemotherapy is recommended, sequential chemotherapy and radiotherapy can be used. Chemotherapy alone is an alternative option.

27.5 Menopause and Vulval/Vaginal Cancer

These are infrequent cancers of postmenopausal women presenting with chronic itching and per vaginal discharge. Diagnosis is usually by office biopsy specimen.

27.6 Menopause and Colorectal Cancer

Data regarding the role of sex hormones in colorectal cancer development are conflicting. Data from clinical trials suggest that hormone therapy reduces the risk of colorectal cancer, while data from prospective cohort studies suggest that circulating oestrogen levels are positively associated with risk of developing colorectal cancer.

Late menopause and age at first childbirth are associated with risk of colorectal cancer [17]. Among women with no history of hormone therapy use, older age at menarche and higher parity are inversely associated with this risk. Greater exposure to endogenous oestrogen may increase the risk of colorectal cancer in postmenopausal women [17].

The WHI trial showed that risk of colorectal cancer was reduced in the combined oestrogen and progestogen arm, though no effect was shown in the oestrogen-alone group. After stopping HRT, over 13 years cumulative follow-up, the risk-reduction with combined oestrogen and progestogen decreased [18].

27.7 Colorectal Cancer Screening Recommendations for Postmenopausal Women

Organisation	Screening population	Screening methods
U.S. Preventive Services Task Force [19]	All adults of age 50–75 years at average risk	Guaiac-based FOBT or FIT annually; multitargeted faecal DNA testing 1–3 yearly; CT colonography or flexible sigmoidoscopy every 5 years; colonoscopy every 10 years; flexible sigmoidoscopy every 10 years with FIT annually
	Healthy adults of 76–85 years age, who have never been screened, if co-morbidities do not limit life expectancy	

Organisation	Screening population	Screening methods
American College of Gastroenterology [20]	Black women aged 45 years or more; all other women aged 50 years or more.	The preferred screening test is colonoscopy every 10 years; alternatives are flexible sigmoidoscopy every 5–10 years and CT colonography every 5 years. If screening methods above are declined, annual FIT is the preferred screening method; alternatively, FOBT or multitargeted faecal DNA testing may be done every 3 years
	Screening obese women of 45 years and above and women with more than a 20 pack-year history of smoking may be cost-effective and beneficial	

Key: *CT* computed tomography, *FIT* faecal immunochemical testing, *FOBT* faecal occult blood testing

27.7.1 Menopause and Breast Cancer

The chances of developing breast cancer increase with age. In addition, some of the drugs used in management of menopausal symptoms may increase or decrease this risk.

Risk Factors for Breast Cancer: About 95% of women diagnosed with breast cancer each year are over age 40 and about 50% are of age 61 and above. Risk of invasive breast cancer is strongly associated with age: ≤39 years: 1 in 210; 40–59 years: 1 in 26; 60–69 years: 1 in 28; ≥70 years: 1 in 15; lifetime risk: 1 in 8 (12.5%) [21].

If an immediate family member (mother, sister or daughter) has had breast cancer, especially if it was at an early age, personal risk is also greater. Women who have had a breast biopsy that shows benign disease are more likely to have breast cancer. Other risk factors include:

- Early menarche (before age 12)
- Late menopause (after age 55)
- First childbirth after age 30
- Nulliparity
- Overweight or obesity after menopause
- Genetic: Mutation of BRCA1 or BRCA2 gene
- Carcinoma in one breast (may develop in the other or recur)
- History of uterine, ovarian or colon cancer

Menopausal hormone replacement therapy (MHRT) except vaginal oestrogens are associated with increased breast cancer risks, which increase steadily with duration of use and reduced after cessation of use and are greater for oestrogen-progestogen than oestrogen-only preparations [22, 23].

27.8 Breast Cancer Screening Guidelines for High-Risk Women

As per American Cancer Society (ACS) screening recommendation [24], women at high risk for breast cancer predicted by certain factors should have a breast MRI and a mammogram annually, starting at age 30. This includes women with:

1. A lifetime risk of breast cancer of 20–25% or greater, according to risk assessment tools based mainly on family history.
2. A known BRCA1 or BRCA2 gene mutation.
3. A first-degree relative with a BRCA1 or BRCA2 gene mutation and have not had genetic testing themselves.
4. Cowden syndrome, Li-Fraumeni syndrome or a first-degree relatives with one of these syndromes.
5. History of radiation therapy to the chest between age of 10 and 30 years.

   The ACS recommends against MRI screening for women whose lifetime risk of breast cancer is <15%.

   There is not enough evidence to recommend for or against yearly MRI screening for women who have a higher lifetime risk based on certain factors, such as:

   (a) Personal history of breast cancer, ductal carcinoma in situ, lobular carcinoma in situ, atypical ductal hyperplasia or atypical lobular hyperplasia.
   (b) Mammogram showing "extremely" or "heterogeneously" dense breasts.

MRI should be, if used, only in addition to and not replacing a screening mammogram; as, albeit an MRI is more likely to detect cancer than mammogram, it may be unable to detect some cancers that a mammogram would do.

27.9 Conclusion

Menopause does not cause cancer, but the risk of developing cancer increases with age. Among gynaecological cancers, cervical cancer is the most common, followed by ovarian and endometrial cancer and rarely vulval and vaginal cancer. Most of these postmenopausal women are oblivious to these malignancies and their symptoms. Also, the non-specific nature of these symptoms lead women to mistake these aberrations as normal part of menopause. Hence, raising awareness, screening and immediate assessment and treatment is vital in menopausal women.

References

1. Desai S, Guddati AK. Bimodal age distribution in cancer incidence. World J Oncol. 2022;13(6):329–36.
2. Burd EM. Human papillomavirus and cervical cancer. Clin Microbiol Rev. 2003;16(1):1–17.

3. Marth C, Landoni F, Mahner S, McCormack M, Gonzalez-Martin A, N. Colombo, on behalf of the ESMO Guidelines Committee. Cervical cancer: ESMO clinical practice guidelines for diagnosis, treatment and follow-up. Ann Oncol. 2017;28(Suppl. 4):iv72–83.
4. Smitha EM, Johnson SR, Ritchiec JM, Feddersen D, Wangd D, Turekd LP, Haugend TH. Persistent HPV infection in postmenopausal age women. Int J Gynaecol Obstet. 2004;87(2):131–7.
5. NHS Cervical Screening Programme. Cervical screening programme, England—2021–2022 [NS].
6. Aggarwal LM, Yeo YC, Ng ZY. HPV independent cervical cancer and its precursor lesion. Obstetr Gynecol. 2023;25:47–58.
7. Ovarian cancer statistics. Ovarian Cancer National Alliance. Available from: www.ovariancancer.org/about-ovarian-cancer/statistics.
8. Colombo N, Sessa C, du Bois A, Ledermann J, McCluggage WG, McNeish I, Morice P, Pignata S, Ray-Coquard I, Vergote I, et al. ESMO–ESGO consensus conference recommendations on ovarian cancer: pathology and molecular biology, early and advanced stages, borderline tumours and recurrent disease. Ann Oncol. 2019;30:672–705.
9. Scully RE, Yong RH, Clement PB. Tumors of the ovary, maldeveloped gonads, fallopian tube and broad ligament. In: Atlas of tumor pathology. 3rd series, fascicle 23. Washington, DC: Armed Forces Institute of Pathology; 1998. p. 1–168.
10. Khatun S, Ferdous J. Menopause and gynecological malignancy, review article. J South Asian Federation Menopause Soc. 2013;1(2):75–9.
11. American College of Obstetricians and Gynecologists. ACOG practical bulletin: clinical management guidelines for obstetrician and gynecologist. Obstetr Gynecol. 2017;130(3):e168–86.
12. Berek JS, Renz M, Kehoe S, Kumar L. Cancer of the ovary, fallopian tube and peritoneum: 2021 update, Fifo cancer report 2021. Int J Gynecol Obstet. 2021;155(Suppl. 1):61–85.
13. The management of ovarian cysts in postmenopausal women. Green Top Guidelines No 34 July 2016.
14. Winter-Roach BA, Kitchener HC, Dickinson HO. Adjuvant (post-surgery) chemotherapy for early stage epithelial ovarian cancer. Cochrane Database Syst Rev. 2009:CD004706.
15. Jones ER, O'Flynn H, Njoku K, et al. Detecting endometrial cancer. Obstetr Gynecol. 2021;23:103–12.
16. Oaknin A, Bosse TJ, Creutzberg CL, Giornelli G, Harter P, Joly F. Endometrial cancer: ESMO clinical practice guideline for diagnosis, treatment and follow-up. Ann Oncol. 2022;33(9)
17. Zervoudakis A, Strickler HD, Park Y, Xue X, Hollenbeck A, Schatzkin A, Gunter MJ. Reproductive history and risk of colorectal cancer in postmenopausal women. J Natl Cancer Inst. 2011;103(10):826–34. https://doi.org/10.1093/jnci/djr101.
18. Prentice RL, Pettinger M, Beresford SA, et al. Colorectal cancer in relation to postmenopausal estrogen and estrogen plus progestin in the Women's Health Initiative clinical trial and observational study. Cancer Epidemiol Biomarkers Prev. 2009;18(5):1531–7. https://doi.org/10.1158/1055-9965.EPI-08-1209. Available from: https://www.ncbi.nlm.nih.gov/pmc/articles/PMC2689377
19. U.S. Preventive Services Task Force. Colorectal cancer: screening. June 2016. https://www.uspreventiveservicestaskforce.org/uspstf/document/UpdateSummaryFinal/colorectal-cancer-screening?ds=1&;s=colorectal%20cancer. Accessed June 21, 2016.
20. Rex DK, Johnson DA, Anderson JC, Schoenfeld PS, Burke CA, Inadomi JM, American College of Gastroenterology. American College of Gastroenterology guidelines for colorectal cancer screening 2009 [published correction appears in Am J Gastroenterol. 2009;104(6):1613]. Am J Gastroenterol. 2009;104(3):739–50.
21. Jemal A, Siegel R, Ward E, Hao Y, Xu J, Murray T, Thun MJ. Cancer statistics, 2008. CA: Cancer J Clin. 2008;58(2):71–96. https://doi.org/10.3322/CA.2007.0010.
22. Beral V, for the Collaborative Group on Hormonal Factors in Breast Cancer. Breast cancer and hormone replacement therapy (HRT): collaborative reanalysis of data from 51 epidemiological studies of 52,705 women with breast cancer and 108,411 women without breast cancer. Breast Cancer Res. 2002;4(Suppl. 1):3. https://doi.org/10.1186/bcr486.

23. Collaborative Group on Hormonal Factors in Breast Cancer. Type and timing of menopausal hormone therapy and breast cancer risk: individual participant meta-analysis of the worldwide epidemiological evidence. Lancet. 2019;394(10204):1159–68. https://doi.org/10.1016/S0140-6736(19)31709-X.
24. Roca SA, Arranz SJ, Laguna AB, Checa VQ, Clar EG. Breast cancer screening in high risk populations. Radiología. 2012;54:490–502.

Genitourinary Syndrome of Menopause 28

Anusha Devalla, Ved Prakash Rao Cheruvu, Pankuri Dubey, and Ruchika Garg

28.1 Introduction

The genitourinary syndrome of menopause (GSM), previously vulvovaginal atrophy, incorporates a spectrum of urogenital & sexual symptoms evolving over the menopausal transition due to underlying hypoestrogenism. Recognizing the need to address the chronic debilitating sequelae of menopause, International Society for the Study of Women's Sexual Health and the North American Menopause Society have introduced a change in the terminology.

This syndrome is seen to affect as many as half of the postmenopausal women and up to 15% of women in perimenopausal period. Clinical features include dryness, burning and irritation in the external genitalia; burning micturition, feeling of urgency, frequent urinary tract infections; and sexual symptoms like discomfort or dyspareunia, dryness, and impaired libido function [1, 2]. The symptoms may cause considerable morbidity and unlike vasomotor symptoms, they do not improve over time if left untreated. The experience of the symptoms may be severely debilitating especially after surgical menopause with abrupt estrogen deprivation with much poorer quality-of-life outcomes [3].

A. Devalla (✉)
Department of Obstetrics and Gynecology, All India Institute of Medical Sciences, Bibinagar, Hyderabad, Telangana, India

V. P. R. Cheruvu
Department of Burns and Plastic Surgery, All India Institute of Medical Sciences, Bhopal, Madhya Pradesh, India

P. Dubey
Department of Obstetrics and Gynecology, All India Institute of Medical Sciences, Rajkot, Gujarat, India

R. Garg
Department Obstetrics and Gynaecology, SN Medical College, Agra, India

R. Garg (ed.), *Management of Menopause*,
https://doi.org/10.1007/978-981-96-0239-1_28

However, GSM remains underreported and underdiagnosed due to variety of reasons. Embarrassment and reluctance to discuss sexual health with clinician, dismissal of the symptoms as a consequence to aging by women themselves, and a general lack of awareness are significant barriers to healthcare seeking behavior in these women [4]. Further, there may be a lack of proactive assessment by clinicians for GSM as part of routine clinical review.

It is important to timely detect and ensure proper patient education regarding GSM to avoid the long-term morbidity. Treatment must be tailored based on clinical profile and severity of symptoms [5].

28.2 Pathophysiology

28.2.1 Development & Premenopausal Physiology

During embryologic development in females, the urogenital sinus and sinovaginal node combine to form the urinary bladder, trigone, entire urethra, vestibule of the vagina, and lower third of vagina. This forms the basis of sharing the estrogen receptor function in the vulvovaginal tissues, pelvic floor musculature, endopelvic fascia, and the lower urinary tract. The endogenous estrogen act on these receptors to maintain the normal physiological mechanisms [6]. Though less studied, androgens too are implicated to have a role in maintenance of normal function & structure of the genitourinary tissues. Receptors for these steroids, especially estrogen, are distributed throughout the vulvovaginal tissues, pelvic floor musculature, endopelvic fascia, and the lower urinary tract.

During the reproductive years, estrogen stimulation helps in the upkeep of these tissues in various ways. This includes production of adequate epithelial collagen content to maintain an appropriate mucosal thickness and elasticity, stimulation of hyaluronic acid and glycogen-rich mucopolysaccharide production to help with surface moisturization, maintenance of optimal blood flow via regional vasculature, and promotion of a healthy vaginal flora. Activated estrogen receptors encourage prolubricative and proelastic function of vaginal epithelium during sexual stimulation. Epithelial proliferation gives rise to rugosity of the vaginal mucosa which increases mechanical compliance, thus improving the libido during sexual stimulation [7].

The characteristic rugated, elastic and thickened vagina with rich glycogen promoting a healthy vaginal flora is due to the local estradiol concentrations. A preponderance of lactobacilli over other polymicrobial organisms is responsible for creating a natural acidic (pH 3.5–4.5) barrier mechanism produced by the conversion of glycogen to lactic acid.

28.2.2 Postmenopausal Physiology

Declining estrogen levels due to ovarian ageing and progressive loss of receptors has both vulvovaginal and urologic effects. Atrophy of the genital tissues occurs due to substantial loss of vascularization and dermal collagen. Vaginal epithelium characteristically appears attenuated, pale, flat, and featureless due to loss of rugosity. Length and elasticity of vagina is also reduced causing frictional trauma and dyspareunia [8]. Hypoestrogenism causes alterations in vaginal microflora and cellular biochemistry appear as well. Accumulation of glycogen in the vaginal epithelial cells is hampered which leads to reduced lactobacilli colonies. This causes change in the pH of vaginal fluid to more than 5, which further promotes overgrowth of skin & rectal flora (Group B streptococcus, staphylococci, gram-negative rods, diphtheroids) inducing local vaginal and urinary tract infections [3].

GSM-associated urge incontinence is the key cause for menopausal recurrent urinary tract infections. Postmenopausal hypoestrogenism decreases receptor-mediated sensory threshold of bladder causing impairment of the bladder neck and urethral closure pressures leading to urge symptoms. In addition, altered connective tissue integrity and urethral sphincter dysfunction contribute to stress incontinence [9, 10].

28.3 Epidemiology

28.3.1 Prevalance

Since the condition remains underreported, it is difficult to estimate the exact prevalence of this condition. However, most menopausal women eventually develop urogenital atrophy which may be symptomatic or asymptomatic. A detailed review on GSM prevalence and treatment observed that 40–60% of the peri- and postmenopausal women report GSM-related concerns with many women describing up to four or five symptoms (32% and 10%, respectively) [11].

28.3.2 Etiology

Declining estrogen levels in peri- and postmenopausal phase remain the key factor in development of GSM. Duration of hypoestrogenism appears to have a direct correlation with severity of symptoms. Besides menopause, other hypoestrogenic states may also cause GSM-like symptoms. These include conditions like primary ovarian insufficiency, bilateral oophorectomy, and iatrogenic causes of ovarian failure or insufficiency due to radiation, chemotherapy, complication of uterine artery embolization, antiestrogenic drugs etc. Postpartum reduction in estrogen levels, especially during lactation may also cause hypoestrogenic symptoms.

28.4 Etiological Risk Factors for Genitourinary Syndrome of Menopause

Surgical menopause secondary to bilateral oophorectomy.
Ovarian failure (drugs/surgery/radiation).
Tobacco smoking/alcoholism.
Decreased sexual activity.
Prolonged immobility and lack of physical exercise.
Nulliparity.

28.5 Clinical Evaluation

Clinical manifestations of GSM are summarized in Fig. 28.1. Symptoms may be due to vulvovaginal, sexual or urinary dysfunction.

Approach to GSM requires proactive assessment by the treating physician as majority of the times there can be sociocultural inhibitions. This leads to frequent self-treatment options making lifestyle changes, for instance, sexual abstinence. Clinical evaluation should include a thorough medical history and a pelvic examination. Diagnosis is clinical and laboratory testing is not usually required.

28.5.1 History

History should include obstetric, menstrual and sexual history with a review of systems to evaluate urogenital symptoms attributable to causes other than peri- or postmenopausal hypoestrogenism. Use of hygiene products which may be possible irritants should be enquired. These include perfumes, deodorants, soaps, powder, lubricants, panty liners, etc. Symptoms related to vulvar pain that may be due to infection or inflammation should be discussed to rule other differentials. Psychological aspects related to appearance of symptoms should also be assessed, e.g., behavioral response to symptoms and quality-of-life measures in sexual health.

28.5.2 Pelvic Examination

Examination may reveal features which include pallor of vulvovaginal tissues, dryness, fissures, tissue fragility, labial fusion, retraction & narrowing of vaginal introitus, absence of vaginal rugosity, prominent urethral meatus, urethral eversion due to loss of collagen support and pelvic organ prolapse. Caution must be exercised to perform a gentle examination; even a slight surface contact or even examiner's hand may cause pain and bleeding. Levator muscles may go into spasm upon contact with the posterior vagina. Vagina may be narrowed and shortened. Cervix may be found flushed with the vaginal vault and fornices obliterated. Examination must be stopped if patient becomes too distressed due to pain or discomfort. Vaginoscopy may be done as an alternative [11].

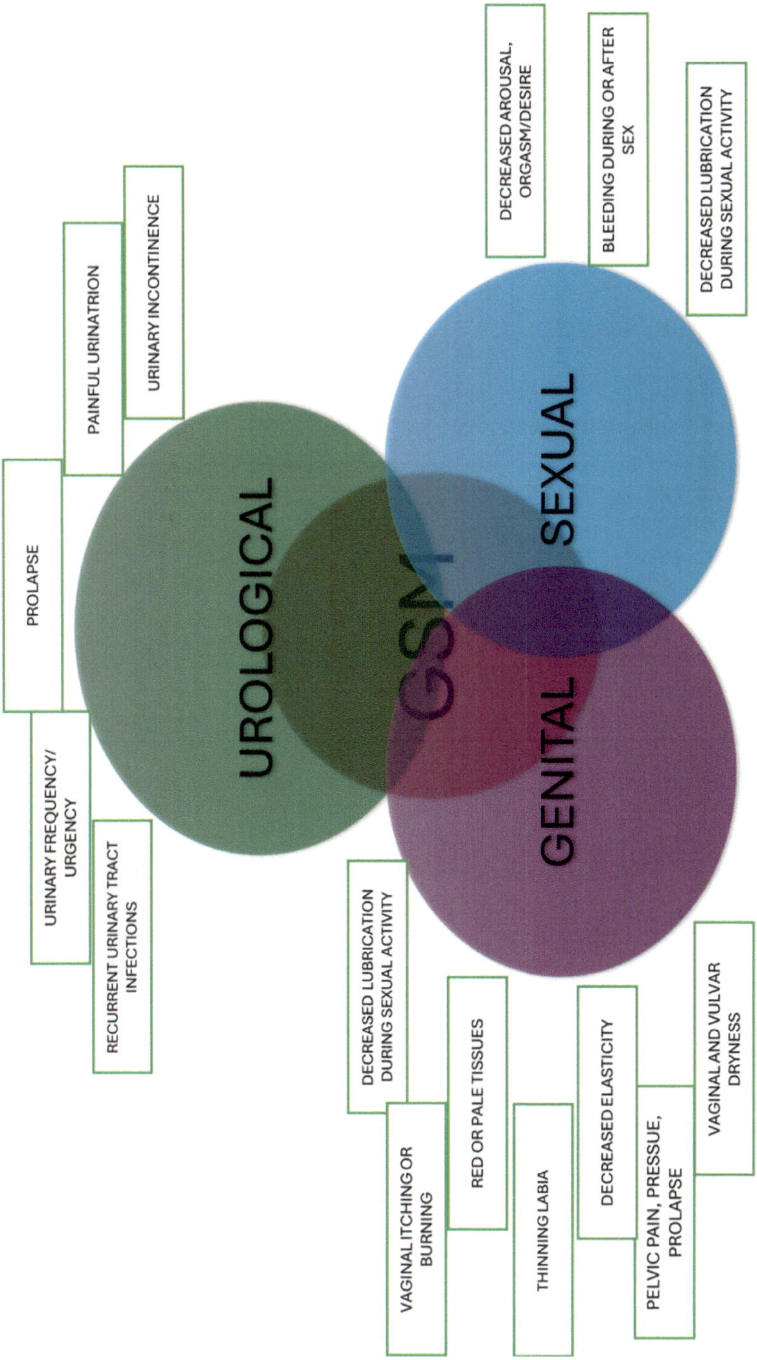

Fig. 28.1 Symptoms of genitourinary syndrome in menopause

28.5.3 Laboratory Investigations

Laboratory tests are not typically required to conclude a diagnosis. Vaginal pH may be tested using a simple pH strip by holding it against the vaginal wall. A raised pH reading (≥5) could suggest vaginal atrophy secondary to hypoestrogenism without the obvious features of infection or seminal secretions in the recent sexual intercourse. Vaginal smear for the assessment of the maturation index describing a progressive increase in parabasal cells with concomitant decrease in the superficial cells signifies hypoestrogenism. Microscopic evaluation of urine and vaginal discharge is pertinent if urinary tract infections (UTI) or vaginitis is suspected.

Complications of GSM [12]:

- Labial atrophy.
- Introital stenosis.
- Retraction of the intravaginal urethra.
- Alkaline pH (>5).
- Ischemia of vaginal trigone.
- Urethral prolapse.
- Genital prolapse.
- Urethral caruncle.

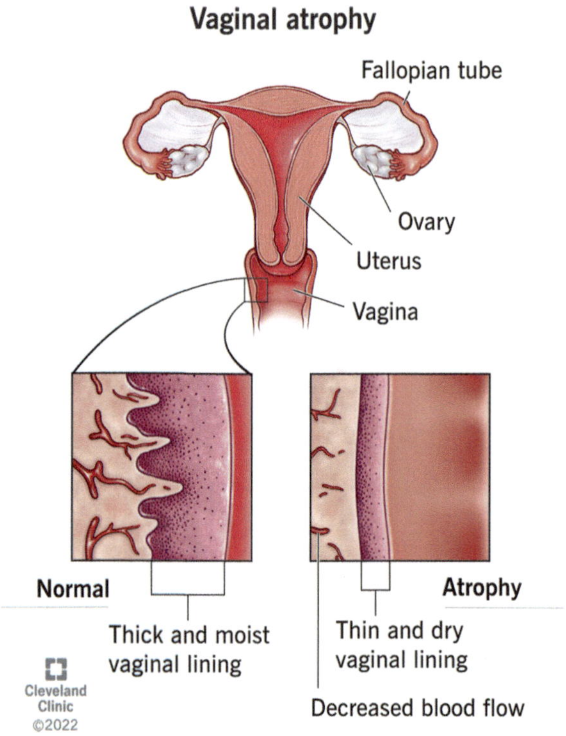

28.6 Investigations

Apart from clinical evaluation, certain tests are required to correlate the physical findings.

1. Cystoscopy:
   - Pale and shortened urethra
   - Squamous metaplasia of trigone
   - Urinary internal and external sphincter dysfunction
   - Reduced bladder compliance
   - Pale trigone
2. Laparoscopy:
   - Pale and atrophic uterus, fallopian tubes and ovaries.
   - Lax ligaments.

28.7 Diagnostic Aid

1. Ultrasound of pelvis (TVS/TAS): An endometrial thickness of ≤5 mm suggests decreased estrogen stimulation.
2. Papanicolou test for cervical cytology.
3. Decreased vaginal maturation index.
4. High vaginal swabs to rule out infections and pH testing (symptomatic pH 5–7).
5. Magnetic resonance imaging/computed tomography scan—pelvic and adnexal abnormalities.

28.8 Differential Diagnosis

1. Infections: Bacterial vaginosis, candidiasis, trichomoniasis.
2. Vaginal stenosis secondary to infection.
3. Foreign matter/piercings/contact irritants, sexual trauma.
4. Precancerous lesions of vulva and vagina.
5. Endocrine disorders—diabetes mellitus, hypothyroidism.
6. Dermatological conditions—lichen sclerosus, lichen planus.

The following are the hormonal and nonhormonal preparations used in the treatment of GSM [13] (Table 28.1):

Table 28.1 Nonhormonal and hormonal treatment options

Formulation	Composition	Dosages
Nonhormonal options		
Lubricants	Water/silicone/ polycarbophil based	
Moisturizers	Hyaluronic acid Polyacrylic acid Polycarbophil-based vaginal moiturizer	5 mg daily for 2 weeks, then 3–5 times per week 3 g daily 2.5 g three times/week
Vaginal suppositories	Vitamins D, E	1000 IU, 30–200 IU respectively
Lidocaine	4% Aqueous lidocaine	Fully saturated cotton ball applied to vulva for 3 min
Hormonal options		
Vaginal cream	Conjugated equine estrogen	Twice weekly 0.5 g intravaginally for moderate-to-severe dyspareunia Dosage regimen of 1 g every night for 2 weeks or 0.5 g two times a week are commonly used
Vaginal cream	Testosterone	300 μg or 150 μg applied daily 300 μg or 150 μg locally daily for 2 weeks, then 3 times a week
Vaginal ring	17 Beta-estradiol	7.5 μg/d for 90 days
Vaginal tablet	Estradiol hemihydrate	10 μg/day for 2 weeks, then 10 μg/day 2 times a week A vaginal insert containing 4 μg is available, although not used in included studies
Vaginal insert	Prasterone	One 6.5 mg vaginal insert once daily

28.9 Treatment of GSM

GSM, being a chronic condition, requires symptomatic prolonged treatment. Nonhormonal local moisturizer preparations are preferred first-line treatment for urogenital symptoms, in the background of estrogen-dependent breast cancer. Estrogen topical creams are effective either alone or in combination with systemic hormone replacement therapy, measured as improvements in vaginal maturation index (VMI). Herbal remedies are an alternative that have been extensively studied but the effect of black cohosh on the vaginal atrophy remains controversial [2]. Besides VMI, local vaginal pH test and cytology may be useful [14]. There is no proven efficacy using these remedies. It is estimated that 10% of women prefer herbal concoctions such as black cohosh, soy foods, comfrey root. They may have an association with vaginal wall remodeling.

Some vitamins such as Vitamins E and D have been used for GSM therapy; Vitamin D may help generate keratinocyte proliferation and differentiation in the vaginal epithelium [15].

28.9.1 Lubricants and Moisturizers

These are preferred first-line treatments for mild vulvovaginal symptoms that are not associated with sexual intercourse. Compounds containing poly-carbophilic-based polymers stick to vaginal walls and can relieve the friction. While using barrier contraceptives, most water-based and silicone-based lubricants are safe to use; oil-based lubricants are not recommended.

Constituents of the moisturizers must mimic the vaginal secretions with respect to osmolality and pH. Usually, they stay for <24-h duration and need daily applications. Hyaluronic acid-based moisturizers have not been found to improve vaginal maturation index. The use of topical lidocaine may have a promising role to relieve superficial dyspareunia.

28.9.2 Estrogen Therapy

Hormonal therapy is considered as first-line option for moderate-to-severe symptoms or where lubricants/moisturizers did not relieve the symptoms. It is important to rule out all risk factors and patient needs to be fully explained about the benefits and risks before prescribing. Local combined with systemic administration of estrogens have proven benefit in rapidly restoring vaginal epithelium and associated vasculature, thereby minimizing the vulvovaginal symptoms.

Although not significant, there is a theoretical risk of high estrogen levels and its proliferative effects on the endometrium. Hence, the lowest effective dose of local estrogens should be advised. According to the North American Menopause society, low-dose vaginal estrogens decreases the vaginal pH, increase the number of vaginal lactobacilli, improve vaginal and urethral cytology, and prevent urinary tract infection.

Upon systemic absorption, it could lead to unwanted side effects such as breast tenderness, breakthrough bleeding, weight gain, and nausea/vomiting due to water retention [16].

The adverse effects due to unopposed estrogen exposure are not usually observed if used up to 6 months. A hormone-free interval followed by resumption is advisable. Increased vaginal secretions are expected side effect with the use of intravaginal applications [17]. Systemic hormone therapy may precipitate stress incontinence and hence not recommended as a solo treatment. Vaginal dehydroepiandrosterone (DHEA) or testosterone can be a useful substitute to patients with low libido and where vaginal estrogens are contraindicated [7, 15].

Contraindications to the Use of ET:

- Confirmed/suspected hormone-sensitive cancer (breast/endometrial).
- Uninvestigated vaginal bleeding.
- Personal history of thromboembolism.
- Metabolic disease.
- Cardiovascular and cerebrovascular disease.
- Liver disease.

- Pregnancy.
- Smoking in those age > 35 years.
- Migraines with neurologic symptoms.
- Acute cholecystitis/cholangitis.

28.9.3 Synthetic Steroid

Tibolone, a potent synthetic steroid, has been found to have estrogenic, androgenic, and progestational activities. It has been used systemically to improve the vaginal maturation index thus reducing vulvovaginal symptoms and improve sex drive. Moreover, urinary urgency and urge incontinence were found to reduce.

28.9.4 Selective Estrogen Receptor Modulators (SERMs)

Recently SERMs like Ospemifene, administered orally, was approved by the Food and Drug Administration in 2013. The drug is found to be efficacious in improving the pH and vaginal wall vasculature in women and can be used as a potential alternative in women with contraindications to starting estrogen therapy [18]. A higher risk of venous thromboembolism must alert its use in individuals with possible risk factors.

Lasofoxifene is another SERM in phase III trials and not yet marketed for the use. This has resulted in significant improvements in vaginal cytology, vaginal pH, and VMI. Further trials are needed for its application in the treatment of GSM [19].

28.9.5 Tissue-Specific Estrogen Complexes—Bazedoxifene (BZA) and Conjugated Estrogens (CEs)

A novel therapy combining an SERM and a conjugated estrogen (tissue-specific estrogen complexes) are equally efficacious to combined hormone replacement therapy [20]. BZA/CE has been in use in postmenopausal women as it is designed to prevent the vasomotor symptoms apart from being safe for the endometrium and breast. It also alleviates the loss of bone mineral density [21].

28.9.6 Laser Therapies

Notably, the use of lasers are an innovative treatment option for GSM introduced in 2014. The Food and Drug Administration has approved the use of fractional microablative carbon-dioxide laser therapy. Although not yet approved, the erbium lasers have been used as a novel technique in refractory symptoms of GSM. These can stimulate the vaginal wall epithelial growth factor along with collagen and extracellular matrix. The timed impulses aim to spread through the vaginal tissue and subsequently raise the local temperature causing remodeling of collagen in the vaginal canal thus giving a "tightening" effect. The effect on improvement of symptoms may last 6 months following treatment. Similar effects have been observed by using low-energy dynamic quadripolar radiofrequency (dqrf) lasers producing remarkable improvements in urinary symptoms and sexual satisfaction rates [22].

28.9.7 Intravaginal Dehydroepiandrosterone

Dehydroepiandrosterone is a steroid hormone intermediate in the biosynthesis pathway for androgen and estrogen synthesis. In concentration of 0.5%, dehydroepiandrosterone increased superficial cell percentage and decreased parabasal cell in the vaginal epithelium, decreased vaginal pH, and decreased superficial dyspareunia.

28.9.8 Oxytocin

Oxytocin, the neuropeptide released by the posterior pituitary gland, where the treated participants reported significant reduction in the GSM symptoms. Additionally, vaginal pH decreased with the use of oxytocin. Additionally, there is no increase in endometrial thickness indicating its possible use where estrogen creams are contraindicated [23].

28.9.9 Homeopathic Remedies

Effects of agrimony, black cohosh, soy, and other phytoestrogens for vaginal dryness and dyspareunia have been studied but no concrete evidence is available to support the beneficial claims.

28.9.10 Lifestyle Modifications

Increased sexual activity has been correlated to improved blood circulation to the vagina and the seminal fluids contain sexual steroids and essential fatty acids, which serve to maintain vaginal tissue and stretching. Masturbation or sex devices can serve similar benefits in individuals without a partner.

Cognitive behavioral therapy and stress-reduction strategies may relieve symptoms. Apart from general well-being, smoking cessation has been observed to cause collagen preservation in the vaginal canal. Importantly, wearing loose clothes can improve local air circulation and discourage microbial growth.

28.10 Conclusion

- GSM needs a careful assessment of the vulvovaginal symptoms and lower urinary tract symptoms secondary to hypoestrogenism.

- This can have a profound impact on quality of life of the woman and needs effective life-long therapy.
- It is a largely underdiagnosed condition, and women show reluctance to consult and take hormone therapy owing to possible side effects and consider it a part of normal aging.
- Nonhormonal moisturizers are usually the first-line treatment in women with vaginal dryness unrelated to the sexual intercourse. It is especially beneficial in patients where vaginal estrogen creams are contraindicated.
- Vaginal estrogens effectively relieve common vulvovaginal symptoms and have additional effects on urinary symptoms such as urinary urgency, frequency or nocturia, stress urinary incontinence (SUI), and recurrent UTIs.

References

1. Portman DJ, Gass MLS, Vulvovaginal Atrophy Terminology Consensus Conference Panel. Genitourinary syndrome of menopause: new terminology for vulvovaginal atrophy from the International Society for the Study of Women's Sexual Health and the North American Menopause Society. Menopause N Y N 2014;21(10):1063–1068.
2. Angelou K, Grigoriadis T, Diakosavvas M, Zacharakis D, Athanasiou S. The genitourinary syndrome of menopause: an overview of the recent data. Cureus. 2020;12(4) Available from: https://www.ncbi.nlm.nih.gov/pmc/articles/PMC7212735/
3. Mac Bride MB, Rhodes DJ, Shuster LT. Vulvovaginal atrophy. Mayo Clin Proc. 2010;85(1):87–94.
4. Kim HK, Kang SY, Chung YJ, Kim JH, Kim MR. The recent review of the genitourinary syndrome of menopause. J Menopausal Med. 2015;21(2):65.
5. Gandhi J, Chen A, Dagur G, Suh Y, Smith N, Cali B, et al. Genitourinary syndrome of menopause: an overview of clinical manifestations, pathophysiology, etiology, evaluation, and management. Am J Obstet Gynecol. 2016;215(6):704–11.
6. Wilson D, Bordoni B. Embryology, mullerian ducts (paramesonephric ducts). In: StatPearls. Treasure Island (FL): StatPearls Publishing; 2024. [cited 2024 Apr 27]. Available from: http://www.ncbi.nlm.nih.gov/books/NBK557727/.
7. North American Menopause Society. The role of local vaginal estrogen for treatment of vaginal atrophy in postmenopausal women: 2007 position statement of The North American Menopause Society. Menopause N Y N. 2007;14(3 Pt 1):355–69. quiz 370–1
8. Nappi RE, Palacios S. Impact of vulvovaginal atrophy on sexual health and quality of life at postmenopause. Climacteric J Int Menopause Soc. 2014;17(1):3–9.
9. Estrogenic action on innate defense mechanisms in the urinary tract—PubMed. [cited 2024 Apr 27]. Available from: https://pubmed.ncbi.nlm.nih.gov/24296328/.
10. Hyun HS, Park BR, Kim YS, Mun ST, Bae DH. Urodynamic characterization of postmenopausal women with stress urinary incontinence: retrospective study in incontinent pre- and post-menopausal women. J Korean Soc Menopause. 2010:148–52.
11. Mili N, Paschou SA, Armeni A, Georgopoulos N, Goulis DG, Lambrinoudaki I. Genitourinary syndrome of menopause: a systematic review on prevalence and treatment. Menopause. 2021;28(6):706.
12. Cleveland Clinic. [cited 2024 May 1]. What is vaginal atrophy (GSM or atrophic vaginitis)? Available from: https://my.clevelandclinic.org/health/diseases/15500-vaginal-atrophy.
13. Da Silva AS, Baines G, Araklitis G, Robinson D, Cardozo L. Modern management of genitourinary syndrome of menopause. Fac Rev. 2021;10:25.

14. Palacios S, Combalia J, Emsellem C, Gaslain Y, Khorsandi D. Therapies for the management of genitourinary syndrome of menopause. Post Reprod Health. 2020;26(1):32–42.
15. North American Menopause Society. Management of symptomatic vulvovaginal atrophy: 2013 position statement of the North American Menopause Society. Menopause N Y N. 2013;20(9):888–902.
16. Ngan HYS, Seckl MJ, Berkowitz RS, Xiang Y, Golfier F, Sekharan PK, et al. Update on the diagnosis and management of gestational trophoblastic disease. Int J Gynaecol Obstet Off Organ Int Fed Gynaecol Obstet. 2018;143(Suppl. 2):79–85.
17. Meta-analysis of estrogen therapy in the management of urogenital atrophy in postmenopausal women: second report of the Hormones and Urogenital Therapy Committee—PubMed. [cited 2024 Apr 27]. Available from: https://pubmed.ncbi.nlm.nih.gov/9764689/.
18. Pinkerton JV, Stanczyk FZ. Clinical effects of selective estrogen receptor modulators on vulvar and vaginal atrophy. Menopause N Y N. 2014;21(3):309–19.
19. North American Menopause Society. The 2012 hormone therapy position statement of: The North American Menopause Society. Menopause N Y N. 2012;19(3):257–71.
20. Mirkin S, Komm BS. Tissue-selective estrogen complexes for postmenopausal women. Maturitas. 2013;76(3):213–20.
21. Vaginal estrogen for genitourinary syndrome of menopause: a systematic review—PubMed. [cited 2024 Apr 27]. Available from: https://pubmed.ncbi.nlm.nih.gov/25415166/.
22. Laser therapy in the treatment of female urinary incontinence and genitourinary syndrome of menopause: an update—PMC. [cited 2024 Apr 27]. Available from: https://www.ncbi.nlm.nih.gov/pmc/articles/PMC6582847/.
23. Intravaginally applied oxytocin improves post-menopausal vaginal atrophy—PMC. [cited 2024 Apr 27]. Available from: https://www.ncbi.nlm.nih.gov/pmc/articles/PMC4566058/.

GPSR Compliance

The European Union's (EU) General Product Safety Regulation (GPSR) is a set of rules that requires consumer products to be safe and our obligations to ensure this.

If you have any concerns about our products, you can contact us on ProductSafety@springernature.com

In case Publisher is established outside the EU, the EU authorized representative is:

Springer Nature Customer Service Center GmbH
Europaplatz 3
69115 Heidelberg, Germany

Batch number: 09363454

Printed by Printforce, the Netherlands